PNDR:
Psychologists' Neuropsychotropic
Drug Reference

Clinical Pharmacology Specialty Texts and References by the Pagliaros

Pharmacologic Aspects of Aging. C. V. Mosby (1983).

Drug Reference Guide to Brand Names and Active Ingredients. C. V. Mosby (1986).

Pharmacologic Aspects of Nursing. C. V. Mosby (1986).

Problems in Pediatric Drug Therapy. Drug Intelligence (1979), (1987), (1995); American Pharmaceutical Association (1996), (in preparation).

Substance Use Among Infants, Children, and Adolescents: Its Nature, Extent, and Effects from Conception to Adulthood. John Wiley & Sons (1996).

The Pharmacologic Basis of Psychotherapeutics: An Introduction for Psychologists. Brunner/Mazel (1998).

PPDR: Psychologists' Psychotropic Drug Reference. Brunner/Mazel (1999).

PNDR: Psychologists' Neuropsychotropic Drug Reference. Brunner/Mazel (1999).

Clinical Pharmacopsychotherapeutics for Psychologists. Brunner/Mazel (in preparation).

Substance Use Among Women: Its Nature, Consequences, and Treatment. Brunner/Mazel (forthcoming).

PNDR:
Psychologists' Neuropsychotropic Drug Reference

by

Louis A. Pagliaro, MS, PharmD, PhD, FPPR
Professor, Department of Educational Psychology and
President, College of Alberta Psychologists

and

Ann Marie Pagliaro, BSN, MSN, PhD Candidate, FPPR
Professor, Faculty of Nursing and
Director, Substance Abusology Research Unit

University of Alberta

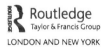

Routledge
Taylor & Francis Group
LONDON AND NEW YORK

PSYCHOLOGISTS' NEUROPSYCHOTROPIC DRUG REFERENCE

First published 1999
by Brunner/Mazel

Published 2014 by Routledge
711 Third Avenue, New York, NY 10017
2 Park Square, Milton Park, Abingdon, Oxfordshire OX14 4RN

First issued in paperback
Routledge is an imprint of the Taylor & Francis Group, an informa business

Cover design by Curtis Tow.

A CIP catalog record for this book is available from the British Library.

Library of Congress Cataloging-in-Publication Data
Pagliaro, Louis A.
      Psychologists' neuropsychotropic drug reference / by Louis A. Pagliaro, Ann Marie Pagliaro.
      p.   cm.
      Includes bibliographical references and index.
      ISBN 0-87630-956-2 (case: alk. paper)
      1. Neuropsychopharmacology—Handbooks, manuals, etc. 2. Psychotropic drugs—Handbooks, manuals, etc.
I. Pagliaro, Ann Marie II. Title.
      [DNLM: 1. Psychotropic Drugs handbooks. 2. Psychopharmacology handbooks. QV 39 P138p 1999]
      RM315.P32526 1999
      615'.788—dc21
      DNLM/DLC
      for Library of Congress   98–32463
                                     CIP

ISBN 978-0-87630-956-8 (hbk)
ISBN 978-1-13800-968-4 (pbk)

Dedication

To improved neuropsychological health among all people and the advancement of prescribing psychology

Contents

Editorial Advisory Committee

Charles A. Faltz, PhD
Director of Professional Affairs
California Psychological Association
Sacramento, California

Samuel A. Feldman, PhD, FAPM, FPPR, FSMI, FACAPP
Board-Certified Diplomat and Fellow and President,
Prescribing Psychologists' Register Inc.
North Miami Beach, Florida

Eldridge E. Fleming, PhD, FPPR
Past-President, Mississippi Psychological Association
Chair, Task Force on Psychopharmacology
Mississippi Psychological Association
Tupelo, Mississippi

Raymond A. Folen, PhD
Chief, Behavioral Medicine and Health Psychology Service
Department of Psychology
Tripler Regional Medical Center
Honolulu, Hawaii

Ronald E. Fox, PhD
Former President, American Psychological Association
Executive Director, Division of Organizational and Management Consulting
Human Resource Consultants
Chapel Hill, North Carolina

Alan R. Gruber, DSW, PhD
Co-Chair, Psychopharmacology Committee
Massachusetts Psychological Association
Neurobehavioral Associates
Hingham, Massachusetts

C. Alan Hopewell, PhD, ABPP
Dallas Neuropsychological Institute, PC
Dallas, Texas

Lawrence E. Klusman, PhD
Former Director, Psychopharmacology Demonstration Project
Department of Psychology
Walter Reed Army Medical Center
Washington, DC
Private Practice
Baton Rouge, Louisiana

Maxine L. Stitzer, PhD
Professor of Psychiatry and Behavioral Science
Johns Hopkins University
Baltimore, Maryland

Michael F. Wesner, PhD
Associate Professor of Psychology
Lakehead University
Thunder Bay, Ontario

Jack G. Wiggins, PhD
Former President, American Psychological Association
Consultant, University of Phoenix
Phoenix, Arizona

James P. Zacny, PhD
Associate Professor
Department of Anesthesia and Critical Care
The University of Chicago
Chicago, Illinois

Preface

The purpose of the *Psychologists' Neuropsychotropic Drug Reference* (*PNDR*) is to provide prescribing psychologists and psychology graduate students with an accurate and authoritative reference for the neuropsychotropic drugs that are commonly available for prescription in North America. The authors strongly believe that *all* clinical, health, and school psychologists should have a knowledge of the therapeutic action of the neuropsychotropics and their associated adverse drug reactions (ADRs) and toxicities, which can be confused with, or exacerbated by, virtually every neurologic and psychologic disorder. This reference text is directed particularly for use by psychologists and psychology graduate students who already have, or are currently developing, their professional expertise and responsibilities in the prescription and management of neuropsychotropic pharmacotherapy alone or in combination with psychotherapy.

The *PNDR* presents, in alphabetical order, detailed drug monographs for over 80 different prescription neuropsychotropic drugs available in North America.[1] Thus, this reference is the most comprehensive neuropsychotropic drug reference designed for psychologists currently available. The neuropsychotropic drugs presented in this text include the anticonvulsants, antiparkinsonians, drugs used to treat vascular headaches (e.g., migraine headache), nootropics (including anti-alzheimer drugs and drugs used to enhance memory and cognitive performance among stroke patients), and the opiate analgesics.[2] Monographs also are provided for both the benzodiazepine and opiate analgesic antagonists. Emphasis is on current approved Food and Drug Administration (FDA) and Health Protection Branch (HPB) guidelines for the prescription of these neuropsychotropics when indicated alone, and as adjunctive pharmacotherapy to, or in combination with, other neuropsychotropics.

Each neuropsychotropic drug monograph is clearly and concisely written to reflect only essential and important data that are commonly required by prescribing psychologists. Monographs are organized by generic name in alphabetical order.[3] Whenever available and appropriate, each monograph includes the following information: phonetic pronunciation guide; up to five common trade or brand names; pharmacologic or therapeutic classification and subclassification; United States Drug Enforcement Agency (USDEA) schedule designations for abuse potential (C-I, "high abuse potential," through C-V, "limited abuse potential"; see Appendix B); approved indications for prescription for neuropsychological disorders by psychologists;[4] recommended

---

[1] The use of fixed-dosage combination psychotropics is not generally recommended because of the lack of flexibility in appropriately adjusting the dosage of the component drugs in order to meet individual patient requirements. However, relevant information regarding the fixed-dosage combination products can be obtained using this text by separately accessing required information for each drug. A notable exception to this rule is the combination of levodopa with a peripheral decarboxylase inhibitor (i.e., benserazide or carbidopa).

[2] See Appendix A for a pharmacologic classification of the neuropsychotropics and a complete listing of the neuropsychotropic drugs for which monographs are included in the *PNDR*.

[3] The generic names used in this text are those that have been officially designated by the United States Adopted Names (USAN) Council. International drug names, such as those used by the British Pharmacopeia (British Adopted Names [BAN]), are cross-referenced for convenience as secondary headings.

[4] The FDA allows physicians to prescribe approved drugs for any indication, whether or not the indication is part of the approved labeling. Thus, a physician could prescribe the antibiotic tetracycline for the treatment of Alzheimer's disease if he or she so wished. In the absence of any scientific data to substantiate the efficacy of tetracycline for the

dosages for adults, women who are pregnant (including FDA pregnancy categories; see Appendix C), women who are breast-feeding, elderly adults, adults who have kidney or liver dysfunction, and children and adolescents; guidelines for the initiation, maintenance, and discontinuation of neuropsychotropic pharmacotherapy; available dosage forms and storage instructions; helpful and important notes regarding methods of administration; proposed mechanism(s) of drug action; pharmacokinetic/pharmacodynamic parameters, including therapeutic drug monitoring (TDM) for specific drugs for which TDM is recommended (e.g., the anticonvulsants); relative contraindications to use; cautions and comments to be considered when prescribing and managing neuropsychotropic pharmacotherapy; clinically significant drug interactions currently reported in the literature; the most commonly occurring adverse drug reactions and their general management; and signs and symptoms of overdosage.[5,6]

The *PNDR* integrates important and essential information for each monograph under these major headings in a specially designed taxonomy. For example, information helpful to prescribing psychologists for making decisions regarding the selection of an appropriate neuropsychotropic drug for the prophylactic or symptomatic management of a particular neuropsychological disorder is found in the section "Approved Indications for Neuropsychological Disorders." Information regarding the recommended dosage and administration of a particular psychotropic drug is included under "Usual Dosage and Administration." Dosage forms and storage considerations are identified in a specific "Available Dosage Forms, Storage, and Compatibility" section in each monograph. Explanations for the action of each neuropsychotropic are included in the section "Proposed Mechanism of Action," and data concerning the absorption, metabolism, and elimination of a particular drug are presented in the "Pharmacokinetic/Pharmacodynamic" section. Other pertinent data are provided in the "Relative Contraindications" and "Cautions and Comments" sections. Each monograph also includes information on the most common adverse drug reactions associated with a particular neuropsychotropic and the signs and symptoms of overdosage. This integrated organization of these clinical neuropsychotropic drug data should greatly facilitate the rapid retrieval of needed information. The use of the *PNDR* should enable prescribing psychologists to develop and enhance their abilities to prescribe, manage, and discontinue safe and effective neuropsychotropic pharmacotherapy.

Each of the monographs has been reviewed for form, style, and content by the members of the Editorial Advisory Committee for this series of texts. The members of this group of distinguished psychologists from across North America have given freely of their time and expertise in order to improve and advance the clinical practice of psychology. We are extremely grateful for their valuable contributions and support. All psychologists, as well as their patients, who will benefit directly from the clinical application of the information and knowledge gained from this

---

treatment of Alzheimer's disease, we would consider this use to be irrational and professionally negligent. Therefore, indications for use, as adjunctive pharmacotherapy for psychological disorders, are limited to those indications that have received FDA and/or HPB approval *and* for which efficacy has been established in the published clinical literature (i.e., for pharmacotherapy that has been empirically validated).

[5] Signs and symptoms of neuropsychotropic overdosages are presented to assist prescribing psychologists in recognizing possible overdosage among their patients so that pharmacotherapy can be appropriately discontinued and patients referred for emergency symptomatic medical management. The clinical management of overdosages is considered to be within the practice realm of medicine. Therefore, a discussion of the actual emergency symptomatic medical management of overdosage (e.g., selection and dosage of specific drugs used to facilitate drug elimination; use of adjunctive measures, such as hemodialysis; support of body systems [e.g., mechanical ventilation; provision of fluids and electrolytes]; and laboratory monitoring parameters) have not been included in this text. Whenever overdosage is *suspected*, clinical psychologists should directly refer their patients for emergency medical evaluation and management.

[6] The data included in these monographs have been derived from several sources including: references listed in the first volume in this series, *The Pharmacologic Basis of Psychotherapeutics: An Introduction for Psychologists*; current (1999) official FDA- and HPB-approved drug monographs for each of the neuropsychotropics listed; previous textbooks by the authors (see listing in the front material for this text); the authors' current graduate lectures for the "Series of Hierarchical Graduate and Post-Graduate Courses in Pharmacopsychology"; and the authors' clinical experiences. These available data were content-analyzed and synthesized into the monographs presented.

and the other texts in this series, owe the Editorial Advisory Committee a profound debt of gratitude. In all cases, responsibility for the completeness and accuracy of the data in this and the other texts in the series remains with the authors.[7]

As previously noted, the neuropsychotropics discussed in the *PNDR* are referred to by their generic (nonproprietary) USAN names. However, psychologists who use brand or trade names may access needed information by consulting the general index located at the end of this reference. All dosages included in the *PNDR* are average dosages derived, utilizing population-based statistical models, from data obtained from sample groups of research subjects and are, therefore, approximate. In all cases, variability in *individual* patient response may necessitate alterations in drug dosages or frequency of dosing. Accepted guidelines for the use of each neuropsychotropic drug, including drug information centers, current manufacturer patient and product package inserts, or other authoritative references, should be consulted whenever there is further question about a particular use or dose of a drug. For example, psychologists who require additional information, or review, concerning the basic principles of clinical pharmacology are referred to the companion volume and first text in this series, *The Pharmacologic Basis of Psychotherapeutics: An Introduction for Psychologists* (Pagliaro & Pagliaro, 1998).[8] Detailed information regarding the psychotropics (i.e., antidepressants, antimanics, antipsychotics, CNS stimulants, opiate analgesics,[9] and sedative hypnotics) is presented in the second volume in this series, *Psychologists' Psychotropic Drug Reference* (L. A. Pagliaro & A. M. Pagliaro, 1999). In addition, psychologists who require additional information or review regarding the indications and use of the psychotropics as adjuncts to psychotherapy and other therapeutic modalities (e.g., biofeedback, electroconvulsive therapy) that are most appropriate for the symptomatic management of specific psychological disorders are referred to the companion volume and fourth text in this series, *Clinical Pharmacopsychotherapeutics for Psychologists* (L. A. Pagliaro & A. M. Pagliaro, in press).[10]

When additional age-specific information regarding pharmacotherapy is required for children and adolescents or the elderly, psychologists are referred to L. A. Pagliaro and A. M. Pagliaro (Eds.), *Problems in Pediatric Drug Therapy* (4th ed., American Pharmaceutical Association, in press), or L. A. Pagliaro and A. M. Pagliaro (Eds.), *Problems in Geriatric Drug Therapy* (in preparation), respectively. For a more detailed discussion of abusable psychotropic exposure and use among infants, children, and adolescents, psychologists are referred to A. M. Pagliaro and L. A. Pagliaro, *Substance Use Among Children and Adolescents: Its Nature, Extent, and Effects from Conception to Adulthood* (New York: John Wiley & Sons, 1996). For further assistance, several appendices, including a list of abbreviations used in the *PNDR*, can be found at the end of this text.

[7] However, readers of this text have a professional responsibility to actively seek and obtain clarification whenever information seems to them to be unclear or incomplete.

[8] *The Pharmacologic Basis of Psychotherapeutics: An Introduction for Psychologists* is the first text in this series from both a temporal publication perspective and a pedagogical hierarchical perspective. For this reason, it is expected that readers of the *PNDR* are already familiar with the terms (e.g., akathisia, anorexiant), concepts (e.g., methods of drug administration; therapeutic drug monitoring), and basic principles of pharmacology (e.g., basic mechanisms of drug action; similarities and differences between and among the various classes of psychotropics). If not, they should first review *The Pharmacologic Basis of Psychotherapeutics: An Introduction for Psychologists*.

See the preface for *The Pharmacologic Basis of Psychotherapeutics*, which has been reproduced in the front material of this text, for further details and information about that text and the series.

[9] The opiate analgesics are discussed in both volumes.

[10] *Clinical Pharmacopsychotherapeutics for Psychologists* discusses, in the context of specific psychological disorders that are amenable to adjunctive pharmacotherapy, the currently available treatment modalities (e.g., alternative, such as acupuncture; medical, such as surgery; and psychological, such as biofeedback, hypnotherapy, pharmacotherapy, and psychotherapy). The treatment modalities are evaluated in terms of their demonstrated efficacy. The criteria and parameters for selecting the best (individual or combination) therapy for specific individual patients are presented with an emphasis upon empirically validated psychotherapeutic modalities.

It is hoped that the information presented in the **PNDR** will better enable prescribing psychologists and graduate psychology students, as they strive to significantly improve neuropsychological health, to provide their patients with the maximal benefits of neuropsychotropic pharmacotherapy with minimal adverse and toxic effects.

LAP/AMP
1999

Preface to *The Pharmacologic Basis of Psychotherapeutics: An Introduction for Psychologists* [a]

We are in a time of significant economic, political, and social change. This time of change is affecting the professional practice of psychology in a variety of ways as traditional disciplinary lines are dissolving and new boundaries are being drawn. Major practice issues, such as prescription and hospital admitting privileges for psychologists, need to be expediently and adequately addressed. Naturally, it is to be expected that some psychologists, perhaps because they are content with the status quo or because they are fearful of change, may wish that things be left as they are. Unfortunately, things cannot be left as they are. As noted by Chesterton almost 90 years ago, "If you leave a thing alone you leave it to a torrent of change" (*Orthodoxy*, 1908). Thus, our only logical and rational alternative is to become involved with the changes and to view the process of change not as a threat but as an opportunity to broaden the professional practice of psychology and, in so doing, improve the health and well-being of people who require psychological services.

As many psychologists have come to realize, appropriate pharmacotherapy can be a useful adjunct to appropriate psychotherapy and, as such, is a welcome tool for psychologists. Certainly, the optimal professional practice of psychology requires, if not prescription privileges for psychologists, at least a minimum significant degree of specialized knowledge about the propensity for psychotropics to affect behavior, cognition, learning, memory, and psychological health. Even those psychologists who choose not to prescribe psychotropics as part of their professional practice require an understanding of the use and effects of these drugs.

Such understanding is essential in order for all psychologists to meet more competently and comprehensively the needs of their patients, many of whom will be prescribed a psychotropic by a family physician or another prescriber (e.g., advanced practice nurse, cardiologist, clinical pharmacist, dentist, or psychiatrist). For example, even psychologists considered to be the best *psychotherapists* in the world would more than likely be unsuccessful in the treatment of a depression if they were unaware that the clinical depression was a direct adverse result of the use of a benzodiazepine (e.g., Ativan®, Halcion®, Valium®) with the adverse drug reaction of depression. In another example, school psychologists, considered to be the best learning specialists in the world, would be unable to plan optimal programs for learning disabled children if they were unaware that the children's learning problems were a direct result of anticonvulsant drug therapy, which some children require for the treatment of seizure disorders, or too high a dosage of methylphenidate (Ritalin®), which is commonly prescribed to children for the treatment of attention-deficit/hyperactivity disorder (A-D/HD). This argument becomes even more relevant when it is recognized that virtually every psychological disorder, whether characterized by DSM-IV or other relevant criteria (e.g., ICD), can have its signs and symptoms mimicked by the adverse drug reactions of the various psychotropics.

---

[a] The preface of the first text in the series of pharmacopsychology texts for psychologists is reproduced here in order to place the current text, which is a continuation of that series, in both historical and pedagogical perspective.

Prescription privileges and related issues are being actively addressed by the profession of psychology in several countries, including Canada, South Africa, New Zealand, and the United Kingdom. In these countries, professional practice acts are increasingly being rewritten to incorporate a *nonexclusive* scope of practice for all of the health professions. By providing "nonexclusive" scopes of practice, these acts appropriately and correctly recognize that no one individual or group exclusively "owns" knowledge of a particular area of mental health practice (e.g., prescription authority). However, nowhere has this issue received more scrutiny and active debate within the profession of psychology than in the United States, where it has received the official endorsement of the American Psychological Association, the largest psychological association in the world. The Foreword of this text, written by Patrick DeLeon and Morgan Sammons, provides a historical overview of the debate and progress surrounding this crucial issue for psychologists.

The Ad Hoc Task Force on Psychopharmacology of the American Psychological Association has recommended three levels of psychopharmacology education. Level 1, "basic psychopharmacology education," would provide a minimal level of psychopharmacology education for all psychologists in clinical practice. Level 2, "collaborative practice," would provide additional education to enable psychologists to participate actively as partners with physicians and other prescribers in determining the need for and the monitoring of psychotropic therapy for patients they "share." Level 3, "prescription privileges," would provide the education necessary for psychologists to have independent psychotropic prescription privileges.

In accordance with these developments in psychology and the need for related formal advanced education, the authors of this text developed, at the University of Alberta, the "Hierarchical Integrated Series of Graduate/Postgraduate Courses in Pharmacopsychology," which they have taught since 1990 to both graduate psychology students and postgraduate psychologists in private practice.[1,2] The development of the "hierarchical series" was based on three basic assumptions: (1) that no single profession or group exclusively "owns" any given knowledge; (2) that psychologists, who as a group are the highest academically prepared health care professionals, are able to comprehend and to apply appropriately in clinical contexts the information and concepts of clinical pharmacology relevant to the promotion of mental health; and (3) that appropriate pharmacotherapy, when prescribed by psychologists, should be used only as an adjunct to appropriate psychotherapy.[3,4]

The current series of textbooks, of which this text is the first, is based on the authors' experience in teaching the hierarchical series of pharmacopsychology courses to a variety of graduate students in psychology and postgraduate psychologists in independent practice in many different settings. The development of this series of textbooks also reflects the authors' concern that psychologists be provided with reference texts that are pharmacologically correct and that specif-

---

[1] Interested readers can contact the authors for a copy of the syllabus "A Hierarchical Integrated Series of Graduate/Postgraduate Courses in Pharmacopsychology."

[2] The "Hierarchical Integrated Series of Graduate/Postgraduate Courses in Pharmacopsychology" was also developed to help psychologists and graduate psychology students become better prepared to more competently perform research in the area of pharmacopsychology. In this regard, the series has become a foundational component of the research program of most of the authors' own doctoral students.

[3] For example, when treating a depressed patient, a psychologist would use appropriate pharmacotherapy to complement or augment established psychotherapy (e.g., cognitive therapy). In this example, if the psychologist believed that psychotherapy was unnecessary and that only pharmacotherapy was required, then the patient should be referred to another prescriber (e.g., advanced practice nurse; family physician; psychiatrist).

[4] The third assumption is predicated upon the following rationale. First, psychotherapy is the core foundational aspect of clinical psychology treatment services (i.e., while psychologists may provide additional forms of treatment, such as biofeedback and hypnotherapy, psychotherapy remains the *raison d'etre* for the existence of clinical psychology as a distinct treatment-providing health care profession). Second, although research studies examining the relative therapeutic benefits of pharmacotherapy and psychotherapy have provided mixed results, a growing consensus is that the appropriate combination of these psychotherapeutic modalities in the treatment of amenable mental disorders leads, overall, to greater success (i.e., better therapeutic outcome) than the use of either modality alone.

ically reflect the expanded professional practice of psychology. Although each of the three initial textbooks in the series can be used alone, they have been developed as a complementary set to delineate the pharmacopsychologic knowledge required for the optimal professional practice of psychology (i.e., basic principles of pharmacotherapy, synopses of psychotropic drugs, and clinical psychopharmacotherapeutics).

The first volume in the series, *The Pharmacologic Basis of Psychotherapeutics: An Introduction for Psychologists*, introduces psychology students and psychologists to the basic principles and concepts of pharmacotherapy. As such, it assumes no prior knowledge of the principles and concepts of pharmacotherapy and should be readily amenable for use by the graduate psychology student or postgraduate psychologist in clinical practice. The second volume in the series, *PPDR: Psychologists' Psychotropic Drug Reference*, provides psychologists with a valuable synopsis of all of the clinically relevant data currently available for each of the psychotropics marketed in North America. These data have been subsumed and arranged within individual drug monographs in order to facilitate the conceptualization and rapid retrieval of desired information when needed. The optimal use of this text requires a knowledge of the basic principles and concepts of psychotherapeutics, discussed in the first volume in the series. The volume in the series, *Clinical Pharmacopsychotherapeutics for Psychologists*, in preparation, will critically discuss each of the major psychological disorders that is amenable to pharmacotherapy as an adjunct to psychotherapy. Thus, emphasis is on the validated effectiveness of these combined therapeutic approaches and related issues, including their empirical validation.[5] The optimal use of this text requires mastery of the information presented in the first and second volumes in the series, which have been designed to facilitate retrieval and review of required material.

Thus, the present volume is the foundational text that provides the pharmacologic basis of psychotherapeutics that is required for optimal use of the second and third volumes in this series. Together, these three volumes reflect all three levels of pharmacopsychology education. *The Pharmacologic Basis of Psychotherapeutics: An Introduction for Psychologists* is divided into six chapters. The Foreword, "Prescription Privileges for Psychologists: An Historical Overview," written by Patrick DeLeon, a champion of prescription drug privileges for psychologists, and Morgan Sammons, one of the first graduates of the Department of Defense Psychopharmacology Fellowship Program, provides a brief history of the major events leading to prescription privileges for psychologists. It also provides a précis of the arguments that have been made both for and against this expanded role for psychologists.[6] Chapter 1, "Introduction to the Basic Principles of Pharmacotherapy," describes and discusses the various purported mechanisms by which psychotropic drugs elicit their effects in the human body. Chapter 2, "The Psychotropics," introduces readers to the psychotropic drugs, including their differentiation according to abuse liability and pharmacologic classification. In addition, an overview of the remaining chapters in the textbook, in terms of their relevance to the central theme of the text and their application to clinical practice, is presented. Chapter 3, "Pharmacokinetics and Pharmacodynamics," deals with the processes of absorption, distribution, and elimination (i.e., metabolism and excretion) of psychotropic drugs from the human body. In addition, the concept of therapeutic drug monitoring (TDM) and the influences of age and disease states on pharmacokinetic and pharmacodynamic processes are presented and discussed. Related mathematical modeling, including graphical representations and formulas, is included. Chapter 4, "Administration of Psychotropics," provides

---

[5]The series of texts focuses exclusively on the therapeutic uses of the psychotropics. Psychologists who require additional specific information regarding the problematic patterns of abusable psychotropic use (i.e., those patterns associated with addiction and habituation) are referred to *Substance Use Among Children and Adolescents: Its Nature, Extent, and Consequences From Conception to Adulthood* (A. M. Pagliaro & L. A. Pagliaro, 1996).

[6]We are extremely grateful to Patrick DeLeon and Morgan Sammons, who took time from extremely busy schedules to write the Foreword for this first text in the "Series."

an overview of the various formulations of psychotropic drugs (e.g., injectables, tablets, transdermal delivery systems) and their methods of administration (e.g., intramuscular injection, oral ingestion). Attention is given to optimizing drug delivery and therapeutic response. Chapter 5, "Adverse Drug Reactions," discusses the nature and extent of adverse drug reactions involving the psychotropic drugs. Adverse drug reactions that mimic the various psychological disorders, including those related to the use of nonpsychotropic drugs (e.g., antibiotics, antiulcer drugs), also are discussed. Several comprehensive tables have been included to facilitate retrieval of relevant information. Chapter 6, "Drug Interactions," discusses the general mechanisms and sites of drug interactions that are known to occur in the human body. Individual monographs for each clinically significant drug interaction known to involve the psychotropics are provided, with attention to the specific nature, mechanisms, and clinical consequences of the drug interactions. Methods used to prevent or manage each of these interactions also are discussed.

As a means for ensuring that each chapter is as comprehensive, well written, and up to date as humanly possible, the chapters have been subjected to a rigorous process of writing and revision. This has been done by the authors taking into consideration their extensive academic and clinical backgrounds, in terms of both clinical pharmacology and psychology, and the related, relevant published literature. In addition, an Editorial Advisory Committee, composed of distinguished academics, researchers, and clinical psychologists from across North America, was established to help to ensure that the focus and leveling of the series of textbooks was appropriately directed to the needs and abilities of graduate psychology students and psychologists.[7] Each chapter has been independently reviewed by several members of the Editorial Advisory Committee, who have given freely of their time and expertise in order to help produce a series of textbooks that should become a proud standard for psychologists. The authors, and all psychology students and psychologists who use these texts, owe a profound debt of gratitude to these advisory committee members.[8]

It is hoped that, by using the information presented in this specially developed series of pharmacopsychology texts, psychologists will be better able to provide their patients who have various psychological disorders with optimal psychotropic pharmacotherapy as an appropriate adjunct to psychotherapy and, thus, optimize the benefit derived by all patients who seek professional treatment from psychologists. In our earnest attempt to provide the best possible series of pharmacopsychology texts for psychologists, we are humbly reminded of the following words and sentiment paraphrased from Adlai Stevenson:

> *We have not done as well as we would have liked to have done,*
> *But we have done our best, honestly and forthrightly.*
> *No one can do more and you (our colleague psychologists)*
> *are entitled to no less.*

LAP/AMP
1998

---

[7]For example, in order to assist with this goal, the Editorial Advisory Committee (EAC) identified terms with which psychologists might not be readily familiar. The most common terms were then defined and arranged in a glossary that can be found in Appendix D at the end of this text.

In relation to leveling, it should be noted that the series, although in many regards introductory to the subject matter, was written for psychologists at a graduate level of education. Therefore, the "series" is significantly more comprehensive and at a higher scholarly level than will be found in related undergraduate texts, including those generally written for medical students.

[8]The responsibility for the completeness and accuracy of all information provided within this text remains with the authors.

Foreword to *The Pharmacologic Basis of Psychotherapeutics: An Introduction for Psychologists*

Prescription Privileges for Psychologists: An Historical Overview

For professional psychology, the prescription privilege agenda began in earnest in the late 1980s. On November 30, 1984 U.S. Senator Daniel K. Inouye addressed the annual meeting of the Hawaii Psychological Association (HPA) and urged them to adopt: "... an entirely new legislative agenda which I think fits very nicely into the theme of your convention: 'Psychology in the 80's: Transcending Traditional Boundaries'. As a United States Senator, I have also been working closely during the past decade with a number of your 'natural allies'. I am particularly thinking of our nation's nurse practitioners, nurse midwives, and optometrists. The members of these professions have been successful to differing degrees in amending their state practice acts to allow them to independently utilize drugs where appropriate.... In my judgment, when you have obtained this statutory authority, you will have really made the big time. Then, you truly will be an autonomous profession and your clients will be well-served" (Inouye, 1984). Interestingly, that same year Richard Samuels, then President of the APA Division of Psychologists in Independent Practice (Division 42), called for a similar policy agenda. These futuristic "calls for action" were enthusiastically heard by many within our professional community but in retrospect, it has become evident that the vast majority of our colleagues had yet to really appreciate the monumental long-term implications for their professional identities, clinical practices, and training institutions (DeLeon, Fox, & Graham, 1991).

In many ways, the maturation of the prescription privilege agenda might well be viewed as being closely related to psychology's gradual emergence over the past several decades as a bona fide health care profession. An increasing number of our colleagues no longer identify with psychology's traditional self-conceptualization of solely being a "mental health specialist." Instead, they are genuinely interested in providing "comprehensive primary care" or working as an integral element of our nation's *health care* system—effectively addressing the psychosocial and behavioral aspects of a wide range of physical ailments (DeLeon, Frank, & Wedding, 1995).

Without question, psychology's status within the health care arena has dramatically increased over the recent years. In our judgment, this evolution (maturation) has been closely related to two distinct clinical developments: the increasing appreciation by medicine of the considerable benefits of the behavioral sciences in general, and the significant successes of the other non-physician disciplines in demonstrating that they do, indeed, provide high quality and cost-effective health services. From our experiences at the national level it has become quite evident that psychology is already intimately involved in a wide range of health initiatives, including serving prominently on the university faculty of a number of professional disciplines—for example, *approximately one* quarter of doctoral level nursing faculty possess degrees in psychology.

Today, nearly a decade and a half since Senator Inouye's initial challenge, there has been considerable progress in the efforts of the various non-physician disciplines to obtain prescriptive authority. Optometry, for example, first obtained this clinical responsibility in the State of Indiana in 1935. Fifty years later, Maryland became the final state in the nation to formally recognize their pharmacological expertise. Nurse practitioners began their quest with the successful passage of legislation in North Carolina in 1975. Today, 48–49 states have enacted legislation providing Advanced Practice Nursing (APN) with prescriptive authority, under various conditions; the movement clearly being towards "physician substitution" statutes (i.e., granting nursing professional autonomy). Similar progress has been made by podiatry (all states), physician assistants (40 states), and pharmacists (seven states). Not surprisingly, every step of the way (with the notable exception of physician assistants) the competing medical specialty groups strenuously opposed the granting of this particular privilege—arguing in essence that if granted, their counterparts would affirmatively "harm" their patients (i.e., that since they did not attend medical school, non-physicians represent definite "public health hazards") (DeLeon & Wiggins, 1996).

From both a public policy and evolutionary perspective, there has also been *remarkable* progress on the prescription agenda within organized psychology (Fox, 1988; Frank, 1992; Pimental, Stout, Hoover, & Kamen, 1997). When one appreciates that the prescription agenda is being primarily advanced by the practice community, rather than by the educational community, the fact that a genuine consensus for obtaining this clinical responsibility has actually evolved, in such a relatively short period of time, is nothing short of amazing. Psychology has never really possessed "homes of its own" where psychology faculty control the day-to-day clinical experiences of their students and where truly comprehensive (including inpatient care) clinical experiences can be provided. Individual clinicians may have obtained considerable "first hand" expertise in utilizing psychopharmacological agents; however, to develop viable, not to mention credible, psychopharmacology training programs a profession must have regular access to those patients who genuinely require these services. That is, the opportunity to provide both didactic and "hands on" expertise must be readily obtainable. Without these necessary resources, it is difficult for psychology faculty who traditionally have been responsible for ensuring that graduate students are competently trained—including "signing off" on internship placements—to feel emotionally comfortable about their potential role (Fox, Schwelitz, & Barclay, 1992). Interestingly, this has not been an issue for the other disciplines.

State Legislative Experiences: During the 1989 legislative session the Hawaii House of Representatives enacted a formal Resolution (H. Res #334-90) calling on the state's Center for Alternative Dispute Resolution to study the prescription issue in depth and report back the following legislative session its policy recommendations. Twenty-nine legislators had signed that resolution and extensive hearings were held in both legislative chambers. In 1993 the Indiana legislature modified its psychology licensure act to authorize prescriptive authority for those psychologists who are "participating in a federal government sponsored training or treatment program." Although this provision of the Indiana statute has not yet been implemented, the affirmative public policy stances taken by the governor (in signing the bill) and the legislature (in passing it) are clear. From our perspective the key policy lesson to be learned from these two examples is that when psychology collectively decides to become involved in the public policy/political process the prescription agenda seems not only reasonable to elected officials, it becomes substantively "doable" (DeLeon, Folen, Jennings, Willis, & Wright, 1991).

Accordingly, over the past several years we have been very pleased to witness an increasing number of prescribing bills being introduced in state legislatures across the nation—resulting in active pro and con lobbying, state association "grass roots" educational campaigns, advocacy positions taken by the popular media, and formal legislative hearings and subsequent (sub)committee votes, etc. (e.g., Hawaii, California, Florida, Louisiana, Missouri, Montana, Oregon, Tennesee). By the mid-1990s approximately 25 states had ongoing prescription privilege task forces. Viable training modules, particularly executive track initiatives targeting practicing clinicians, are actively being established. Internal psychological association surveys continue to demonstrate that initially approximately one third of the membership are supportive while another third possesses serious reservations. As the state association becomes more engaged in the policy debate, however, subsequent surveys soon find that 70–80 percent of the membership are supportive. Again, however, it is important to appreciate that, as we have indicated, even these evolving training programs are often a direct result of concerted action taken by the state psychological association elected leadership rather than spontaneous generation by our traditional training institutions.

Developments Within the APA Governance: In August 1995 the APA Council of Representatives, which is the highest governance body within the Association, formally endorsed the inclusion of prescription privileges as being appropriately within the "scope of practice" of professional psychology. This action by the Council was predicated upon a foundation carefully developed over the previous decade which involved numerous discussions between representatives from the practice, educational, and scientific communities. In many ways, the Council's action may be seen as merely reaffirming a policy first endorsed in 1986 (and authored at that time by those actively seeking policy support for the prescription privilege movement) which had expressly proclaimed that the practice of psychology was to include the use of physical, as well as purely psychological interventions (Cullen & Newman, 1997).

Five years earlier the APA 1990 Council of Representatives had voted to establish a Task Force on Psychopharmacology. This task force submitted a formal report to the Council that recommended the development of three levels of psychopharmacological training. Their report ultimately formed the basis for further action by Council in 1996 solidifying psychology's proactive stance when the Council took the additional step of formally endorsing both model prescription legislation and a model comprehensive curriculum training module.

The curriculum recommended by the Council to those interested in pursuing the prescription agenda consisted of 300 contact hours of didactic instruction in five core content areas: neurosciences; pharmacology and psychopharmacology; physiology and pathophysiology; physical and laboratory assessment; and clinical pharmacotherapeutics. A clinical practicum involving supervised medication treatment of at least 100 patients in both inpatient and outpatient settings was also recommended. The model legislation would authorize the state licensing board to deem (i.e., certify) those competent to possess independent prescribing authority. The board of medicine was not to be involved in determining psychology's clinical competence (i.e., the substitution rather than physician-extender model would be pursued).

We would note in passing that one indication of the extent to which some psychologists perceive expansion into the prescription arena as an extraordinarily significant change in psychology's history (and core definition) is the fact that to our knowledge this is the only time in our profession's history that the APA Council of Representatives ever felt it appropriate (or necessary) to expressly take a policy position on whether a particular clinical technique or modality should be considered within psychology's scope of practice. Historically, the key policy notion has always been to rely upon state licensing boards to ensure that sufficient and relevant training be available; i.e., that the particular clinical function being considered would be within the technical competence of the individual practitioner.

In informal discussions with those who have been intimately involved during this period in shaping APA's policy position on the prescriptive agenda, it would definitely appear that the seminal event which served to crystallize the underlying issues for psychology's governance leadership and ultimately galvanize the professional community behind the movement was the special retreat held by the Board of Professional Affairs (BPA) under the leadership of Norma Simon in

November 1989. After extensive consultation with relevant experts, including psychologists who were intimately involved in the landmark Department of Defense (DoD) psychopharmacology training program, BPA unanimously concluded that: "BPA strongly endorses the immediate research and study intervention feasibility and curricula development in psychopharmacology for psychologists in order to provide broader service to the public and to address more effectively the public's psychological and mental health needs. And BPA strongly recommends moving to the highest APA priority a focused attention to the responsibility of preparing the profession of psychology to address the current and future needs of the public for psychologically managed psychopharmacological interventions."

The following year under future APA President Bob Resnick's leadership, BPA further recommended to the Board of Directors that a special task force on psychopharmacology be established. The APA Board of Directors concurred and recommended that the Council of Representatives fund such a task force out of its coming year's contingency funds—thus effectively setting the stage for a true policy debate at the highest level. As we have indicated, that August after extensive discussion in which at least seventeen members of Council expressed a wide range of views—including the possible impact on the homeless, women's health care, the elderly, rural America, and psychology's historical ability to develop responsive and responsible training programs—the Council voted *in favor* of establishing the historic task force 118-2. An outcome that in all candor, no one could have predicted. The actual motion adopted stated: "To determine the advisability and feasibility of psychopharmacology prescription privileges for psychologists, an APA Task Force on Psychopharmacology be formed with the following charge: 1) To involve relevant constituencies and Divisions in this process in conjunction with the Education, Science, and Practice Directorates. 2) To determine the competency criteria necessary for training of psychologists to practice the highest quality patient care without adverse consequences for patients. 3) To develop alternative curricular models necessary to achieve the above, and to consider data-based evaluation of such training and evaluate the pros & cons of each training model. This task force shall be comprised of 7 members representing a range of scientific, educational, and clinical practice expertise and should report to the APA Board of Directors and the APA Council of Representatives. . . ." It should be clear from the actual language of the Council's action that throughout the process there really has been considerable involvement of all aspects of the APA governance. The Committee for the Advancement of Professional Practice (CAPP) and the Board of Educational Affairs (BEA), and particularly its Committee on Continuing Education, have also been actively and formally involved. Similarly, the leadership of the Board of Scientific Affairs (BSA) played a major role and the concerns expressed by the Board for the Advancement of Psychology in the Public Interest (BAPPI) regarding the historic over-reliance upon psychotropic medications with women and people of color were noted. We really do want to stress the extent to which throughout the association's deliberation process the widest range of views have been heard and addressed.

Health Policy Formulation—The Demonstration Approach: Very few psychologists appreciate the extent to which our nation has a rich history at both the state and federal level of systematically testing out potentially innovative and viable health care programs, including the non-traditional utilization of health professional expertise. In many ways, for example, the history of the phenomenal growth of advanced practice nursing epitomizes this notion. Under our system of constitutional "checks and balances," the various governmental entities at both the state and federal level possess the inherent authority to experiment with expanded scopes of professional practice, notwithstanding statutory limits for the private sector under the provisions of relevant licensing acts. Simply stated, unless expressly enacted into public law, there is no limit on the ability of state health departments or the various federal services to utilize their employees in whatever manner they deem appropriate. In essence, government in its role as a "provider of care" has tremendous flexibility in accomplishing that mission—government does provide a "living laboratory" for innovation.

In the mid-1970s the State of California utilized its health professions demonstration authority to explore the extent to which non-physician health care providers might properly be eventually authorized to possess prescriptive authority, and under what conditions. In November of 1982 the state issued a formal report, *Prescribing and Dispensing Pilot Projects,* in which it was noted that: "None of the projects, to date, have received the intense scrutiny that these 10 prescribing and dispensing projects have received. Over 1 million patients have been seen by these prescribing and dispensing (non-physicians) trainees over the past three years. At least 50 percent of these patients have had drugs prescribed for them or dispensed to them by these professionals" (State of California, p. i). The principle teaching methods used by project staff were lectures and seminars, varying from 16 hours to 95 hours in length. Further, only 56 percent of the trainees had graduated from an academic program with a bachelor's degree or higher. Clearly these trainees possessed considerably less formal education than doctoral level psychologists. All involved in the programs (including supervising physicians) were definitely comfortable with the quality of health care provided. The state authorities found the project to be cost-effective, even when the costs of physician supervision and pharmacist consultation were considered.

The Fiscal Year 1989 Department of Defense Appropriations bill (P.L. 100-463) directed that the administration establish a demonstration pilot training project under which military psychologists could be trained and authorized to issue appropriate psychotropic medications under certain circumstances. The actual training began in August 1991 with four participants in a special 3-year postdoctoral fellowship program consisting of two years of didactic course work at the DoD Uniformed Services University of the Health Sciences, to be followed by one year of clinical "hands on" experience at Walter Reed Army Medical Center. As the training matured and began to systematically take into account the academic and clinical backgrounds of the psychologists Fellows, subsequent classes received one year of didactic work and one year of "hands on" clinical training. By the summer of 1997 ten Fellows had graduated from the program (Sammons & Brown, 1997; Sammons, Sexton, & Meredith, 1996).

It would be a tremendous understatement to suggest that the DoD initiative was controversial, particularly to organized psychiatry. From its inception, the Department contracted for an independent evaluation and two additional external evaluations were also conducted. The latter two studies conflicted as to whether the training program was fundamentally cost-effective. However, even the more critical General Accounting Office (GAO) report concluded that: "DoD has demonstrated that it can train clinical psychologists to prescribe psychotropic medication, and these psychologists have shown that they can provide this service in the MHSS [Military Health Services System]" (U.S. GAO, 1997, p. 20). At organized psychiatry's urging the National Defense Authorization Act for Fiscal Year 1996 (P.L. 104-106) had expressly prohibited the enrollment of any new Fellows in the program; however, organized psychology has been actively seeking a legislative remedy to this particular prohibition. The bottom line is that DoD did clearly demonstrate that it can train military psychologists to safely and competently provide psychotropic medications, notwithstanding the proffered and highly emotional "public health hazard" allegations of psychiatry.

Where From Here?—Although it is always difficult to predict with any sense of accuracy the future of the legislative and/or public policy process, there is no question in our minds that it is only a matter of time—and at that, a relatively brief period of time—before psychology attains its first legislative prescriptive privilege success at the state level. Over the years various federal psychologists have reported that even without formal training they have personally made the clinical decisions as to which psychopharmacological drugs should be taken by their patients; *that is, our colleagues within the federal system have, and do, functionally and legally prescribe,* notwithstanding psychiatry's objections and protestations to the contrary. In at least one agency, the Indian Health Service (IHS) hospital bylaws and central office policy memorandums formally recognized this practice.

Not surprisingly, the DoD psychopharmacology training program objectively demonstrated that it is possible to train psychologists to utilize psychopharmacological agents responsibly. Each of the ten Fellows has expressed to us their confidence that the quality of their clinical services has been excellent and that possessing this clinical expertise has opened up entirely new clinical responsibilities. The concern expressed by some of our psychology colleagues that possessing prescription privileges would cause psychology's clinicians to lose their fundamental behavioral science (and psychology) identity simply has not happened. Instead, the Fellows all enthusiastically describe the clinical advantages to their patients of their fundamental psychological orientation to the use of psychotropic medications. And, we would again reiterate that psychiatry's proffered "public health hazard" allegations have had no basis in fact (DeLeon, Sammons, & Fox, 1995)!

In our judgment, an important historical aspect to the prescription privilege movement has been the necessity to date of developing post-doctoral training modules, targeted towards practicing clinicians. These colleagues are already licensed to independently "diagnose and treat" patients and the additional psychopharmacology training has essentially enhanced their clinical capacities while allowing them to retain their fundamental behavioral science and psychology identity. What will be the long term effect on the profession, if eventually, the decision is made to incorporate prescription training at the predoctoral level is admittedly unclear and only time will tell (DeLeon, Sammons, & Sexton, 1995).

Today there are a number of different training programs being established across the country, some of which interestingly rely considerably upon professional nursing's expertise. As our nation's educational institutions become more attuned to the implications of the rapidly evolving advances within the communications field and as the health care industry itself becomes more responsive to the advances evolving within computer technology, one must expect that these will have a major impact upon prescribing practices. How these changes will affect psychology's presence can not be known at this time. For example, will the ready availability of telemedicine services provide psychology with a greater capacity to obtain supervision experiences for its rural practitioners, or will this technology instead serve to undercut psychology's increased access argument before state legislatures? Or perchance, will technological advances instead open up new markets for psychopharmacological consultation services with prescribing rural primary care physicians and nurse practitioners (DeLeon et al., 1996)?

There are many public and professional policy issues for professional psychology to systematically address as we continue to expand into the prescription arena. What will be the probable impact on interdisciplinary relationships, how (if at all) should our ethical standards be modified, etc.? We are confident that as long as the profession ensures that providing high quality patient care remains the highest priority, that our educational and professional institutions will in the long run be able to address these new challenges with distinction (Lorion, Iscoe, DeLeon, & VandenBos, 1996).

The views expressed in this Foreword are those of the individual authors and not those of the APA, the U.S. Navy, or the Department of Defense.

Pat DeLeon
APA Recording Secretary
and
Morgan Sammons
DoD Psychopharmacology Fellow

References

Cullen, E. A., & Newman, R. (1997). In pursuit of prescription privileges. *Professional Psychology: Research and Practice, 28*(2), 101–106.

DeLeon, P. H., Folen, R. A., Jennings, F. L., Willis, D. J., & Wright, R. H. (1991). The case for prescription privileges: A logical evolution of professional practice. *Journal of Clinical Child Psychology, 20*(3), 254–267.

DeLeon, P. H., Fox, R. E., & Graham, S. R. (1991). Prescription privileges: Psychology's next frontier? *American Psychologist, 46*, 384–393.

DeLeon, P. H., Frank, R. G., & Wedding, D. (1995). Health psychology and public policy: The political process. *Health Psychology, 14*(6), 493–499.

DeLeon, P. H., Howell, W. C., Newman, R. S., Brown, A. B., Keita, G. P., & Sexton, J. L. (1996). Expanding roles in the twenty-first century. In R. J. Resnick & R. H. Rozensky (Eds.), *Health psychology through the life span: Practice and research opportunities* (pp. 427–453). Washington, DC: American Psychological Association.

DeLeon, P. H., Sammons, M. T., & Fox, R. E. (1995, November). A commentary: Canada is not that far north. *Canadian Psychology, 36*(4), 320–326.

DeLeon, P. H., Sammons, M. T., & Sexton, J. L. (1995). Focusing on society's real needs: Responsibility and prescription privileges? *American Psychologist, 50*(12), 1022–1032.

DeLeon, P. H., & Wiggins, J. G. (1996). Prescription privileges for psychologists. *American Psychologist, 51*(3), 225–229.

Fox, R. E. (1988). Prescription privileges: Their implications for the practice of psychology. *Psychotherapy, 25*(4), 501–507.

Fox, R. E., Schwelitz, F. D., & Barclay, A. G. (1992). A proposed curriculum for psychopharmacology training for professional psychologists. *Professional Psychology: Research and Practice, 23*(3), 216–219.

Frank, R. G. (1992). Prescription privileges for psychologists: Now is the time. *Physical Medicine and Rehabilitation: State of the Art Reviews, 6*(3), 565–571.

Inouye, D. K. (1984, November). Invited address at the Hawaii Psychological Association Annual Convention, Honolulu.

Lorion, R. P., Iscoe, I., DeLeon, P. H., & VandenBos, G. R. (Eds.). (1996). *Psychology and public policy: Balancing public service and professional need.* Washington, DC: American Psychological Association.

Pimental, P. A., Stout, C. E., Hoover, M. C., & Kamen, G. B. (1997). Changing psychologists' opinions about prescriptive authority: A little information goes a long way. *Professional Psychology: Research and Practice, 28*(2), 123–127.

Sammons, M. T., & Brown, A. B. (1997). The Department of Defense psychopharmacology demonstration project: An evolving program for postdoctoral education in psychology. *Professional Psychology: Research and Practice, 28*(2), 107–112.

Sammons, M. T., Sexton, J. L., & Meredith, J. M. (1996). Science-based training in psychopharmacology: How much is enough? *American Psychologist, 51*, 230–234.

State of California, Office of Statewide Health Planning and Development, Division of Health Professions Development. (1982, November). *Prescribing and dispensing pilot projects* (Final report to the legislature and to the healing arts licensing boards). Sacramento, CA: Author.

U.S. General Accounting Office (GAO) (1997). *Defense health care: Need for more prescribing psychologists is not adequately justified.* (GAO/HEHS-97-83). Washington, DC: U.S. Government Printing Office.

Acknowledgment

The authors gratefully acknowledge the assistance of a number of people whose concerted efforts made this text and this series of texts possible. First, Herb Reich, for bringing us together with the publisher, Brunner/Mazel (a member of the Taylor & Francis Group). What began as a working relationship several books ago, has developed into a wonderful friendship. Next, we again would like to thank the members of the Editorial Advisory Committee for their continued help and encouragement. A deep expression of gratitude also is extended to Marilynn J. Wood, Dean, Faculty of Nursing, for her support of our textbook writing during an era of diminishing academic resources. We also would like to thank Leona B. Laird for her typing of seemingly countless revisions. Last, but certainly not least, we would like to formally acknowledge and extend our sincerest thanks to all at Brunner/Mazel, particularly Bernadette Capelle, Alison Labbate, and Laura Haefner. Their faith in us and this series of new textbooks for psychologists, their commitment to excellence in publishing, and their continuing assistance and support at every phase of this project have been invaluable.

To our colleagues in psychology, we would like to extend a *special acknowledgment*. The positive feedback that we have received concerning the previous texts in this series has furthered our personal and professional dedication and resolve to continue to provide the very best pharmacopsychology references that are humanly possible. Hopefully, our efforts will be of some assistance to those exceptional leaders in our field, such as Pat DeLeon and Sam Feldman, in the continuing struggle to obtain prescription privileges for psychologists, and also to our fellow practicing psychologists in their earnest attempt to provide the very best professional psychological services possible.

Neuropsychotropic
Drug
Monographs

ACETAZOLAMIDE

(a set a zole′ a mide)

TRADE NAME

Diamox®

CLASSIFICATION

Anticonvulsant (carbonic anhydrase inhibitor)

APPROVED INDICATIONS FOR NEUROPSYCHOLOGICAL DISORDERS

Adjunctive pharmacotherapy for the *prophylactic* management of:

- seizure disorders: absence (petit mal) seizures. Acetazolamide also is indicated for other various forms of seizure disorders.

USUAL DOSAGE AND ADMINISTRATION

Seizure Disorders: Absence (Petit Mal) Seizures

Adults: 8 to 30 mg/kg daily orally in three or four divided doses

MAXIMUM: 1 gram daily orally. Dosages exceeding 1 gram daily do *not* appear to provide any additional efficacy and are *not* recommended.

Women who are, or who may become, pregnant: FDA Pregnancy Category C. Safety and efficacy of acetazolamide pharmacotherapy for women who are pregnant have not been established. Avoid prescribing acetazolamide pharmacotherapy to women who are pregnant. If acetazolamide pharmacotherapy is required, advise patients of potential benefits and possible risk to themselves and the embryo, fetus, or neonate. Collaboration with the patient's obstetrician is indicated.

Women who are breast-feeding: Safety and efficacy of acetazolamide pharmacotherapy for women who are breast-feeding and their neonates and infants have not been established. Acetazolamide is excreted in small amounts in breast milk. However, significant adverse reactions to acetazolamide are unlikely among breast-fed neonates and infants. Collaboration with the patient's pediatrician is indicated.

For details and discussion regarding related basic principles of clinical pharmacology, readers are referred to the first text in this series, *The Pharmacologic Basis of Psychotherapeutics: An Introduction for Psychologists.*

Elderly adults: See "Adults."

Children and adolescents younger than 18 years of age: See "Adults."

Notes, Seizure Disorders: Absence (Petit Mal) Seizures

Acetazolamide is prescribed as adjunctive pharmacotherapy. Tolerance to its anticonvulsant action develops relatively quickly, and, thus, prevents its use for long-term, continuous pharmacotherapy. However, full efficacy is generally quickly restored after a temporary disruption of acetazolamide pharmacotherapy.

AVAILABLE DOSAGE FORMS, STORAGE, AND COMPATIBILITY

Capsules, oral extended-release: 500 mg
Injectable, intravenous: 500 mg/vial (sterile dry powder. See "Notes")
Tablets, oral: 125, 250 mg

Notes

Acetazolamide oral tablets: Diamox® tablets contain povidone. Some patients may be hypersensitive to povidone.

Acetazolamide injectable: The acetazolamide injectable formulation is indicated for intravenous use only. The injectable formulation must be reconstituted prior to use with a minimum of 5 ml of sterile water for injection in order to produce an injectable solution containing *no more than* 100 mg of acetazolamide/ml. The injectable solution should be used within 24 hours after reconstitution because it contains no preservatives. Any unused injectable solution should be safely and appropriately discarded within 24 hours after reconstitution.

General instructions for patients: Instruct patients who are receiving acetazolamide to

- safely store acetazolamide oral capsules and tablets out of the reach of children in child-resistant containers at controlled room temperature (15° to 30°C; 59° to 86°F).
- obtain an available patient information sheet regarding acetazolamide pharmacotherapy from their pharmacist at the time that their prescription is dispensed. Encourage patients to clarify any questions that they may have regarding acetazolamide pharmacotherapy with their pharmacist or, if needed, to consult their prescribing psychologist.

PROPOSED MECHANISM OF ACTION

The exact mechanism of acetazolamide's anticonvulsant action has not yet been fully determined. However, it appears to be associated with the following mechanisms: 1) the production of metabolic acidosis; 2) mediation through an adrenergic mechanism; and 3) carbonic anhydrase inhibition within the brain and resultant increased carbon dioxide tension. Acetazolamide also decreases the formation of cerebrospinal fluid. However, the relevance of this effect to acetazolamide's anticonvulsant action has not been determined.

PHARMACOKINETICS/PHARMACODYNAMICS

Acetazolamide is well absorbed from the GI tract after oral ingestion. Peak blood concentrations are achieved within 1 to 3 hours. Acetazolamide is distributed throughout the body and crosses the placenta. It is excreted 100% in unchanged form in the urine. Additional data are not available.

RELATIVE CONTRAINDICATIONS

Adrenocortical insufficiency
Hyperchloremic acidosis
Hypersensitivity to acetazolamide, other carbonic anhydrase inhibitors, or sulfonamides (acetazolamide is a nonbacteriostatic sulfonamide derivative)
Hypokalemia (low serum potassium concentration)
Hyponatremia (low serum sodium concentration)
Kidney dysfunction, severe
Liver dysfunction, particularly cirrhosis

CAUTIONS AND COMMENTS

Prescribe acetazolamide pharmacotherapy cautiously to patients who

- have severe respiratory impairment (e.g., advanced pulmonary disease, chronic obstructive pulmonary disease [asthma, bronchitis, emphysema], pulmonary infection, pulmonary obstruction). Acetazolamide pharmacotherapy may precipitate or exacerbate respiratory acidosis among these patients.
- have diabetes mellitus. Acetazolamide pharmacotherapy may cause hyperglycemia and glycosuria. Thus, blood and urine glucose should be monitored closely among these patients.
- have gout. Acetazolamide pharmacotherapy decreases uric acid excretion and may, thus, aggravate gout.

Caution patients who are receiving acetazolamide pharmacotherapy against

- performing activities that require alertness, judgment, or physical coordination (e.g., driving an automobile, operating dangerous equipment, supervising children) until their response to acetazolamide pharmacotherapy is known. Acetazolamide may adversely affect these mental and physical functions.

CLINICALLY SIGNIFICANT DRUG INTERACTIONS

Concurrent acetazolamide pharmacotherapy and the following may result in clinically significant drug interactions:

Aspirin Pharmacotherapy

High dosage aspirin pharmacotherapy, such as is commonly used for the treatment of rheumatoid arthritis, may potentiate acetazolamide's adverse drug reactions.

Diuretic Pharmacotherapy

Concurrent acetazolamide pharmacotherapy may augment by way of its own diuretic actions the effects of other drugs that have diuretic actions (e.g., furosemide [Lasix®], hydrochlorothiazide [hydroDIURIL®]).

Lithium Pharmacotherapy

Acetazolamide pharmacotherapy increases the renal excretion of lithium (Lithane®). Monitor lithium blood concentrations and individual patient response whenever concurrent acetazolamide pharmacotherapy is initiated, adjusted, or discontinued.

Pharmacotherapy With Drugs That Are Weak Acids or Weak Bases

Acetazolamide alkalinizes the urine. Thus, the renal excretion of drugs that are weak acids (e.g., phenobarbital [Luminal®], salicylates) is *increased*, while the renal excretion of drugs that are weak bases (e.g., amphetamines, procainamide [Pronestyl®], quinidine [Biquin®]) is *decreased*.

ADVERSE DRUG REACTIONS

Acetazolamide pharmacotherapy has been commonly associated with diarrhea, frequent urination (polyuria), hearing dysfunction (including ringing in the ears [tinnitus]), loss of appetite (anorexia), nausea, paresthesias (particularly a tingling sensation in the extremities), and vomiting. Acetazolamide pharmacotherapy also has been associated with the following ADRs, listed according to body system.

CNS: confusion, depression, drowsiness, fatigue, headache, and sedation
Cutaneous: rash and skin eruptions, including exfoliative dermatitis. These reactions are generally associated with hypersensitivity reactions.
Hematologic: bone marrow suppression, including agranulocytosis, aplastic anemia, hemolytic anemia, leukopenia, and thrombocytopenia. Bone marrow suppression is *potentially fatal*.
Musculoskeletal: muscular weakness
Ophthalmic: myopia (transient)
Renal: crystalluria, dysuria, and renal colic
Miscellaneous: growth suppression (among children), metabolic acidosis, and weight loss

OVERDOSAGE

Data regarding acetazolamide overdosage are not available. In the absence of such data, acetazolamide overdosage should be treated with symptomatic medical support of body systems with attention to increasing acetazolamide elimination. There is no known antidote.

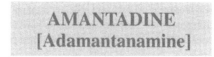

AMANTADINE
[Adamantanamine]

(a man' ta deen)

TRADE NAMES

Endantadine®
Symmetrel®

CLASSIFICATION

Antiparkinsonian (adamantane derivative)

APPROVED INDICATIONS FOR NEUROPSYCHOLOGICAL DISORDERS

Pharmacotherapy for the symptomatic management of:

- Parkinson's disease: drug-induced and idiopathic. Amantadine pharmacotherapy is in-dicated for the symptomatic management of parkinsonian-like extrapyramidal reactions among patients who are receiving antipsychotic pharmacotherapy when a reduction in the patient's antipsychotic dosage has been unsuccessful for the management of these re-actions. Amantadine pharmacotherapy should be discontinued appropriately, as soon as therapeutic benefit (i.e., management of parkinsonian-like extrapyramidal reactions) has been achieved.

USUAL DOSAGE AND ADMINISTRATION

Parkinson's Disease, Drug-Induced and Idiopathic

Adults: 200 mg daily orally in two divided doses

MAXIMUM: 400 mg daily orally in divided doses

Women who are, or who may become, pregnant: FDA Pregnancy Category C. Safety and efficacy of amantadine pharmacotherapy for women who are pregnant have not been estab-lished. Although risk generally appears to be low, avoid prescribing amantadine pharmacotherapy to women who are pregnant. If amantadine pharmacotherapy is required, advise patients of po-tential benefits and possible risks to themselves and the embryo, fetus, or neonate. Collaboration with the patient's obstetrician is indicated.

For details and discussion regarding related basic principles of clinical pharmacology, readers are referred to the first text in this series, *The Pharmacologic Basis of Psychotherapeutics: An Introduction for Psychologists.*

Women who are breast-feeding: Safety and efficacy of amantadine pharmacotherapy for women who are breast-feeding and their neonates and infants have not been established. Amantadine is excreted in low concentrations in breast milk. Avoid prescribing amantadine pharmacotherapy to women who are breast-feeding. If amantadine pharmacotherapy is required, breast-feeding should be discontinued. If desired, lactation may be maintained and breast-feeding resumed following the discontinuation of short-term amantadine pharmacotherapy. Collaboration with the patient's pediatrician is indicated.

Elderly, frail, or debilitated patients and those who have kidney dysfunction: Initially, 100 mg daily orally in a single dose or two divided doses. Gradually increase the dosage if needed, according to individual patient response. Generally prescribe lower dosages for elderly, frail, or debilitated patients, particularly those who have congestive heart failure, orthostatic (postural) hypotension, or peripheral edema. These patients may be more sensitive to the pharmacologic actions of amantadine than are younger or healthier adult patients.

Also prescribe lower dosages of amantadine for patients who have kidney dysfunction. Prescribe dosages for these patients according to their individual rates of creatinine clearance. See the table "Amantadine Dosage for Patients Who Have Kidney Dysfunction."

Amantadine dosage for patients who have kidney dysfunction.

Creatinine clearance (ml/minute/1.73m^2)	Amantadine dosage
$\geqslant$80	200 mg daily orally in two divided doses
60 to 79	200 mg orally once every other day alternating with 100 mg orally once every other day
40 to 59	100 mg daily orally
30 to 39	200 mg orally twice weekly
20 to 29	100 mg orally three times weekly
10 to 19	200 mg orally once every seven days alternating with 100 mg orally once every seven days

Children younger than 1 year of age: Safety and efficacy of amantadine pharmacotherapy for children who are younger than 1 year of age have not been established. Amantadine pharmacotherapy is *not* recommended for this age group.

Notes, Parkinson's Disease, Drug-Induced or Idiopathic

Prescribe the smallest quantity of amantadine that is consistent with the patient's requirements and convenience. A small number of patients who were receiving amantadine pharmacotherapy have attempted suicide by means of amantadine overdosage. See "Cautions and Comments." Adjunctive psychotherapy or other pharmacotherapy may be indicated following individual evaluation for mood or other mental disorders.

Discontinuing amantadine pharmacotherapy: *Avoid* the abrupt discontinuation of amantadine pharmacotherapy among patients who have idiopathic or drug-induced Parkinson's disease. The abrupt discontinuation of amantadine pharmacotherapy among patients who have idiopathic Parkinson's disease has been associated with parkinsonian crisis (i.e., sudden, marked clinical deterioration). The abrupt discontinuation of amantadine pharmacotherapy also has been associated with the neuroleptic malignant syndrome among patients who were receiving amantadine pharmacotherapy for the symptomatic management of parkinsonian-like extrapyramidal reactions related to their antipsychotic pharmacotherapy. Whenever possible, gradually discontinue amantadine pharmacotherapy for these patients.

AVAILABLE DOSAGE FORMS, STORAGE, AND COMPATIBILITY

Capsules, oral: 100 mg
Solution, oral: 10 mg/ml
Syrup, oral: 10 mg/ml

Notes

General instructions for patients: Instruct patients who are receiving amantadine pharmacotherapy to

- ingest each dose of the amantadine oral capsules, solution, or syrup with food to decrease associated GI irritation.
- safely store amantadine oral dosage forms out of the reach of children in tightly closed, child-resistant containers at controlled room temperature (15° to 30°C; 59° to 86°F). Instruct patients to store amantadine oral capsules and oral solution in light-resistant containers.
- obtain an available patient information sheet regarding amantadine pharmacotherapy from their pharmacist at the time that their prescription is dispensed. Encourage patients to clarify any questions that they may have regarding amantadine pharmacotherapy with their pharmacist or, if needed, to consult their prescribing psychologist.

PROPOSED MECHANISM OF ACTION

The exact mechanism of action of amantadine for the symptomatic management of Parkinson's disease is unknown. Available data suggest that amantadine may elicit its actions by one or more of the following mechanisms: 1) release of catecholamines, including dopamine, from peripheral nerve storage sites; 2) blocking the re-uptake of dopamine into presynaptic neurons; and 3) direct stimulation of postsynaptic receptors.

PHARMACOKINETICS/PHARMACODYNAMICS

Amantadine is well but variably absorbed (i.e., 50% to 90%) from the GI tract following oral ingestion. Peak blood concentrations are achieved within 1 to 4 hours. Amantadine is widely distributed and achieves cerebrospinal fluid concentrations equal to approximately one-half of the blood concentrations. It is ~67% bound to plasma proteins and has an apparent volume of distribution of ~7 liters/kg. Small amounts of amantadine are excreted in breast milk. Large amounts of amantadine are found in the saliva and in nasal excretions. Amantadine is not metabolized. It is excreted primarily in unchanged form (~90%) in the urine. Acidification of the urine increases the rate of amantadine urinary excretion. The mean half-life of elimination is approximately 16 hours (range: 9 to 37 hours). The total body clearance ranges from 0.2 to 0.3 liters/hour/kg.

RELATIVE CONTRAINDICATIONS

Hypersensitivity to amantadine

CAUTIONS AND COMMENTS

Prescribe amantadine pharmacotherapy cautiously to patients who

- have histories of schizophrenia and other psychotic disorders, including those associated with problematic patterns of abusable psychotropic use (i.e., substance use disorders). Amantadine pharmacotherapy may initiate or exacerbate the signs and symptoms of psychosis (e.g., feelings of depersonalization, hallucinations, paranoia) among these patients.
- have histories of seizure disorders. Patients who have seizure disorders appear to be at risk for experiencing an increased incidence of seizures during amantadine pharmacotherapy. Initially prescribe lower dosages for these patients and monitor these patients closely for seizure activity.
- have histories of suicide attempts or suicide ideation. Amantadine pharmacotherapy rarely has been associated with an increased incidence of suicide ideation and attempts. A causal mechanism for this increased incidence has not been established clearly.
- have kidney dysfunction. Amantadine is excreted almost completely in unchanged form in the urine. These patients are at risk for amantadine toxicity. See the "Elderly, Frail, and Debilitated Patients and Those Who Have Kidney Dysfunction" subsection of "Usual Dosage and Administration." Also see "Notes, Parkinson's Disease, Drug-Induced or Idiopathic."

Caution patients who are receiving amantadine pharmacotherapy against

- performing activities that require alertness, judgment, or physical coordination (e.g., driving an automobile, operating dangerous equipment, supervising children) until their response to amantadine pharmacotherapy is known. Amantadine may adversely affect these mental and physical functions by means of its CNS actions and effects on vision (e.g., blurred vision).

In addition to this general precaution, caution patients who are receiving amantadine pharmacotherapy to

- inform their prescribing psychologist if they begin or discontinue any other pharmacotherapy while receiving amantadine pharmacotherapy.

CLINICALLY SIGNIFICANT DRUG INTERACTIONS

Concurrent amantadine pharmacotherapy and the following may result in clinically significant drug interactions:

Pharmacotherapy With CNS Stimulants

Concurrent amantadine and CNS stimulant (e.g., amphetamine, cocaine, methylphenidate [Ritalin®]) pharmacotherapy may result in additive CNS stimulant actions and, thus, excessive CNS stimulation.

Pharmacotherapy With Anticholinergics and Other Drugs That Produce Anticholinergic Actions

Concurrent amantadine pharmacotherapy with anticholinergics (e.g., atropine) and other drugs that produce anticholinergic actions (e.g., phenothiazines, TCAs) may result in additive anticholinergic actions. Concurrent amantadine and atropine pharmacotherapy has resulted in atropinism. Atropinism is characterized by such signs and symptoms as hallucinations and nocturnal mental confusion.

ADVERSE DRUG REACTIONS

Amantadine pharmacotherapy has been commonly associated with anxiety, dizziness, impaired concentration, insomnia, lightheadedness, and nausea. It also has been associated with the following ADRs, listed according to body system:

Cardiovascular: congestive heart failure and postural hypotension
CNS: agitation, delusions, depression, drowsiness, hallucinations (visual), headache, hyperkinesia, illusions, incoordination (ataxia), irritability, mental confusion, nervousness, slurred speech, somnolence, and tremor
Cutaneous: peripheral edema; semi-permanent bluish mottling of the hands, legs, and skin (livedo reticularis); and rash
Genitourinary: urinary retention
GI: constipation, dry mouth, loss of appetite (anorexia), and vomiting
Ophthalmic: blurred vision, corneal edema, light sensitivity, optic nerve palsy, and punctate subepithelial corneal opacity
Respiratory: dry nasal passages and shortness of breath (dyspnea)
Miscellaneous: decreased sex drive and fatigue

OVERDOSAGE

Amantadine overdosage may be fatal. Signs and symptoms of amantadine overdosage include CNS toxicity (e.g., aggressive behavior, coma, confusion, hallucinations, hyperkinesia, psychosis), hypertension, kidney dysfunction, respiratory dysfunction, and tachycardia. Amantadine overdosage requires emergency symptomatic medical support of body systems with attention to *increasing amantadine* elimination. There is no known antidote.

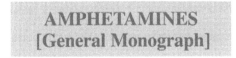

AMPHETAMINES
[General Monograph]

(am fet′ a meens)

GENERIC NAMES

For trade names, see individual drug monographs.

Amphetamines, mixed*
Dextroamphetamine
Methamphetamine

CLASSIFICATION

CNS stimulant (amphetamine) (C-II)

See also individual amphetamine monographs

APPROVED INDICATIONS FOR NEUROPSYCHOLOGICAL DISORDERS[1]

Pharmacotherapy for the symptomatic management of:

- sleep disorders: narcolepsy

USUAL DOSAGE AND ADMINISTRATION

Sleep Disorders: Narcolepsy

Adults: See individual amphetamine monographs.

Women who are, or who may become, pregnant: FDA Pregnancy Category C. Safety and efficacy of amphetamine pharmacotherapy for women who are pregnant have not been established. Avoid prescribing amphetamine pharmacotherapy to women who are pregnant. If amphetamine pharmacotherapy is required, advise patients of potential benefits and possible risks to themselves and the embryo, fetus, or neonate. Collaboration with the patient's obstetrician is indicated.

---

[1] For information and discussion of the use of the amphetamines as adjunctive pharmacotherapy for the symptomatic management of mental disorders (e.g., attention-deficit/hyperactivity disorder, eating disorders [exogenous obesity]), readers are referred to the related text in this series, *PPDR: Psychologists' Psychotropic Drug Reference* (L. A. Pagliaro & A. M. Pagliaro, 1999).

For details and discussion regarding related basic principles of clinical pharmacology, readers are referred to the first text in this series, *The Pharmacologic Basis of Psychotherapeutics: An Introduction for Psychologists.*

Women who are breast-feeding: Safety and efficacy of amphetamine pharmacotherapy for women who are breast-feeding and their neonates and infants have not been established. Amphetamines are excreted into breast milk. Neonates and infants may display expected pharmacologic effects (e.g., irritability, weight loss). Avoid prescribing amphetamine pharmacotherapy to women who are breast-feeding. If amphetamine pharmacotherapy is required, breast-feeding should be discontinued. Collaboration with the patient's pediatrician is indicated.

Elderly, frail, or debilitated patients: Generally prescribe lower dosages for elderly, frail, or debilitated patients. Gradually increase the dosage, if needed, according to individual patient response. These patients may be more sensitive to the pharmacologic actions of the amphetamines than are younger or healthier adult patients.

Children and adolescents: Dosages for children and adolescents generally should not exceed adult dosages, except where specifically indicated. See individual amphetamine monographs.

Notes, Sleep Disorders: Narcolepsy

Initiating amphetamine pharmacotherapy: Before prescribing amphetamine pharmacotherapy for the symptomatic management of narcolepsy,

- assure an accurate diagnosis of narcolepsy. Narcolepsy should be appropriately differentiated from other causes of hypersomnia. Depression, exhaustion, neurotic fatigue, sleep apnea, and sleepiness are differentiated from narcolepsy by evaluation of the circumstances of sleep, duration of signs and symptoms, lack of cataplexy (momentary paralysis without loss of consciousness occurring in association with sudden emotional reactions), and evaluation of general mental status.
- refer patients to their advanced practice nurse, family physician, or a specialist (neurologist) for medical evaluation of their general physical health and body system function. Attention should also be given to ruling out any medical disorders (e.g., encephalitis, tumor of the hypothalamus) that may mimic the signs and symptoms of narcolepsy.
- identify any problematic patterns of abusable psychotropic use, including any heavy alcohol, opiate, or sedative-hypnotic use.
- note any previous amphetamine or other related pharmacotherapy (e.g., methylphenidate pharmacotherapy) and the patient's response.
- identify possible hypersensitivity to amphetamines or other sympathomimetics and note any contraindications, cautions, and potential drug interactions.
- assess the patient's abilities to manage his or her amphetamine pharmacotherapy. Children will generally require parental guidance and supervision. Assure that adequate and appropriate assistance is available for children when doses are required during the day while at school.
- assure that patients and their parents, or legal guardians as appropriate, are provided with realistic information regarding the benefits of amphetamine pharmacotherapy for the symptomatic management of narcolepsy and have an understanding of the planned course of amphetamine pharmacotherapy. Patients should know

  - that amphetamines may cause addiction or habituation.
  - that dosage selection depends on several factors, such as age, gender, weight, metabolism, and response to previous amphetamine or related pharmacotherapy.
  - that the prescribed pharmacotherapy can be enhanced by concurrent participation in psychotherapy and other therapy. Patients, as appropriate, should be encouraged

to ask questions about the therapeutic plan as active consumers of comprehensive neuropsychologic services.

- the exact name of the amphetamine prescribed, its general action, purpose, dosage, storage, administration, associated contraindications, cautions, ADRs, and signs and symptoms of overdosage. They should know how to monitor therapeutic response and know which signs and symptoms indicate that the prescribing psychologist should be contacted or that emergency medical care should be obtained.
- the names of support groups for patients who have narcolepsy and their family members. Direct patients and their family members, as appropriate, to available support groups for additional help. Involve patients and their family members, as appropriate, in treatment planning whenever possible and provide them with adequate evaluation of the patient's progress.

Maintaining amphetamine pharmacotherapy:

- Monitor patients for initial and continued therapeutic response to amphetamine pharmacotherapy as denoted by decreased frequency or severity of signs and symptoms of narcolepsy.
- Monitor patients for ADRs, particularly overstimulation (e.g., insomnia, irritability).
- Assist patients to manage common or troublesome ADRs such as weight loss. Advise patients, as appropriate, to follow a balanced diet and exercise program to maintain their normal weight, to monitor their daily caloric intake, and to eat nutritious low-calorie snack foods. Collaboration with the patient's advanced practice nurse or a nutritional consultant (e.g., dietitian) may be required.
- Periodically interrupt amphetamine pharmacotherapy (at least once annually) to determine if signs and symptoms warrant the continuation of amphetamine pharmacotherapy for the symptomatic management of narcolepsy.

Discontinuing amphetamine pharmacotherapy: Abrupt discontinuation of amphetamine pharmacotherapy following long-term high-dosage pharmacotherapy, or regular personal use, may result in extreme fatigue, mental depression, and sleep pattern changes on EEG. Gradually discontinue long-term amphetamine pharmacotherapy, or regular personal use. See "Cautions and Comments."

AVAILABLE DOSAGE FORMS, STORAGE, AND COMPATIBILITY

Various oral formulations are available for patients who require amphetamine pharmacotherapy for the symptomatic management of narcolepsy. See individual amphetamine monographs.

Notes

General instructions for patients: Instruct patients who are receiving amphetamine pharmacotherapy to

- safely store amphetamine oral capsules and tablets out of the reach of children in child-resistant containers.

• obtain an available patient information sheet regarding amphetamine pharmacotherapy from their pharmacist at the time that their prescription is dispensed. Encourage patients (or parents/legal guardians when patients are children) to clarify any questions that they may have regarding amphetamine pharmacotherapy with their pharmacist or, if needed, to consult their prescribing psychologist.

PROPOSED MECHANISM OF ACTION

Chemically, the amphetamines are members of the phenylisopropylamine family. They are non-catechol, sympathomimetic amines. When compared to epinephrine and other catecholamines, the amphetamines produce greater CNS stimulation. As such, the amphetamines are indirect-acting CNS stimulants. They stimulate the release of biogenic amines (e.g., dopamine, norepinephrine, and serotonin) from presynaptic nerve terminal storage vesicles and/or inhibit their re-uptake. These actions result in expected pharmacologic effects, including abnormal dilation of the pupils (mydriasis), bronchodilation, CNS stimulation, contraction of the urinary bladder sphincter, increased blood pressure, and loss of appetite (anorexia). The amphetamines also inhibit, to varying degrees, monoamine oxidase. However, the clinical significance of this action has not yet been clearly established. The exact mechanism of action of the amphetamines when prescribed for the symptomatic management of narcolepsy is related to their CNS stimulant actions.

PHARMACOKINETICS/PHARMACODYNAMICS

The amphetamines are readily absorbed following oral ingestion. They are widely distributed in body tissues, with the highest concentrations in the CNS. Urinary excretion is pH dependent. Amphetamine elimination is increased in acidic urine and decreased in alkaline urine.

See individual amphetamine monographs.

RELATIVE CONTRAINDICATIONS

Addiction or habituation to amphetamines or other abusable psychotropics, history of
Agitation
Arteriosclerosis, advanced
Breast-feeding
Hypersensitivity to amphetamines or other sympathomimetic amines
Hypertension, moderate to severe
Hyperthyroidism
MAOI pharmacotherapy, concurrent or within 14 days. Concurrent pharmacotherapy has been associated with the development of the potentially fatal serotonin syndrome.
Pregnancy, particularly the first trimester

CAUTIONS AND COMMENTS

The amphetamines are addicting and habituating. Tachyphylaxis and tolerance have been demonstrated for all drugs in this class. Patients have reportedly increased their dosage to many times the recommended dosage. Thus, the amphetamines require cautious prescription with attention to abuse potential. Prescribe the lowest effective dosage and the smallest amount for dispensing at one time to minimize the possible development of problematic patterns of use. Although an amphetamine withdrawal syndrome has not been specifically identified, abrupt discontinuation following long-term, high-dosage pharmacotherapy, or regular personal use, may result in extreme fatigue, mental depression, and sleep pattern changes on EEG. Signs and symptoms of long-term, high-dosage pharmacotherapy, or regular personal use, include agitation, cardiomyopathy, dermatoses (severe), hallucinations, hyperactivity, insomnia (marked), irritability, paranoia and personality changes. One of the most severe signs and symptoms is psychosis. Amphetamine psychosis is often clinically indistinguishable from schizophrenia. Amphetamine psychosis also may occur with excessive short-term personal use (i.e., "amphetamine run").

Prescribe amphetamine pharmacotherapy cautiously to patients who

- have hypertension, including mild hypertension. Amphetamine pharmacotherapy may increase blood pressure excessively among these patients.
- have insulin-dependent diabetes mellitus and also are receiving concurrent dietary restrictions. Psychological disturbances have been reported among these patients. Insulin requirements also may be altered.

Caution patients who are receiving amphetamine pharmacotherapy against

- performing activities that require alertness, judgment, and physical coordination (e.g., driving an automobile, operating dangerous equipment, supervising children) until their response to amphetamine pharmacotherapy is known.
- giving, selling, or trading the amphetamine to any relatives, friends, or others.

In addition to these general precautions, caution patients to

- carry a card indicating that they are receiving amphetamine pharmacotherapy in case of an emergency. The card also should include other relevant information, such as the name of the family member to contact in case of an emergency and the name of the prescribing psychologist.
- inform their advanced practice nurse, dentist, family physician, or other health care providers that they are receiving amphetamine pharmacotherapy.

In addition to these general precautions for patients, caution women to

- inform their prescribing psychologist if they become or intend to become pregnant while receiving amphetamine pharmacotherapy so that the safe discontinuation of their pharmacotherapy can be considered and planned.

CLINICALLY SIGNIFICANT DRUG INTERACTIONS

Concurrent amphetamine pharmacotherapy and the following may result in clinically significant drug interactions:

Antihypertensive Pharmacotherapy

Amphetamines may decrease the hypotensive action of antihypertensive drugs (e.g., guanethidine [Ismelin®]).

MAOI Pharmacotherapy

See "Relative Contraindications."

Pharmacotherapy With Drugs That Acidify the Urine

Urinary acidifiers (e.g., ammonium chloride) decrease amphetamine blood concentrations by increasing the renal excretion of the amphetamine.

Pharmacotherapy With Drugs That Alkalinize the Urine

Urinary alkalinizers (e.g., acetazolamide [Diamox®] or sodium bicarbonate) increase amphetamine blood concentrations by decreasing the renal excretion of the amphetamine.

TCA Pharmacotherapy

Amphetamines may potentiate the actions of the TCAs.

ADVERSE DRUG REACTIONS

Amphetamine pharmacotherapy has been associated with the following ADRs, listed according to body system:

Cardiovascular: increased blood pressure (hypertension) and heart rate (tachycardia)
CNS: dizziness, euphoria, headache, insomnia, irritability, nervousness, psychosis, restlessness, tics, and tremor
Cutaneous: flushing
GI: abdominal cramps, constipation, diarrhea, dry mouth, loss of appetite (anorexia), nausea, vomiting, and weight loss
Metabolic/Endocrine: see "Genitourinary"
Ocular: abnormal dilation of the pupils (mydriasis) and blurred vision
Miscellaneous: chills and increased sex drive

OVERDOSAGE

Signs and symptoms of acute amphetamine overdosage include the following: agitation, constipation, hallucinations, panic, paranoia, overstimulation, restlessness, rapid respirations (tachypnea), and tremor. Depression and fatigue usually follow the CNS stimulation. Other signs and symptoms include abdominal cramps, circulatory collapse, diarrhea, dysrhythmias, hypertension or hypotension, nausea, and vomiting. Hyperpyrexia (i.e., elevated body temperature) and rhabdomyolysis (i.e., an acute, sometimes fatal reaction caused by the destruction of skeletal muscle) can result in other complications. Fatal amphetamine overdosage usually is preceded by convulsions and coma. Acute amphetamine overdosage requires emergency symptomatic medical support of body systems with attention to increasing amphetamine elimination. There is no known antidote.

AMPHETAMINES, MIXED*

(am fet′ a meens)

TRADE NAME

Adderall®

CLASSIFICATION

CNS stimulant (amphetamine) (C-II)

See also "Amphetamines, General Monograph."

APPROVED INDICATIONS FOR NEUROPSYCHOLOGICAL DISORDERS

Pharmacotherapy for the symptomatic management of:

- sleep disorders: narcolepsy

USUAL DOSAGE AND ADMINISTRATION

Sleep Disorders: Narcolepsy

Adults: 15 to 60 mg daily orally in a single or divided dose

Women who are, or who may become, pregnant: FDA Pregnancy Category C. Safety and efficacy of mixed amphetamines pharmacotherapy for women who are pregnant have not been established. Data implicating amphetamines in fetal harm (i.e., birth defects) have been inconsistent and inconclusive. Neonates born to mothers who are addicted to amphetamines have an increased risk for premature delivery and low birth weight. During the neonatal period, these neonates also may display signs and symptoms of the amphetamine withdrawal syndrome, including agitation and lassitude. Avoid prescribing mixed amphetamines pharmacotherapy to women who are pregnant. If mixed amphetamines pharmacotherapy is required, advise patients of potential benefits and possible risks to themselves and the embryo, fetus, or neonate. Collaboration with the patient's obstetrician is indicated.

Women who are breast-feeding: Safety and efficacy of mixed amphetamines pharmacotherapy for women who are breast-feeding and their neonates and infants have not been established. Amphetamines are excreted into breast milk. Avoid prescribing mixed amphetamines pharmacotherapy to women who are breast-feeding. If mixed amphetamines pharmacotherapy is required, breast-feeding should be discontinued. Collaboration with the patient's pediatrician may be indicated.

For details and discussion regarding related basic principles of clinical pharmacology, readers are referred to the first text in this series, *The Pharmacologic Basis of Psychotherapeutics: An Introduction for Psychologists.*

Children 6 to 12 years of age: Initially, 5 mg daily orally in a single dose upon awakening in the morning. Increase the daily dosage at weekly intervals by 5 mg until optimal therapeutic benefit is achieved. Note that narcolepsy seldom occurs among children who are younger than 12 years of age.

Children 12 years of age and older: Initially, 10 mg daily orally in a single dose upon awakening in the morning. Increase the daily dosage at weekly intervals by 10 mg until optimal therapeutic benefit is achieved.

Notes, Narcolepsy

Prescribe the lowest effective dosage. Adjust the dosage according to individual patient response. Late evening doses should be avoided because of associated insomnia.

AVAILABLE DOSAGE FORMS, STORAGE, AND COMPATIBILITY

Tablets, oral: 5, 10, 20, 30 mg

Notes

Each mixed amphetamines tablet contains	5-mg tablet	10-mg tablet	20-mg tablet	30-mg tablet
amphetamine aspartate	1.25 mg	2.5 mg	5 mg	7.5 mg
amphetamine sulfate	1.25 mg	2.5 mg	5 mg	7.5 mg
dextroamphetamine saccharate	1.25 mg	2.5 mg	5 mg	7.5 mg
dextroamphetamine sulfate	1.25 mg	2.5 mg	5 mg	7.5 mg
Total amphetamine base equivalent	3.13 mg	6.3 mg	12.6 mg	18.8 mg

General instructions for patients: Instruct patients who are receiving mixed amphetamines pharmacotherapy to

- safely store mixed amphetamines oral tablets out of the reach of children in tightly closed, child- and light-resistant containers at controlled room temperature (15° to 30°C; 59° to 86°F).
- obtain an available patient information sheet regarding mixed amphetamines pharmacotherapy from their pharmacist at the time that their prescription is dispensed. Encourage patients to clarify any questions that they may have regarding mixed amphetamines pharmacotherapy with their pharmacist or, if needed, to consult their prescribing psychologist.

PROPOSED MECHANISM OF ACTION

The mixed amphetamines are members of the amphetamine group of sympathomimetic amines that have CNS stimulant action (see "Amphetamines, General Monograph"). Peripheral actions include elevation of systolic and diastolic blood pressures and weak bronchodilator and respiratory stimulant action. The mixed amphetamines appear to primarily elicit their stimulant actions by increasing the release of norepinephrine from presynaptic storage vesicles in central adrenergic neurons. A direct effect on α- and β-adrenergic receptors, inhibition of the enzyme amine oxidase, and the release of dopamine also may be involved. However, the exact mechanism of action has not yet been fully determined.

PHARMACOKINETICS/PHARMACODYNAMICS

Data are not available. See "Amphetamines, General Monograph."

RELATIVE CONTRAINDICATIONS

Addiction and habituation to amphetamines or other abusable psychotropics, history of
Agitation
Arteriosclerosis, advanced
Glaucoma
Heart disease, symptomatic
Hypersensitivity to amphetamines or other sympathomimetic amines (e.g., ephedrine)
Hypertension, moderate to severe
Hyperthyroidism
MAOI pharmacotherapy, concurrent or within 14 days. Mixed amphetamines and MAOI
pharmacotherapy, concurrent or within 14 days, may result in hypertensive crisis.

CAUTIONS AND COMMENTS

Amphetamines have a high abuse potential. Prescribe mixed amphetamines pharmacotherapy cautiously for the symptomatic management of narcolepsy. Long-term mixed amphetamines pharmacotherapy, or regular personal use, may lead to addiction and habituation. Thus, attention must be given to the possibility that some patients may become addicted or habituated to mixed amphetamines as a result of their pharmacotherapy. Attention also must be given to the possibility that some patients may seek mixed amphetamines prescriptions to support their addiction or habituation to amphetamines or other CNS stimulants.

The amphetamines have been associated with problematic patterns of use since their synthesis, including patterns of abuse and compulsive use. Reportedly, patients have increased their dosage to many times the usual recommended dosage. The signs and symptoms of amphetamine toxicity or intoxication include agitation, hallucinations, hyperactivity, irritability, marked insomnia, paranoia, personality changes, psychosis, and severe dermatoses. Psychosis is probably one of the most severe signs and symptoms of amphetamine intoxication and is often clinically indistinguishable from paranoid schizophrenia.

Abrupt discontinuation of high-dosage, long-term mixed amphetamines pharmacotherapy, or regular personal use, may result in the amphetamine withdrawal syndrome. Signs and symptoms of this syndrome include abnormal changes in EEG during sleep, fatigue, and mental depression. Prescribe mixed amphetamines pharmacotherapy cautiously and monitor patients closely. Limit prescriptions to the smallest amount that is feasible for dispensing at one time to minimize the possible development of problematic patterns of use.

Prescribe mixed amphetamines pharmacotherapy cautiously to patients who

- have histories of cardiovascular disorders, including mild hypertension. Amphetamine pharmacotherapy has been associated with cardiac dysrhythmias and increased hypertension among these patients.
- have histories of schizophrenia or other psychotic disorders, particularly children. Amphetamine pharmacotherapy for children who have psychotic disorders may exacerbate the signs and symptoms of behavior disturbance and thought disorder. Amphetamines reportedly exacerbate motor and phonic tics and Tourette's disorder (Gilles de la Tourette's syndrome). Clinical assessment of children for tics and Gilles de la Tourette's syndrome should precede the prescription of mixed amphetamines pharmacotherapy.

Caution patients who are receiving mixed amphetamines pharmacotherapy against

- performing activities that require alertness, judgment, or physical coordination (e.g., driving an automobile, operating dangerous equipment, supervising children) until their response to mixed amphetamines is known. The mixed amphetamines may adversely affect these mental and physical functions.

In addition to these general precautions, caution patients who are receiving mixed amphetamines to

- inform their prescribing psychologist if they begin or discontinue any other pharmacotherapy while receiving mixed amphetamines pharmacotherapy.

CLINICALLY SIGNIFICANT DRUG INTERACTIONS

Concurrent mixed amphetamines pharmacotherapy and the following may result in clinically significant drug interactions:

Guanethidine Pharmacotherapy

Mixed amphetamines pharmacotherapy may decrease the neuronal uptake of guanethidine (Ismelin®) and, thus, decrease its antihypertensive action. An adjustment in the guanethidine dosage may be required. Collaboration with the prescriber of the guanethidine is indicated.

Insulin Pharmacotherapy

Mixed amphetamines pharmacotherapy may alter the insulin requirements of patients who have insulin-dependent diabetes mellitus, particularly those patients who also have a restricted-calorie diet.

MAOI Pharmacotherapy

Mixed amphetamines may interact with MAOIs (e.g., phenelzine [Nardil®]) and cause the release of large amounts of catecholamines. This interaction may result in hypertensive crisis, characterized by severe headache and hypertension. Thus, mixed amphetamines pharmacotherapy, concurrent or within 14 days of MAOI pharmacotherapy, is contraindicated.

Pharmacotherapy With Drugs That Acidify the Urine

Concurrent mixed amphetamines pharmacotherapy with drugs that acidify the urine (e.g., ammonium chloride) may increase the urinary excretion of mixed amphetamines.

Pharmacotherapy With Drugs That Alkalinize the Urine

Concurrent mixed amphetamines pharmacotherapy with drugs that alkalinize the urine (e.g., acetazolamide [Diamox®] or sodium bicarbonate) may decrease the urinary excretion of mixed amphetamines.

Phenothiazine Pharmacotherapy

Concurrent mixed amphetamines and phenothiazine pharmacotherapy can result in the diminished action of the mixed amphetamines. Phenothiazines antagonize the CNS stimulatory actions of the amphetamines.

TCA Pharmacotherapy

Concurrent mixed amphetamines and TCA pharmacotherapy may result in the potentiation of CNS stimulant actions. As with other amphetamine or sympathomimetic pharmacotherapy, monitor patients closely and adjust the dosage of both drugs carefully when concurrent pharmacotherapy is required.

See also "Amphetamines, General Monograph."

ADVERSE DRUG REACTIONS

Mixed amphetamines pharmacotherapy has been associated with the following ADRs, listed according to body system:

Cardiovascular: increased blood pressure, palpitations, and tachycardia
CNS: dizziness, dysphoria, euphoria, headache, insomnia, and overstimulation. Rarely, psychotic episodes have been reported among patients who were receiving mixed amphetamines pharmacotherapy at recommended dosages.
Cutaneous: hives (urticaria)
Genitourinary: changes in sex drive and impotence
GI: constipation, diarrhea, dry mouth, loss of appetite (anorexia), nausea, and unpleasant taste
Metabolic/Endocrine: weight loss
Musculoskeletal: restlessness and tremor. Suppression of growth also has been reported among children who have received long-term mixed amphetamines pharmacotherapy.

See also "Amphetamines, General Monograph."

OVERDOSAGE

Signs and symptoms of mixed amphetamines overdosage include: assaultiveness, cardiovascular reactions (e.g., dysrhythmias, hypertension or hypotension, and circulatory collapse), confusion, GI complaints (e.g., abdominal cramps, diarrhea, nausea, and vomiting), hallucinations, hyperpyrexia (abnormal elevation of body temperature), hyperreflexia, panic, rapid respirations, restlessness, rhabdomyolysis, and tremor. Depression and fatigue usually follow the central stimulation. Fatal amphetamine overdosage usually terminates in convulsions and coma.

Mixed amphetamines overdosage requires emergency symptomatic medical support of body systems with attention to increasing mixed amphetamines elimination. There is no known antidote. Chlorpromazine pharmacotherapy may be of benefit because it blocks dopamine and norepinephrine re-uptake, which inhibits the central stimulant actions of the amphetamines.

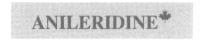

ANILERIDINE

(an i leer′ i deen)

TRADE NAME

Leritine®

CLASSIFICATION

Opiate analgesic (C: "not established")

See also "Opiate Analgesics, General Monograph."

APPROVED INDICATIONS FOR NEUROPSYCHOLOGICAL DISORDERS

Adjunctive pharmacotherapy for the symptomatic management of:

• pain disorders: acute pain, moderate to severe

USUAL DOSAGE AND ADMINISTRATION

Moderate to Severe Pain

Adults: 25 to 50 mg orally every six hours, as needed; *or* 25 to 75 mg intramuscularly or subcutaneously every four to six hours, as needed. More frequent dosing may be required for the symptomatic management of severe pain. However, hospitalization is required unless adequate monitoring and assistance is available in the home setting.

MAXIMUM: 200 mg daily

Women who are, or who may become, pregnant: FDA Pregnancy Category "not established." Safety and efficacy of anileridine pharmacotherapy for women who are pregnant have not been established. Avoid prescribing anileridine pharmacotherapy to women who are pregnant. If anileridine pharmacotherapy is required, advise patients of potential benefits and possible risks to themselves and the embryo, fetus, or neonate. Collaboration with the patient's obstetrician is indicated.

Women who are breast-feeding: Safety and efficacy of anileridine pharmacotherapy for women who are breast-feeding and their neonates and infants have not been established. Avoid prescribing anileridine to women who are breast-feeding. If anileridine pharmacotherapy is required, breast-feeding probably should be discontinued. Collaboration with the patient's pediatrician may be required.

For details and discussion regarding related basic principles of clinical pharmacology, readers are referred to the first text in this series, *The Pharmacologic Basis of Psychotherapeutics: An Introduction for Psychologists.*

Elderly, frail, or debilitated patients and those who have respiratory dysfunction: Prescribe anileridine pharmacotherapy cautiously to elderly, frail, or debilitated patients. Respiratory depression occurs most frequently among these patients and those who have respiratory dysfunction accompanied with hypoxia or hypercapnia. These medical disorders may be further compromised by even moderate therapeutic dosages of anileridine. Collaboration with the patient's family physician or a respiratory specialist is indicated.

Children younger than 12 years of age: Safety and efficacy of anileridine pharmacotherapy for children who are younger than 12 years of age have not been established. Anileridine pharmacotherapy is *not* recommended for this age group.

Notes, Acute Pain: Moderate to Severe

Anileridine injectable pharmacotherapy: The injectable formulation of anileridine is for intramuscular or subcutaneous injection. Generally, intravenous injection is *not* recommended. Rapid intravenous injection of a dose greater than 10 mg has been associated with apnea, hypotension, and cardiac arrest.

AVAILABLE DOSAGE FORMS, STORAGE, AND COMPATIBILITY

Injectable, intramuscular or subcutaneous: 25 mg/ml ampules
Tablets, oral: 25 mg

Notes

The anileridine injectable formulation contains sodium bisulfite. Sulfites have been associated with hypersensitivity reactions, including anaphylactic reactions, among susceptible patients. Although relatively uncommon, these reactions appear to occur with a higher incidence among patients who have asthma.

General instructions for patients: Instruct patients who are receiving anileridine pharmacotherapy to

- safely store anileridine oral tablets out of the reach of children in tightly closed, child- and light-resistant containers.
- obtain an available patient information sheet regarding anileridine pharmacotherapy from their pharmacist at the time that their prescription is dispensed. Encourage patients to clarify any questions that they may have regarding anileridine pharmacotherapy with their pharmacist or, if needed, to consult their prescribing psychologist.

PROPOSED MECHANISM OF ACTION

Anileridine is a relatively strong, centrally acting, synthetic opiate analgesic. Although the exact mechanism of action is not yet fully understood, anileridine appears to elicit its analgesic action primarily by binding to the endorphin receptors in the CNS. See also "Opiate Analgesics, General Monograph."

PHARMACOKINETICS/PHARMACODYNAMICS

Anileridine is well absorbed after oral ingestion and intramuscular and subcutaneous injection. Its onset of analgesic action is generally within 15 minutes. Its duration of action is approximately 2 to 3 hours. Anileridine is virtually completely metabolized in the liver. Only a small amount is excreted in unchanged form in the urine. Additional data are not available.

RELATIVE CONTRAINDICATIONS

Hypersensitivity to anileridine
Respiratory depression, including that associated with head injury or brain tumor

CAUTIONS AND COMMENTS

Anileridine is addicting and habituating. Anileridine can counteract the morphine withdrawal syndrome. Long-term anileridine pharmacotherapy over 2 to 3 weeks has been associated with addiction and habituation equal to that of morphine. Only prescribe anileridine pharmacotherapy when required for the symptomatic management of acute moderate to severe pain and do not prolong pharmacotherapy unnecessarily.

Prescribe anileridine pharmacotherapy cautiously to patients who

- have acute alcoholism, delirium tremens, or seizures.
- have Addison's disease (i.e., medical disorder associated with a deficiency in the secretion of adrenocortical hormones).
- are receiving MAOI pharmacotherapy.
- have CNS depression or coma, or are in shock. Anileridine's respiratory depressant action may further reduce the circulating blood volume, cardiac output, and blood pressure among these patients. If severe respiratory depression and circulatory collapse are eminent, the opiate antagonist, naloxone (Narcan®), may assist in counteracting these effects.
- have head injuries or other conditions associated with increased intracranial pressure. Anileridine pharmacotherapy can further increase intracranial pressure among these patients.
- have liver dysfunction (severe). The metabolism of anileridine may be decreased among these patients and result in toxicity. Extreme caution is recommended.
- have myxedema (i.e., medical disorder associated with dysfunction of the thyroid gland).

CLINICALLY SIGNIFICANT DRUG INTERACTIONS

Concurrent anileridine pharmacotherapy and the following may result in clinically significant drug interactions:

Alcohol Use

Concurrent alcohol use may increase the CNS depressant action of anileridine. Advise patients to avoid, or limit, their use of alcohol while receiving anileridine pharmacotherapy.

Pharmacotherapy with CNS Depressants and Other Drugs That Produce CNS Depression

Concurrent anileridine pharmacotherapy and pharmacotherapy with other opiate analgesics, sedative-hypnotics, or other drugs that produce CNS depression (e.g., antihistamines, phenothiazines, TCAs) may cause additive CNS, respiratory, or circulatory depression.

See also "Opiate Analgesics, General Monograph."

ADVERSE DRUG REACTIONS

Respiratory depression and, to a lesser extent, circulatory depression are the most serious ADRs associated with anileridine pharmacotherapy. Anileridine pharmacotherapy also has been associated with the following ADRs, listed according to body system:

Cardiovascular: bradycardia and hypotension (transient, slight)
CNS: dizziness, euphoria, excitement, nervousness, and restlessness
Cutaneous: sweating (excessive)
GI: dry mouth, nausea, and vomiting
Ocular: visual difficulty
Miscellaneous: sensation of warmth

See also "Opiate Analgesics, General Monograph."

OVERDOSAGE

The signs and symptoms of anileridine overdosage include severe respiratory depression with circulatory depression and related sequelae. Anileridine overdosage requires emergency symptomatic medical support of body systems with attention to increasing anileridine elimination and maintaining respiratory function. Respiratory depression can be treated with the opiate antagonist, naloxone (Narcan®). The use of an opiate antagonist may precipitate an acute opiate withdrawal syndrome among patients who are addicted to opiate analgesics. The severity of this syndrome depends on the amount of opiate analgesic used, the duration of long-term use, and the amount of antagonist injected.

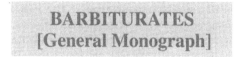
BARBITURATES
[General Monograph]

(bar bit′ oo rates)

GENERIC NAMES

For trade names, see individual drug monographs.

Mephobarbital
Phenobarbital
Primidone

CLASSIFICATION

Anticonvulsant (sedative-hypnotic) (barbiturate) (C-II, C-III)

See also individual barbiturate monographs.

APPROVED INDICATIONS FOR NEUROPSYCHOLOGICAL DISORDERS[2]

Pharmacotherapy for the prophylactic and symptomatic management of:

- seizure disorders: partial and tonic-clonic seizures. Although all barbiturates can be of therapeutic value for the symptomatic management of seizure disorders, only mepho-barbital, phenobarbital, and primidone generally are indicated for the prophylactic management of seizure disorders; the others are not. These barbiturates generally are thera-peutically effective as anticonvulsants in subhypnotic dosages. For example, amobarbital (Amytal®) or secobarbital (Seconal®) injectable pharmacotherapy may be prescribed oc-casionally to terminate an acute seizure episode. However, the required dose generally is high enough to induce hypnosis (i.e., to put the patient to sleep).

USUAL DOSAGE AND ADMINISTRATION

Seizure Disorders: Partial and Tonic-Clonic Seizures

Adults: See individual barbiturate monographs.

[2]For discussion of the use of the barbiturates as adjunctive pharmacotherapy for the symptomatic management of mental disorders (e.g., anxiety disorders, sleep disorders) the reader is referred to the related text in this series, *PPDR: Psychologists' Psychotropic Drug Reference* (L. A. Pagliaro & A. M. Pagliaro, 1999).

For details and discussion regarding related basic principles of clinical pharmacology, readers are referred to the first text in this series, *The Pharmacologic Basis of Psychotherapeutics: An Introduction for Psychologists.*

Women who are, or who may become, pregnant: FDA Pregnancy Category D. Barbiturate pharmacotherapy during pregnancy has been associated with congenital malformations (i.e., birth defects). Following oral ingestion, barbiturates readily cross the placental barrier and are distributed throughout the placenta and embryonic and fetal tissues. The highest concentration is found in the brain and liver.

Barbiturate pharmacotherapy, or regular personal use, during pregnancy has been associated with a significantly increased incidence of hemorrhagic disease of the newborn. Generally, this disorder is readily correctable with appropriate vitamin K_1 (phytonadione) pharmacotherapy for the neonate. Neonates born to mothers who received barbiturate pharmacotherapy, or personally used barbiturates, throughout the last trimester of pregnancy also may display signs and symptoms of the barbiturate withdrawal syndrome. These signs and symptoms include irritability and seizures. A delayed onset of the signs and symptoms of the barbiturate withdrawal syndrome may occur for up to 14 days after delivery.

Do *not* prescribe barbiturate pharmacotherapy to women who are pregnant. If barbiturate pharmacotherapy is required, advise patients of the potential benefits and possible risks to themselves and the embryo, fetus, or neonate. Collaboration with the patient's obstetrician and pediatrician is required.

Women who are breast-feeding: Safety and efficacy of barbiturate pharmacotherapy for women who are breast-feeding and their neonates and infants have not been established. Small amounts of barbiturates are excreted in breast milk. Breast milk concentrations may be sufficient to cause expected pharmacologic actions among breast-fed neonates and infants, including drowsiness and lethargy. Concentrations also may be sufficient both to cause addiction among breast-fed neonates and infants and to stimulate hepatic microsomal enzyme metabolism. Avoid prescribing barbiturate pharmacotherapy to women who are breast-feeding. If barbiturate pharmacotherapy is required, breast-feeding should be discontinued because of the potential for these ADRs among breast-fed neonates and infants. Collaboration with the patient's pediatrician is indicated.

Elderly, frail, or debilitated patients and those who have kidney or liver dysfunction: Generally prescribe lower dosages of the barbiturates for elderly, frail, and debilitated patients. Gradually increase the dosage, if needed, according to individual patient response. These patients may be more sensitive to the CNS depressant action of the barbiturates than are younger or healthier adult patients. Elderly, frail, or debilitated patients may react to barbiturate pharmacotherapy with marked confusion, depression, or excitement. Lower dosages also should be prescribed for patients who have kidney or liver dysfunction.

Children: See individual barbiturate monographs.

Notes, Seizure Disorders: Partial and Tonic-Clonic Seizures

Initiating barbiturate pharmacotherapy: *Before* prescribing barbiturate pharmacotherapy for the prophylactic and symptomatic management of the seizure disorder,

- assure an accurate diagnosis of partial or tonic-clonic seizures.
- assess the patient's perception of his or her seizure disorder and the need for barbiturate pharmacotherapy.
- identify any previous problematic patterns of abusable psychotropic use, including any heavy alcohol, barbiturate, or benzodiazepine use.

- note any previous barbiturate or other anticonvulsant pharmacotherapy for the prophylactic or symptomatic management of seizure disorders and the patient's response.
- identify possible hypersensitivity to the barbiturates and potential contraindications, cautions, and drug interactions.
- assess the patient's abilities to manage his or her barbiturate pharmacotherapy.

Encourage patients to ask questions regarding their barbiturate pharmacotherapy as active consumers of comprehensive neuropsychologic services. They should know the exact name of their prescribed barbiturate and its general action, purpose, dosage, storage, and administration. They also should be advised in relation to associated potential ADRs. They should know how to monitor therapeutic response, identify and manage common ADRs, and identify the signs and symptoms that indicate that the prescribing psychologist should be contacted or emergency medical evaluation sought. Also, direct patients and their families, as appropriate, to available support groups (e.g., Epilepsy Society) for additional help.

Maintaining barbiturate pharmacotherapy: Prescribing psychologists should do the following in regard to appropriately managing barbiturate pharmacotherapy for the prophylactic and symptomatic management of seizure disorders:

- Monitor patients for the desired therapeutic response to the prescribed barbiturate pharmacotherapy (i.e., prevention or control of seizures).
- Avoid concurrent use of interacting drugs.
- Monitor patients for ADRs, particularly over-sedation, which can result in falls and other accidents. Assure that safety precautions (e.g., supervised ambulation or tobacco smoking) are implemented, as needed. Elderly, frail, or debilitated patients or those who have histories of chronic alcoholism may be particularly sensitive to the barbiturates.

Discontinuing barbiturate pharmacotherapy: Abrupt discontinuation of long-term barbiturate pharmacotherapy, or regular personal use, may result in the barbiturate withdrawal syndrome. Signs and symptoms of the barbiturate withdrawal syndrome, which may be fatal, include convulsions and delirium. Gradually discontinue barbiturate pharmacotherapy for patients who have received long-term barbiturate pharmacotherapy or who have personally used excessive dosages over long periods of time.

AVAILABLE DOSAGE FORMS, STORAGE, AND COMPATIBILITY

The barbiturates are available in various dosage forms, including oral tablets and capsules, injectables for intramuscular or intravenous use, and rectal suppositories. See individual barbiturate monographs.

Notes

General instructions for patients: Instruct patients who are receiving barbiturate pharmacotherapy to

- safely store barbiturate formulations out of the reach of children in child-resistant containers. See individual barbiturate monographs.

- obtain an available patient information sheet regarding barbiturate pharmacotherapy from their pharmacist at the time that their prescription is dispensed. Encourage patients to clarify any questions that they may have regarding barbiturate pharmacotherapy with their pharmacist or, if needed, to consult their prescribing psychologist.

PROPOSED MECHANISM OF ACTION

Chemically, the barbiturates are members of the family of substituted pyrimidines. They are structurally derived from barbituric acid, which has no intrinsic CNS activity of its own. The barbiturates depress the sensory cortex, decrease motor activity, and alter cerebellar function. In addition, they can produce, through their dose-related CNS action, all levels of CNS depression ranging from mild sedation and hypnosis to anesthesia, deep coma, and death.

The exact proposed mechanism of action of the barbiturates for the prophylactic and symptomatic management of seizure disorders has not yet been fully determined. However, the anticonvulsant action of the barbiturates appears to involve binding to barbiturate receptors within the GABA receptor complex. This binding results in the retention of GABA at its receptor and an increased influx of chloride ions through the associated chloride channels. These actions produce neuronal inhibition and a resultant reduction in both monosynaptic and polysynaptic nerve transmission. These actions, in turn, increase the seizure threshold and, thus, also directly contribute to the anticonvulsant action of the barbiturates.

PHARMACOKINETICS/PHARMACODYNAMICS

Barbiturates display wide variability in regard to absorption following oral ingestion. The onset of action generally occurs within 10 to 60 minutes. They are rapidly distributed to all body fluids and tissues and attain high concentrations in the brain, kidneys, and liver because they are weak acids. However, their lipid solubility is the main factor for their wide distribution. Barbiturates are bound to plasma and tissue proteins. The degree of binding associated with the various barbiturates also is a direct function of their lipid solubility. Thiopental, which is used as a general anesthetic, is the most lipid-soluble barbiturate and is ~65% plasma protein bound. The duration of action of the barbiturates, which is related to the rate by which they are distributed throughout the body, varies among patients and in the same patient from time to time. Barbiturates have been classified as short-acting (e.g., 6 to 8 hours for thiopental), intermediate-acting (e.g., 8 to 12 hours for secobarbital, which is used as an anxiolytic and sedative-hypnotic), and long-acting (e.g., 12 to 48 hours for phenobarbital). They are metabolized primarily by the hepatic microsomal enzyme system. Their metabolites are excreted in the urine and, to a lesser extent, in the feces. The inactive metabolites are excreted as conjugates of glucuronic acid.

See also individual barbiturate monographs.

RELATIVE CONTRAINDICATIONS

Hepatic coma
Hypersensitivity to barbiturates
Porphyria, history of latent or manifest

CAUTIONS AND COMMENTS

Barbiturates are addicting and habituating. Addiction and habituation have been particularly associated with long-term, high-dosage pharmacotherapy or regular personal use. The signs and symptoms of acute barbiturate intoxication include unsteady gate, slurred speech, and sustained nystagmus. Signs and symptoms of chronic barbiturate intoxication include confusion, poor judgment, irritability, insomnia, and somatic complaints. Signs and symptoms are similar to those associated with chronic alcoholism. In this regard, if a patient appears intoxicated with alcohol to a degree that is radically disproportionate to his or her blood alcohol concentration, barbiturate intoxication should be suspected. The lethal dose (LD_{50}) of barbiturates is greatly reduced when alcohol is ingested concurrently.

The abrupt discontinuation of barbiturate use among patients who are addicted to barbiturates may be fatal. Signs and symptoms of withdrawal may appear 8 to 12 hours after the last use of a barbiturate. These signs and symptoms generally occur in the following order: anxiety, muscle twitching, tremor of the hands and fingers, progressive weakness, dizziness, distortion in visual perception, nausea and vomiting, insomnia, and postural hypotension. More severe signs and symptoms of barbiturate withdrawal include convulsions and delirium. These signs and symptoms may occur within 16 hours of the last use of a barbiturate and may last up to 5 days. The intensity of these signs and symptoms declines gradually over approximately 15 days. Patients who are susceptible to barbiturate addiction and habituation usually have histories of problematic patterns of alcohol, amphetamine, opiate analgesic, or other abusable psychotropic use.

Barbiturate addiction and habituation is associated with the regular long-term use of a barbiturate in amounts generally exceeding recommended therapeutic dosages. People who have problematic patterns of barbiturate use may have: a strong desire or need to continue using the barbiturate; a tendency to increase the dose and decrease the dosing interval; habituation characterized by a craving to use the barbiturate; and a desire for or an appreciation of its actions. They also have a need for increasingly higher dosages to prevent the barbiturate withdrawal syndrome, the signs and symptoms of which are immediately relieved by the use of the barbiturate. Barbiturate addiction and habituation generally require cautious and gradual discontinuation of the barbiturate.

Prescribe barbiturate pharmacotherapy cautiously to patients who

- have acute or chronic pain. Paradoxical excitement may occur among these patients. Barbiturate pharmacotherapy also may mask the signs and symptoms important for the monitoring of their pain management.
- have depression or histories of attempted suicide.
- have histories of problematic patterns of abusable psychotropic use. Patients who become addicted and habituated to barbiturates may increase the dosage or decrease the dosage interval without consulting with their prescribing psychologist. To minimize the possible development of addiction and habituation, prescribe the smallest quantity of barbiturates feasible for dispensing (i.e., limit the prescribed quantity to the amount required between appointments).
- have histories of severe respiratory dysfunction. Therapeutic dosages of barbiturates have been associated with changes in respiratory function among normal subjects. However, high therapeutic dosages among patients who have chronic obstructive lung disease (e.g., asthma, bronchitis, emphysema) may result in respiratory distress. Barbiturate overdosage also may result in respiratory distress. The barbiturates depress alveolar ventilation and decrease hypoxic drive. These actions may result in respiratory acidosis. Generally, apnea does not occur unless another CNS depressant (e.g., alcohol or an opiate analgesic) has been used concurrently.

- have sleep apnea. Avoid prescribing barbiturates to these patients. If barbiturate pharmacotherapy is required, prescribe the lowest effective dosage. Monitor patients for potential exacerbation of sleep apnea.

Caution patients who are receiving barbiturate pharmacotherapy against

- drinking alcohol or using other drugs that produce CNS depression. Barbiturates may produce drowsiness and other effects that may be potentiated by these drugs. Advise patients to report the use of any other drugs (prescription or nonprescription) while receiving barbiturate pharmacotherapy.
- exceeding the prescribed dosage, decreasing the dosing interval, or using the barbiturate for a longer period of time than prescribed. Advise patients regarding the addiction and habituation potential of the barbiturates.
- giving, selling, or trading their barbiturate to any relatives, friends, or others.
- performing activities that require alertness, judgment, and physical coordination (e.g., driving an automobile, operating dangerous equipment, supervising children) until their response to barbiturate pharmacotherapy is known. The CNS depressant action of the barbiturates may adversely affect these mental and physical functions.

In addition to these general precautions for patients, caution women to

- inform their prescribing psychologist if they become or intend to become pregnant while receiving barbiturate pharmacotherapy so that their pharmacotherapy can be safely discontinued.

CLINICALLY SIGNIFICANT DRUG INTERACTIONS

Most of the clinically significant drug interactions involving the barbiturates have occurred with phenobarbital. However, these data appear to be applicable to mephobarbital and primidone, as well as the other barbiturates, because of their general chemical and pharmacological similarities.

Concurrent barbiturate pharmacotherapy and the following may result in clinically significant drug interactions:

Alcohol Use

Concurrent alcohol use may increase the CNS depressant action of the barbiturates. Advise patients to avoid, or limit, their use of alcohol while receiving barbiturate pharmacotherapy.

Anticoagulant (Oral) Pharmacotherapy

Barbiturates can induce the hepatic microsomal enzymes and, thus, increase the metabolism of oral anticoagulants (e.g., warfarin [Coumadin®]). This interaction may result in a decreased anticoagulant response. Patients who are stabilized on oral anticoagulant pharmacotherapy may require dosage adjustments if concurrent barbiturate pharmacotherapy is initiated or discontinued. Collaboration with the prescriber of the anticoagulant is indicated.

Corticosteroid Pharmacotherapy

Barbiturates appear to increase the metabolism of exogenous corticosteroids, probably through the induction of hepatic microsomal enzymes. Patients who have been stabilized on corticosteroid pharmacotherapy may require dosage adjustments if concurrent barbiturate pharmacotherapy is initiated or discontinued. Collaboration with the prescriber of the corticosteroid is indicated.

Disulfiram Pharmacotherapy

Disulfiram (Antabuse®) pharmacotherapy may decrease the metabolism of the barbiturates. This interaction may increase the incidence and severity of the ADRs associated with the barbiturates.

Estrogen Pharmacotherapy

Concurrent phenobarbital pharmacotherapy may decrease the action of the estrogen present in oral contraceptives by increasing the hepatic metabolism of the estrogen. This interaction may result in contraception failure. Alternative contraception may be required. Collaboration with the prescriber of the oral contraceptive is indicated. See "Pharmacotherapy With Drugs That Are Metabolized Primarily by the Liver."

Pharmacotherapy With CNS Depressants and Other Drugs That Produce CNS Depression

Concurrent barbiturate pharmacotherapy and pharmacotherapy with opiate analgesics, other sedative-hypnotics, or other drugs that produce CNS depression (e.g., antihistamines, phenothiazines, TCAs) may produce additive CNS depression.

Pharmacotherapy With Drugs That Are Metabolized Primarily by the Liver

Barbiturates do not impair normal liver function. However, they may induce the production of liver microsomal enzymes, and, thus, alter the metabolism of drugs that are primarily metabolized by the liver (e.g., anticoagulants [oral], corticosteroids, estrogens). Thus, concurrent barbiturate pharmacotherapy may affect pharmacotherapy with drugs that are susceptible to hepatic microsomal enzyme metabolism. This potential interaction may require therapeutic drug monitoring to determine the need to adjust the dosages of these drugs. Collaboration with other prescribers may be required.

Phenytoin Pharmacotherapy

Barbiturates appear to have variable effects on phenytoin (Dilantin®). When concurrent barbiturate and phenytoin pharmacotherapy is required, monitor the blood concentrations of both drugs and adjust the dosages, as needed.

Valproic Acid Pharmacotherapy

Valproic acid and its derivatives (i.e., divalproex sodium, sodium valproate) appear to decrease barbiturate metabolism. When concurrent pharmacotherapy is required, monitor barbiturate blood concentrations and adjust the dosage, as needed.

See also individual barbiturate monographs.

ADVERSE DRUG REACTIONS

Barbiturate pharmacotherapy for the prophylactic and symptomatic management of seizure disorders has been commonly associated with severe drowsiness (somnolence). Among some patients, particularly those who are elderly, barbiturates reportedly produce excitement rather than drowsiness. Barbiturate pharmacotherapy also has been associated with the following ADRs, listed according to body system:

Cardiovascular: bradycardia, fainting (syncope), and hypotension

CNS: anxiety, abnormal thinking, agitation, confusion, depression, dizziness, headache, hallucinations (visual), incoordination (ataxia), insomnia, lethargy, mental depression, nightmares, and paradoxic excitement (hyperactivity), particularly among children, the elderly, and patients who have severe pain. Barbiturate pharmacotherapy also is associated with impaired memory and reduced performance on neuropsychologic tests.

Cutaneous: angioedema (hives and edema involving areas of the skin, mucous membranes, or body organs), exfoliative dermatitis (Stevens–Johnson syndrome), and rash (particularly with mephobarbital and phenobarbital)

GI: constipation, diarrhea, nausea, and vomiting

Hematologic: megaloblastic anemia (following long-term phenobarbital pharmacotherapy, or regular personal use)

Musculoskeletal: abnormally increased muscular movement and physical activity (hyperkinesia), joint pain (arthralgia), and muscle pain (myalgia)

Respiratory: apnea, bronchospasm, coughing, hypoventilation, and laryngospasm. *Note*: The ADRs affecting the respiratory system are generally associated with either overdosage or too-rapid intravenous injection of the barbiturate injectable formulations.

Miscellaneous: fever

See also individual barbiturate monographs.

OVERDOSAGE

The ingestion of 1 gram (1,000 milligrams) of most barbiturates generally produces serious overdosage among adults. The signs and symptoms of barbiturate overdosage may be confused with alcohol intoxication or various neurological disorders. Generally, the ingestion of 2 to 10 grams of barbiturates is fatal. The signs and symptoms of acute barbiturate overdosage include CNS and respiratory depression, which may progress to Cheyne–Stokes respirations, areflexia, slightly constricted pupils (in severe overdosage, pupils may show paralytic dilation), decreased urine production (oliguria), tachycardia, hypotension, lowered body temperature, and coma. A typical shock syndrome (i.e., apnea, circulatory collapse, respiratory arrest, and death) may occur. In addition to other complications (e.g., pneumonia), extreme barbiturate overdosage may result in the cessation of all electrical activity in the brain. This effect is reportedly fully reversible unless hypoxic damage has occurred. Barbiturate overdosage requires emergency symptomatic medical support of body systems with attention to increasing barbiturate elimination. There is no known antidote.

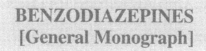
BENZODIAZEPINES
[General Monograph]

(ben zoe dye az' e peens)

GENERIC NAMES

For trade names, see individual benzodiazepine monographs.[3]

    Chlordiazepoxide
    Clonazepam
    Clorazepate
    Diazepam
    Lorazepam
    Nitrazepam

CLASSIFICATION

Anticonvulsant (sedative-hypnotic) (benzodiazepine) (C-IV)

See also individual benzodiazepine monographs.

APPROVED INDICATIONS FOR NEUROPSYCHOLOGICAL DISORDERS[4]

Pharmacotherapy for the prophylactic and symptomatic management of:

- seizure disorders. Benzodiazepine pharmacotherapy is indicated for the prevention and treatment of absence seizures, akinetic seizures, myoclonic seizures, status epilepticus, and seizures associated with the acute alcohol withdrawal syndrome. In regard to the latter, long-acting benzodiazepines, such as chlordiazepoxide and diazepam, are preferred.

See individual benzodiazepine monographs.

---

[3] Although several other benzodiazepines are commercially available in North America (see *PPDR: Psychologists' Psychotropic Drug Reference* [L. A. Pagliaro & A. M. Pagliaro, 1999]), their use is *not* approved for the prophylactic or symptomatic management of the various neuropsychological disorders (e.g., seizure disorders).

[4] For discussion of the use of the benzodiazepines as adjunctive pharmacotherapy for the symptomatic management of anxiety disorders and sleep disorders (i.e., insomnia), readers are referred to the related text in this series, *PPDR: Psychologists' Psychotropic Drug Reference* (L. A. Pagliaro & A. M. Pagliaro, 1999).

For details and discussion regarding related basic principles of clinical pharmacology, readers are referred to the first text in this series, *The Pharmacologic Basis of Psychotherapeutics: An Introduction for Psychologists.*

USUAL DOSAGE AND ADMINISTRATION

Seizures Disorders

Adults:　See individual benzodiazepine monographs.

Women who are, or who may become, pregnant:　FDA Pregnancy Category D. Safety and efficacy of benzodiazepine pharmacotherapy for women who are pregnant have not been established. The benzodiazepines readily cross the placental barrier and often achieve fetal blood concentrations that are equal to or higher than maternal blood concentrations. Avoid prescribing benzodiazepine pharmacotherapy to women who are pregnant. If benzodiazepine pharmacotherapy is required, advise patients of potential benefits and possible risks to themselves and the embryo, fetus, or neonate. Collaboration with the patient's obstetrician is indicated. See also individual benzodiazepine monographs.

Women who are breast-feeding:　Safety and efficacy of benzodiazepine pharmacotherapy for women who are breast-feeding and their neonates and infants have not been established. Benzodiazepines are excreted in breast milk, generally in concentrations sufficient to cause sedation and potential addiction among breast-fed neonates and infants. Avoid prescribing benzodiazepine pharmacotherapy to women who are breast-feeding. If benzodiazepine pharmacotherapy is required, breast-feeding probably should be discontinued. If desired, lactation may be maintained and breast-feeding resumed following the discontinuation of short-term benzodiazepine pharmacotherapy.

Elderly, frail, or debilitated patients:　Generally prescribe lower dosages for elderly, frail, or debilitated patients. Gradually increase the dosage, if needed, according to individual patient response. These patients may be more sensitive to the pharmacologic actions of the benzodiazepines than are younger or healthier adult patients. Chlordiazepoxide, clonazepam, clorazepate, diazepam, and nitrazepam (lorazepam is conjugated and excreted in the urine) generally have prolonged half-lives of elimination among these patients. See also individual benzodiazepine monographs.

Children and adolescents:　When prescribed for children and adolescents for the prophylactic and symptomatic management of seizure disorders, benzodiazepine dosages generally should *not* exceed the usual recommended adult dosages, except where specifically indicated. See individual benzodiazepine monographs.

Notes, Seizure Disorders

Generally prescribe the lowest effective dosage to avoid over-sedation and other associated ADRs. These ADRs may be particularly problematic for elderly, frail, or debilitated patients. Adjust the dosage according to individual patient response. See individual benzodiazepine monographs.

Benzodiazepine injectable pharmacotherapy:　Benzodiazepine injectable pharmacotherapy is associated with apnea, bradycardia, cardiac arrest, and hypotension, particularly among elderly, frail, or debilitated patients or those who have cardiovascular or respiratory disorders. An increased incidence of these ADRs is associated with high dosages and rapid intravenous injection.

Initiating benzodiazepine pharmacotherapy: *Before* prescribing benzodiazepine pharmacotherapy for the prophylactic or symptomatic management of seizure disorders,

- assure an accurate diagnosis of the seizure disorder.
- assess the patient's perception of his or her seizure disorder and the need for benzodiazepine pharmacotherapy.
- identify any previous problematic patterns of abusable psychotropic use, including any heavy alcohol, barbiturate, benzodiazepine, or other sedative-hypnotic use.
- note any previous benzodiazepine or other anticonvulsant pharmacotherapy and the patient's response.
- identify possible hypersensitivity to the benzodiazepines and potential contraindications, cautions, and drug interactions.
- assess the patient's ability to manage his or her benzodiazepine pharmacotherapy.
- assure that patients have an understanding regarding the course of their prescribed pharmacotherapy. Patients should be made aware that benzodiazepines may cause addiction and habituation. In addition, they should know the exact name of the benzodiazepine required, its general action, purpose, dosage, storage, and administration. They should know how to monitor therapeutic response, identify and manage common ADRs, and identify signs and symptoms that indicate that the prescribing psychologist should be contacted or emergency medical services be sought. Direct patients and their families, as appropriate, to available support groups (e.g., Epileptic Society) for additional help.

Maintaining benzodiazepine pharmacotherapy

- Monitor for therapeutic response to benzodiazepine pharmacotherapy (e.g., absence of, or a significant reduction in, seizure activity).
- Monitor patients for common ADRs. Elderly, frail, or debilitated patients and patients who have histories of chronic alcoholism may be particularly sensitive to the sedative effects and postural (orthostatic) hypotension associated with benzodiazepine pharmacotherapy. These ADRs may result in falls or other accidents among these patients. Advise patients, or their family members as appropriate, to implement appropriate safety precautions (e.g., supervised ambulation, supervised tobacco smoking), as needed.
- Avoid prescribing concurrent pharmacotherapy with interacting drugs (see "Clinically Significant Drug Interactions").

Discontinuing benzodiazepine pharmacotherapy: A benzodiazepine withdrawal syndrome has been associated with the abrupt discontinuation of long-term benzodiazepine pharmacotherapy and regular personal use. Signs and symptoms of the withdrawal syndrome range from mild dysphoria and insomnia to more severe signs and symptoms that include abdominal and muscle cramps, sweating, tremors, convulsions, and vomiting. Signs and symptoms of the benzodiazepine withdrawal syndrome have included life-threatening seizures at dosages within the recommended range for some benzodiazepines (e.g., alprazolam [Xanax®]). The severity of the withdrawal syndrome and its duration appear to be related to the dosage and duration of benzodiazepine pharmacotherapy or regular personal use.

Signs and symptoms of the benzodiazepine withdrawal syndrome have been associated with rapid reductions in dosage and abrupt discontinuation of pharmacotherapy. Avoid rapid reductions in dosage and abrupt discontinuation of benzodiazepine pharmacotherapy. Patients who have histories of seizure disorders are at particular risk for the withdrawal syndrome. Closely monitor patients who require dosage reductions or the discontinuation of benzodiazepine pharmacotherapy. The signs and symptoms of benzodiazepine withdrawal may be managed by the reinstitution of benzodiazepine pharmacotherapy. The dosage should be sufficient to relieve the signs and symptoms of withdrawal.

AVAILABLE DOSAGE FORMS, STORAGE, AND COMPATIBILITY

Notes

The benzodiazepines are available in various oral, injectable, rectal, and sublingual formulations. See individual benzodiazepine monographs.

General instructions for patients: Instruct patients who are receiving benzodiazepine pharmacotherapy to

- safely store their prescribed benzodiazepine dosage formulation out of the reach of children in child-resistant containers.
- obtain an available patient information sheet regarding benzodiazepine pharmacotherapy from their pharmacist at the time that their prescription is dispensed. Encourage patients to clarify any questions that they may have regarding benzodiazepine pharmacotherapy with their pharmacist or, if needed, to consult their prescribing psychologist.

See also individual benzodiazepine monographs.

PROPOSED MECHANISM OF ACTION

The benzodiazepines cause a dose-related CNS depression ranging from mild impairment of cognitive and psychomotor functions to hypnosis. The exact mechanism of action for their anticonvulsant action has not yet been fully determined. However, benzodiazepines appear to act at the benzodiazepine receptors (i.e., BZD-1 and BZD-2). These receptors are found at several sites within the CNS, particularly in the cerebral cortex and the limbic system. The benzodiazepine receptors are found primarily in conjunction with the GABA receptor complex and predominantly in association with the $GABA_{(A)}$ receptor. Thus, it appears that the benzodiazepines elicit their pharmacologic actions by potentiating the actions of GABA, a major inhibitory neurotransmitter, within the CNS. In relation to their anticonvulsant action, the benzodiazepines appear to augment presynaptic inhibition. Thus, they suppress seizure activity, but do not abolish the originating abnormal discharge from the seizure foci.

PHARMACOKINETICS/PHARMACODYNAMICS

The benzodiazepines are generally well absorbed following oral ingestion. The ingestion of food can sometimes delay the rate of absorption, but does not generally affect the extent of absorption. The benzodiazepines are highly bound to plasma proteins and are widely distributed throughout body tissues. Some benzodiazepines (e.g., flurazepam [Dalmane®]) undergo extensive first-pass hepatic metabolism. The benzodiazepines and their metabolites readily cross the blood–brain and placental barriers and are excreted in breast milk.

Most benzodiazepines are mainly metabolized by the hepatic microsomal enzyme system. Therefore, liver dysfunction may significantly affect the metabolism of most benzodiazepines and predispose patients who have liver dysfunction to benzodiazepine toxicity. However, exceptions include lorazepam (Ativan®), oxazepam (Serax®), and temazepam (Restoril®). These benzodiazepines are metabolized primarily by urinary conjugation to more water-soluble (i.e., polar) glucuronide derivatives that subsequently are excreted in the urine.

On the basis of their durations of action, the benzodiazepines commonly are classified as: short-acting (e.g., triazolam [Halcion®]); intermediate-acting (e.g., alprazolam [Xanax®], bromazepam [Lectopam®], lorazepam [Ativan®], oxazepam [Serax®], and temazepam [Restoril®]); and long-acting (e.g., chlordiazepoxide [Librium®], clorazepate [Tranzene®], diazepam [Valium®], and flurazepam [Dalmane®]). The duration of action is generally well correlated with the volume of distribution of the various benzodiazepines which, in turn, is correlated with their degree of lipid solubility.

See individual benzodiazepine monographs.

RELATIVE CONTRAINDICATIONS

Alcohol intoxication, acute with depressed cardiovascular and respiratory function
Depression
Glaucoma, acute narrow-angle. This contraindication is noted by most drug manufacturers. However, the benzodiazepines do *not* increase intraocular pressure nor do they possess anticholinergic activity. In addition, glaucoma has *not* been directly associated with benzodiazepine pharmacotherapy.
Hypersensitivity to any of the benzodiazepines
Pain, severe and uncontrolled
Pregnancy
Respiratory depression, severe

See also individual benzodiazepine monographs.

CAUTIONS AND COMMENTS

The benzodiazepines are addicting and habituating. Addiction and habituation are generally associated with long-term, high-dosage pharmacotherapy, or regular personal use. Addiction and habituation may be more commonly observed among patients who have histories of problematic patterns of alcohol or other abusable psychotropic use. These patients may have considerable difficulty decreasing their dosages and discontinuing their benzodiazepine pharmacotherapy, particularly long-term, high-dosage pharmacotherapy.

Paradoxical exacerbation of seizures, although uncommon, has been associated with benzodiazepine pharmacotherapy. Approximately 6% of patients receiving oral benzodiazepine pharmacotherapy, particularly clonazepam pharmacotherapy, may experience a worsening of their seizure disorder. In addition, intravenous benzodiazepine pharmacotherapy has been associated with the precipitation of tonic status epilepticus, particularly among children who have Lennox–Gastaut Syndrome. Monitor all patients who are prescribed benzodiazepine pharmacotherapy for the prophylactic or symptomatic management of seizure disorders for paradoxical exacerbation of their seizure disorders.

Prescribe benzodiazepine pharmacotherapy cautiously to patients who

- have histories of chronic alcoholism. A decreased benzodiazepine elimination rate (increased plasma half-life) has been observed among these patients. This decreased elimination rate has been related to the liver dysfunction commonly associated with chronic alcoholism (i.e., alcoholic cirrhosis).

- have histories of problematic patterns of alcohol or other abusable psychotropic use. These patients require careful monitoring for the development of problematic patterns of benzodiazepine use.
- have histories of severe respiratory dysfunction. Therapeutic dosages of benzodiazepines have been associated with changes in respiratory function among normal subjects. High therapeutic dosages among patients who have chronic obstructive lung disease (e.g., asthma, bronchitis, emphysema) may result in respiratory distress. Benzodiazepine overdosage also may result in respiratory distress. The benzodiazepines depress alveolar ventilation and decrease hypoxic drive, resulting in respiratory acidosis. Generally, apnea does not occur unless other CNS depressants (e.g., alcohol, opiate analgesics) have been used concurrently.
- have kidney or liver dysfunction. The elimination of benzodiazepines may be slowed among these patients, resulting in toxicity.
- have sleep apnea. Avoid prescribing benzodiazepines for these patients. If benzodiazepine pharmacotherapy is required, prescribe the lowest effective dosage. Monitor patients for potential exacerbation of sleep apnea.

Caution patients who are receiving benzodiazepine pharmacotherapy against

- abruptly discontinuing benzodiazepine pharmacotherapy or regular personal use. Abrupt discontinuation of benzodiazepine pharmacotherapy, particularly long-term, high-dosage pharmacotherapy, or regular personal use, may result in the benzodiazepine withdrawal syndrome.
- drinking alcohol or using other drugs that have CNS depressant actions. The concurrent use of alcohol or other drugs that depress the CNS can result in severe CNS depression.
- giving, selling, or trading their benzodiazepine to any friends, relatives, or others.
- increasing their dosage or using the benzodiazepine more often, or for a longer period of time, than prescribed. Long-term regular personal use of benzodiazepines may result in addiction and habituation.
- performing activities that require alertness, judgment, and physical coordination (e.g., driving an automobile, operating dangerous equipment, supervising children) until their response to benzodiazepine pharmacotherapy is known. The benzodiazepines have CNS depressant actions that may affect these mental and physical functions.

In addition to these general precautions, caution patients who are receiving benzodiazepine pharmacotherapy to

- inform their advanced practice nurse, dentist, family physician, and other prescribers that they are receiving benzodiazepine pharmacotherapy.

CLINICALLY SIGNIFICANT DRUG INTERACTIONS

Concurrent benzodiazepine pharmacotherapy and the following may result in clinically significant drug interactions:

Alcohol Use

Concurrent alcohol use may increase the CNS depressant action of the benzodiazepines. Advise patients to avoid, or limit, their use of alcohol while receiving benzodiazepine pharmacotherapy.

Disulfiram Pharmacotherapy

Concurrent disulfiram (Antabuse®) pharmacotherapy may inhibit the metabolism of the benzodiazepines. This interaction may result in an increase in the incidence and severity of the ADRs associated with benzodiazepine pharmacotherapy.

Pharmacotherapy With CNS Depressants and Other Drugs That Produce CNS Depression

Concurrent benzodiazepine pharmacotherapy and pharmacotherapy with opiate analgesics, other sedative-hypnotics, and other drugs that produce CNS depression (e.g., antihistamines, phenothiazines, TCAs) may result in severe additive CNS depression.

Pharmacotherapy With Drugs and Beverages and Foods That Inhibit Hepatic Microsomal Enzyme Metabolism, Particularly Isoenzyme CYP3A4

Hepatic microsomal enzyme inhibitors (e.g., cimetidine [Tagamet®], diltiazem [Cardizem®], erythromycin [E-Mycin®], fluoxetine [Prozac®], fluvoxamine [Luvox®], grapefruit juice, itraconazole [Sporanex®], ketoconazole [Nizoral®], miconazole [Micatin®], nefazodone [Serzone®], omeprazole [Prilosec®], and quinidine [Biquin®]) may decrease benzodiazepine metabolism. This interaction may increase benzodiazepine blood concentrations (sometimes severalfold) and associated CNS depression (e.g., confusion, dizziness, drowsiness, somnolence).

Ritonavir Pharmacotherapy

Ritonavir (Norvir®), an antiretroviral drug indicated for the pharmacologic management of HIV infection, may significantly inhibit the hepatic microsomal enzyme metabolism of the benzodiazepines that are highly metabolized by the liver (i.e., alprazolam [Xanax®], clorazepate [Tranxene®], diazepam [Valium®], flurazepam [Dalmane®], midazolam [Versed®], and triazolam [Halcion®]). This interaction may result in severe sedation and respiratory depression. Concurrent benzodiazepine and ritonavir pharmacotherapy with the highly metabolized benzodiazepines is ***contraindicated***. Concurrent pharmacotherapy with the other benzodiazepines (e.g., oxazepam [Serax®]) also probably should be avoided among patients who are receiving ritonavir pharmacotherapy. If concurrent pharmacotherapy with these other benzodiazepines cannot be avoided, monitor patients carefully for excessive CNS and respiratory depression. Adjust the benzodiazepine dosage according to individual patient response.

Tobacco Smoking

Concurrent tobacco smoking may increase the metabolism of the benzodiazepines. Patients who smoke tobacco may require higher dosages of the benzodiazepines.

See also individual benzodiazepine monographs.

ADVERSE DRUG REACTIONS

Benzodiazepine pharmacotherapy commonly has been associated with confusion, depression, and incoordination (ataxia). See individual benzodiazepine monographs.

OVERDOSAGE

Signs and symptoms of benzodiazepine overdosage include coma, confusion, diminished reflexes, incoordination, and somnolence. Benzodiazepine overdosage is generally not fatal because benzodiazepines possess a high LD_{50}. However, death commonly occurs when benzodiazepines are used in combination with alcohol. Benzodiazepine overdosage requires emergency symptomatic medical support of body systems with attention to increasing benzodiazepine elimination. The benzodiazepine receptor antagonist, flumazenil (Anexate®, Romazicon®), may be required. See the flumazenil monograph.

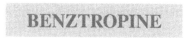

BENZTROPINE

(benz′ troe peen)

TRADE NAME

Cogentin®

CLASSIFICATION

Antiparkinsonian (tertiary amine antimuscarinic)

APPROVED INDICATIONS FOR NEUROPSYCHOLOGICAL DISORDERS

Pharmacotherapy for the symptomatic management of:

- Parkinson's disease: drug-induced and idiopathic

USUAL DOSAGE AND ADMINISTRATION

Parkinson's Disease: Drug-Induced and Idiopathic

Adults: Initially, 2 mg daily orally in a single dose 30 minutes before retiring for bed in the evening. Gradually increase the daily dosage, as needed, by 0.5-mg increments at five-day intervals according to individual patient response.

MAXIMUM: 6 mg daily orally in a single dose or two divided doses

Women who are, or who may become, pregnant: FDA Pregnancy Category C. Safety and efficacy of benztropine pharmacotherapy for women who are pregnant have not been established. Avoid prescribing benztropine pharmacotherapy to women who are pregnant. If benztropine pharmacotherapy is required, advise patients of potential benefits and possible risks to themselves and the embryo, fetus, or neonate. Collaboration with the patient's obstetrician is indicated.

Women who are breast-feeding: Safety and efficacy of benztropine pharmacotherapy for women who are breast-feeding and their neonates and infants have not been established. Avoid prescribing benztropine pharmacotherapy to women who are breast-feeding. If benztropine pharmacotherapy is required, breast-feeding probably should be discontinued. If desired, lactation may be maintained and breast-feeding resumed following the discontinuation of short-term benztropine pharmacotherapy. Collaboration with the patient's pediatrician is indicated.

For details and discussion regarding related basic principles of clinical pharmacology, readers are referred to the first text in this series, *The Pharmacologic Basis of Psychotherapeutics: An Introduction for Psychologists.*

Elderly, frail, or debilitated patients and those who have less than average body weight: Initially, 1 mg daily orally in a single dose or two divided doses. Gradually increase the dosage if needed, according to individual patient response. Generally prescribe lower dosages for elderly, frail, or debilitated patients and those who have less than average body weight. These patients may be more sensitive to the pharmacologic actions of benztropine than are younger or healthier adult patients.

Infants and children younger than 3 years of age: Safety and efficacy of benztropine pharmacotherapy for infants and children who are younger than 3 years of age have not been established. Benztropine pharmacotherapy is *not* recommended for this age group.

Notes, Parkinson's Disease

The acute extrapyramidal reactions generally associated with the initiation of antipsychotic pharmacotherapy are generally transient. Therefore, the need for benztropine pharmacotherapy when prescribed for the symptomatic management of drug-induced Parkinson's disease–like extrapyramidal reactions should be reevaluated after ~2 weeks.

Benztropine injectable pharmacotherapy: The injectable formulation of benztropine rarely is used except in cases of acute dystonic reactions or when the benztropine oral tablets are contraindicated (e.g., when patients are agitated or confused or have nausea and vomiting). When benztropine injectable pharmacotherapy is required, the intramuscular route of administration usually is used because it is more convenient and the onset of action is reportedly similar to intravenous administration. The intravenous route rarely is used.

AVAILABLE DOSAGE FORMS, STORAGE, AND COMPATIBILITY

Injectable, intramuscular or intravenous: 1 mg/ml
Tablets, oral: 0.5, 1, 2 mg

Notes

Benztropine injectable pharmacotherapy: The benztropine injectable formulation contains sodium metabisulfite. Sulfites have been associated with hypersensitivity reactions, including anaphylactic reactions, among susceptible patients. Although relatively uncommon, these reactions appear to occur with a higher incidence among patients who have asthma.

General instructions for patients: Instruct patients who are receiving benztropine pharmacotherapy to

- safely store benztropine oral tablets out of the reach of children in tightly closed, light- and child-resistant containers at controlled room temperature (15° to 25°C; 59° to 77°F).
- obtain an available patient information sheet regarding benztropine pharmacotherapy from their pharmacist at the time that their prescription is dispensed. Encourage patients to clarify any questions that they may have regarding benztropine pharmacotherapy with their pharmacist or, if needed, to consult their prescribing psychologist.

PROPOSED MECHANISM OF ACTION

The exact mechanism of the antiparkinsonian action associated with benztropine is unknown. However, the mechanism of action may be directly related to its anticholinergic activity. Benztropine blocks cholinergic receptors in the basal ganglia.

PHARMACOKINETICS/PHARMACODYNAMICS

The onset of action of benztropine following oral ingestion is between 1 and 2 hours. When injected intramuscularly or intravenously, the onset of action is within minutes. Additional data are not available.

RELATIVE CONTRAINDICATIONS

Angle-closure (narrow-angle) glaucoma
Hypersensitivity to benztropine
Tardive dyskinesia. Benztropine generally is ineffective for the symptomatic management of tardive dyskinesia and may actually aggravate or unmask the signs and symptoms of this movement disorder.

CAUTIONS AND COMMENTS

Prescribe benztropine pharmacotherapy cautiously to patients who

- have chronic medical or psychological disorders.
- are receiving pharmacotherapy with other drugs that produce anticholinergic actions. Benztropine can cause inhibition of normal perspiration (anhidrosis), resulting in hyperthermia, particularly during hot weather. Severe anhidrosis and fatal hyperthermia have been associated with benztropine pharmacotherapy.

Caution patients who are receiving benztropine pharmacotherapy against

- performing activities that require alertness, judgment, or physical coordination (e.g., driving an automobile, operating dangerous equipment, supervising children) until their response to benztropine pharmacotherapy is known. Benztropine may adversely affect these mental and physical functions.

In addition to this general precaution, caution patients to

- inform their prescribing psychologist if they begin or discontinue any other pharmacotherapy while receiving benztropine pharmacotherapy.

CLINICALLY SIGNIFICANT DRUG INTERACTIONS

Concurrent benztropine pharmacotherapy and the following may result in clinically significant drug interactions:

Pharmacotherapy With Anticholinergics and Other Drugs That Produce Anticholinergic Actions

Concurrent benztropine pharmacotherapy and pharmacotherapy with anticholinergics (e.g., atropine) and other drugs that produce anticholinergic actions (e.g., phenothiazines, TCAs) may result in serious and potentially fatal additive anticholinergic toxicity. Signs and symptoms of anticholinergic toxicity may include heat intolerance, hyperthermia, and paralytic ileus. Instruct patients who require this combination of pharmacotherapy to immediately notify their prescribing psychologist if they have constipation, fever, or heat intolerance.

ADVERSE DRUG REACTIONS

Benztropine pharmacotherapy has been commonly associated with ADRs related to its anticholinergic actions. These ADRs are usually dose related and can be reduced or eliminated by decreasing the dosage of benztropine. These and other ADRs are listed according to body system:

Cardiovascular: increased heart rate (tachycardia)
CNS: depression, impaired memory, mental confusion, and nervousness
Cutaneous: impaired ability to perspire normally (anhidrosis) and skin rash
Genitourinary: urinary retention
GI: constipation, dry mouth (may be severe enough to interfere with swallowing or speaking), nausea, and, rarely, paralytic ileus
Musculoskeletal: weakness
Ophthalmic: blurred vision and dilation of the pupils (mydriasis)
Miscellaneous: fever (hyperthermia) and heat stroke

OVERDOSAGE

Signs and symptoms of benztropine overdosage may include the following: clumsiness; CNS depression; confusion; dryness and flushing of the skin; nervousness; shortness of breath; severe dryness of the mouth, nose, and throat; tachycardia; toxic psychosis; and a sensation of warmth. Suspected or actual benztropine overdosage requires emergency symptomatic medical support of body systems with attention to increasing benztropine elimination. Although physostigmine (Antilirium®) is an antidote, it is *not* generally recommended for the treatment of anticholinergic toxicity because of the following: 1) the ADRs associated with its use (e.g., asystole, seizures); and 2) its relative contraindication for use among patients who have asthma, cardiovascular disease, gangrene, and mechanical obstruction of the gastrointestinal or genitourinary tracts.

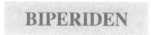
BIPERIDEN

(bye per′ i den)

TRADE NAME

Akineton®

CLASSIFICATION

Antiparkinsonian (tertiary amine antimuscarinic)

APPROVED INDICATIONS FOR NEUROPSYCHOLOGICAL DISORDERS

Pharmacotherapy for the symptomatic management of:

• Parkinson's disease: drug-induced and idiopathic

USUAL DOSAGE AND ADMINISTRATION

Parkinson's Disease: Drug-Induced and Idiopathic

Adults: 4 to 8 mg daily orally in two to four divided doses

MAXIMUM: 16 mg daily orally

Women who are, or who may become, pregnant: FDA Pregnancy Category C. Safety and efficacy of biperiden pharmacotherapy for women who are pregnant have not been established. Avoid prescribing biperiden pharmacotherapy to women who are pregnant. If biperiden pharmacotherapy is required, advise patients of potential benefits and possible risks to themselves and the embryo, fetus, or neonate. Collaboration with the patient's obstetrician is indicated.

Women who are breast-feeding: Safety and efficacy of biperiden pharmacotherapy for women who are breast-feeding and their neonates and infants have not been established. However, biperiden is excreted in breast milk and can achieve concentrations equivalent to those obtained in the maternal blood. Avoid prescribing biperiden pharmacotherapy to women who are breast-feeding. If biperiden pharmacotherapy is required, breast-feeding probably should be discontinued. Collaboration with the patient's pediatrician may be required.

For details and discussion regarding related basic principles of clinical pharmacology, readers are referred to the first text in this series, *The Pharmacologic Basis of Psychotherapeutics: An Introduction for Psychologists.*

Elderly, frail, or debilitated patients: Generally prescribe lower dosages for elderly, frail, or debilitated patients. These patients may be more sensitive to the pharmacologic actions of biperiden than are younger or healthier adult patients. Gradually increase the dosage if needed, according to individual patient response.

Children and adolescents younger than 18 years of age: Safety and efficacy of biperiden pharmacotherapy for children and adolescents who are younger than 18 years of age have not been established. Biperiden pharmacotherapy is *not* recommended for this age group.

Notes, Parkinson's Disease: Drug-Induced and Idiopathic

Biperiden injectable pharmacotherapy: Biperiden injectable pharmacotherapy usually is reserved for the treatment of acute dystonic reactions (e.g., oculogyric crisis, spasmodic torticollis). The usual adult dose is 2 mg intramuscularly or intravenously. This dose may be repeated every 30 minutes to a maximum of four consecutive doses in a 24-hour period.

Discontinuing biperiden pharmacotherapy: Avoid discontinuing biperiden pharmacotherapy abruptly. The abrupt discontinuation of biperiden pharmacotherapy has been associated with rebound cholinergic activity. Whenever possible, discontinue biperiden pharmacotherapy gradually.

AVAILABLE DOSAGE FORMS, STORAGE, AND COMPATIBILITY

Injectable, intramuscular or intravenous: 5 mg/ml
Tablets, oral: 2 mg

Notes

General instructions for patients: Instruct patients who are receiving biperiden pharmacotherapy to

- ingest each dose of the biperiden oral tablets with food to decrease associated gastric irritation.
- safely store biperiden oral tablets out of the reach of children in tightly closed, light- and child-resistant containers at controlled room temperature (15° to 30°C; 59° to 86°F).
- obtain an available patient information sheet regarding biperiden pharmacotherapy from their pharmacist at the time that their prescription is dispensed. Encourage patients to clarify any questions that they may have regarding biperiden pharmacotherapy with their pharmacist or, if needed, to consult their prescribing psychologist.

PROPOSED MECHANISM OF ACTION

The exact mechanism of antiparkinsonian action of biperiden is unknown. However, it is believed to be directly related to its central anticholinergic activity (i.e., competitive antagonism of acetylcholine at the cholinergic receptors within the corpus striatum).

PHARMACOKINETICS/PHARMACODYNAMICS

Biperiden achieves peak blood levels within ~1.5 hours after oral ingestion. The absolute bioavailability of the oral tablets is ~33% because of extensive first-pass liver metabolism ($F = 0.33$). Plasma protein binding is high (94%). The mean half-life of elimination is 30 hours (range: 24 to 38 hours). Additional data are not available.

RELATIVE CONTRAINDICATIONS

Angle-closure (narrow-angle) glaucoma
Bowel obstruction
Hypersensitivity to biperiden
Megacolon
Prostate adenoma
Stenosis of the GI tract
Tachycardia

CAUTIONS AND COMMENTS

Caution patients who are receiving biperiden pharmacotherapy against

- drinking alcohol while receiving biperiden pharmacotherapy.
- performing activities that require alertness, judgment, or physical coordination (e.g., driving an automobile, operating dangerous equipment, supervising children) until their response to biperiden pharmacotherapy is known. Biperiden may cause blurred vision and drowsiness and may thus adversely affect these mental and physical functions.

In addition to these general precautions, caution patients to

- inform their prescribing psychologist if they begin or discontinue any other pharmacotherapy while receiving biperiden pharmacotherapy.

CLINICALLY SIGNIFICANT DRUG INTERACTIONS

Concurrent biperiden pharmacotherapy and the following may result in clinically significant drug interactions:

Pharmacotherapy With Anticholinergics and Other Drugs That Produce Anticholinergic Actions

Concurrent biperiden pharmacotherapy with anticholinergics (e.g., atropine) and other drugs that produce anticholinergic actions (e.g., meperidine [Demerol®], phenothiazines, TCAs) may result in additive anticholinergic actions and possible toxicity.

ADVERSE DRUG REACTIONS

Biperiden pharmacotherapy has been commonly associated with blurred vision and a dry mouth. It also has been associated with the following ADRs, listed according to body system:

Cardiovascular: increased heart rate (tachycardia)
CNS: disorientation, dizziness, drowsiness, hallucinations (rare), and mental confusion
Cutaneous: decreased perspiration (hypohidrosis) and skin rash
Genitourinary: urinary retention
GI: constipation and gastric irritation

OVERDOSAGE

Signs and symptoms of biperiden overdosage include agitation, anxiety, confusion, delirium, dilated pupils, disorientation, dry mouth, hallucinations, illusions, incoherence, incoordination (ataxia), loss of memory, paranoia, and tachycardia. Acute overdosage may progress to stupor, coma, cardiac and respiratory arrest, and coma. Thus, suspected or actual biperiden overdosage requires emergency symptomatic medical support of body systems with attention to increasing biperiden elimination. The acetylcholine esterase inhibitor, physostigmine (Antilirium®), has been used as an antidote. However, the use of physostigmine for the symptomatic management of biperiden overdosage is controversial. Physostigmine is generally *not* recommended for the treatment of anticholinergic toxicity because of the following: 1) the ADRs associated with its use (e.g., asystole, seizures); and 2) its relative contraindication for use among patients who have asthma, cardiovascular disease, gangrene, and mechanical obstruction of the gastrointestinal or genitourinary tracts.

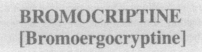

BROMOCRIPTINE
[Bromoergocryptine]

(broe moe krip′ teen)

TRADE NAME

Parlodel®

CLASSIFICATION

Antiparkinsonian (ergot alkaloid derivative)

APPROVED INDICATIONS FOR NEUROPSYCHOLOGICAL DISORDERS

Adjunctive pharmacotherapy for the symptomatic management of:

- Parkinson's disease: idiopathic. Usually, bromocriptine pharmacotherapy is prescribed for this indication as adjunctive pharmacotherapy to levodopa pharmacotherapy. See "Notes, Parkinson's Disease: Idiopathic."

USUAL DOSAGE AND ADMINISTRATION

Parkinson's Disease: Idiopathic

Adults: Initially, 2.5 mg daily orally in two divided doses with meals. Gradually increase the daily dosage by 2.5-mg increments at fourteen-day intervals, according to individual patient response. Dosage increases may be made until desired therapeutic benefit is achieved or dose-limiting ADRs are observed.

MAXIMUM: 100 mg daily orally

Women who are, or who may become, pregnant: FDA Pregnancy Category B. Safety and efficacy of bromocriptine pharmacotherapy for women who are pregnant have not been established. Avoid prescribing bromocriptine pharmacotherapy to women who are pregnant. If bromocriptine pharmacotherapy is required, advise patients of potential benefits and possible risks to themselves and the embryo, fetus, or neonate. Collaboration with the patient's obstetrician or pediatrician is indicated.

For details and discussion regarding related basic principles of clinical pharmacology, readers are referred to the first text in this series, *The Pharmacologic Basis of Psychotherapeutics: An Introduction for Psychologists.*

Women who are breast-feeding: Do not prescribe bromocriptine pharmacotherapy to women who are breast-feeding. Bromocriptine prevents or suppresses lactation. Therefore, bromocriptine pharmacotherapy for the symptomatic management of Parkinson's disease is contraindicated for women who are breast-feeding their infants.

Elderly, frail, or debilitated patients: Initially, 1.25 mg orally 30 minutes before retiring for bed in the evening in order to minimize associated ADRs. May then prescribe the usual adult dosage, according to individual patient response.

Adult patients who have liver dysfunction: Lower dosages of bromocriptine may be required for patients who have liver dysfunction. See "Pharmacokinetics/Pharmacodynamics."

Children and adolescents younger than 15 years of age: Safety and efficacy of bromocriptine pharmacotherapy for children and adolescents who are younger than 15 years of age have not been established. Bromocriptine pharmacotherapy is *not* recommended for this age group.

Notes, Parkinson's Disease: Idiopathic

Usually, bromocriptine pharmacotherapy is prescribed as adjunctive pharmacotherapy to levodopa pharmacotherapy. Adjunctive bromocriptine and levodopa pharmacotherapy allows the prescription of lower dosages of levodopa and, consequently, significantly fewer levodopa-associated ADRs.

Maintaining bromocriptine pharmacotherapy: Safety and efficacy of long-term (i.e., over 2 years) bromocriptine pharmacotherapy for the symptomatic management of idiopathic Parkinson's disease have not been clearly established.

Discontinuing bromocriptine pharmacotherapy: Avoid the abrupt discontinuation of bromocriptine pharmacotherapy among patients who have idiopathic Parkinson's disease. Abrupt discontinuation of pharmacotherapy may result in an exacerbation of the signs and symptoms of this neuropsychologic disorder.

AVAILABLE DOSAGE FORMS, STORAGE, AND COMPATIBILITY

Capsules, oral: 5 mg
Tablets, oral (Parlodel Snap Tabs®): 2.5 mg

Notes

The bromocriptine oral capsules may contain sodium metabisulfite. Sulfites have been associated with hypersensitivity reactions, including anaphylactic reactions, among susceptible patients. Although relatively uncommon, these reactions appear to occur with a higher incidence among patients who have asthma.

General instructions for patients: Instruct patients who are receiving bromocriptine pharmacotherapy to

- ingest each dose of the bromocriptine oral capsules and tablets with food to decrease associated gastric irritation.
- safely store bromocriptine oral capsules and tablets out of the reach of children in tightly closed, light- and child-resistant containers at controlled room temperature (15° to 25°C; 59° to 77°F).
- obtain an available patient information sheet regarding bromocriptine pharmacotherapy from their pharmacist at the time that their prescription is dispensed. Encourage patients to clarify any questions that they may have regarding bromocriptine pharmacotherapy with their pharmacist or, if needed, to consult their prescribing psychologist.

PROPOSED MECHANISM OF ACTION

The exact mechanism of antiparkinsonian action of bromocriptine is unknown. However, it is believed to be related to activation by bromocriptine of dopaminergic (D2) receptors in the nigrostriatal pathway of the CNS.

PHARMACOKINETICS/PHARMACODYNAMICS

Bromocriptine is rapidly and moderately well absorbed (~75%) following oral ingestion. However, its total bioavailability is low ($F = 0.06$) because of significant first-pass hepatic metabolism. Plasma protein binding is high (92% to 96%) and the apparent volume of distribution is ~2 liters/kg. Bromocriptine is almost completely metabolized in the liver with ~2% excreted in unchanged form in the urine. It has a half-life of elimination of ~48 hours. The pharmacokinetics and pharmacodynamics of bromocriptine are subject to significant interindividual variability. Additional data are not available.

RELATIVE CONTRAINDICATIONS

Hypersensitivity to ergot alkaloids
Hypertension, uncontrolled
Toxemia of pregnancy

CAUTIONS AND COMMENTS

Prescribe bromocriptine pharmacotherapy cautiously to patients who

- have mild dementia. High dosages of bromocriptine may cause confusion and significantly aggravate cognitive functioning among these patients.

Caution patients who are receiving bromocriptine pharmacotherapy against

- performing activities that require alertness, judgment, or physical coordination (e.g., driving an automobile, operating dangerous equipment, supervising children) until their response to bromocriptine pharmacotherapy is known. Bromocriptine may cause dizziness and other ADRs that may adversely affect these mental and physical functions.

In addition to this general precaution, caution patients to

- inform their prescribing psychologist if they begin or discontinue any other pharmacotherapy while receiving bromocriptine pharmacotherapy.

CLINICALLY SIGNIFICANT DRUG INTERACTIONS

Concurrent bromocriptine pharmacotherapy and the following may result in clinically significant drug interactions:

Alcohol Use

Bromocriptine, particularly at higher dosages, may augment or exacerbate the actions of alcohol. Advise patients to avoid, or limit, their use of alcohol while receiving bromocriptine pharmacotherapy.

ADVERSE DRUG REACTIONS

Bromocriptine pharmacotherapy has been commonly associated with abdominal pain, constipation, diarrhea, headache, nausea, and vomiting. It also has been associated with the following ADRs, listed according to body system:

Cardiovascular: low blood pressure (hypotension) and abnormally rapid heart rate (tachycardia)

CNS: aggressive behavior, anxiety, delusions, depression, dizziness, drowsiness, faintness, fatigue, hallucinations, insomnia, lightheadedness, mania, mental confusion, migraine, paranoia, and sedation

Cutaneous: itchy hives (urticaria) and skin rashes

GI: dry mouth, indigestion, loss of appetite (anorexia), and a metallic taste

Musculoskeletal: leg cramps

Ophthalmic: blurred vision, burning and discomfort of the eyes, and double vision (diplopia)

Respiratory: nasal congestion and, rarely, shortness of breath (dyspnea)

Miscellaneous: rarely, ergotism and retroperitoneal fibrosis (associated with long-term bromocriptine pharmacotherapy)

OVERDOSAGE

Signs and symptoms of bromocriptine overdosage include dizziness, hallucinations, nausea, severe hypotension, and vomiting. Although no deaths have been directly associated with bromocriptine overdosage, suspected or actual bromocriptine overdosage requires emergency symptomatic medical support of body systems with attention to increasing bromocriptine elimination. There is no known antidote.

BUPRENORPHINE*

(byoo pre nor′ feen)

TRADE NAME

Buprenex®

CLASSIFICATION

Opiate analgesic (mixed agonist/antagonist) (C-V)

See also "Opiate Analgesics, General Monograph."

APPROVED INDICATIONS FOR NEUROPSYCHOLOGICAL DISORDERS

Adjunctive pharmacotherapy for the symptomatic management of:

- pain disorders: pain, moderate to severe

USUAL DOSAGE AND ADMINISTRATION

Moderate to Severe Pain

Adults: 0.3 mg intramuscularly or intravenously every six hours, as needed. May repeat the 0.3-mg dose, if needed, 30 to 60 minutes after the initial dose. Inject intramuscularly into a large healthy muscle site (e.g., dorsogluteal). Slowly inject intravenously over at least two minutes. Extreme caution is required with intravenous injection, particularly with the initial dose, until patient response to intravenous buprenorphine pharmacotherapy is known.

Some patients may require single doses of up to 0.6 mg depending on the severity of the pain and their individual response. Inject this dose only intramuscularly. Do *not* inject this dose intravenously. Single doses exceeding 0.3 mg are *not* recommended for patients who are at increased risk for respiratory depression (e.g., elderly, frail, or debilitated patients, or those who have respiratory dysfunction).

MAXIMUM: 0.6 mg/dose

Women who are, or who may become, pregnant: FDA Pregnancy Category C. Safety and efficacy of buprenorphine pharmacotherapy for women who are pregnant have not been established. Avoid prescribing buprenorphine pharmacotherapy to women who are pregnant. If buprenorphine pharmacothcrapy is required, advise patients of potential benefits and possible

---

For details and discussion regarding related basic principles of clinical pharmacology, readers are referred to the first text in this series, *The Pharmacologic Basis of Psychotherapeutics: An Introduction for Psychologists.*

risks to themselves and the embryo, fetus, or neonate (see also "Opiate Analgesics, General Monograph"). Prescribe buprenorphine pharmacotherapy during pregnancy only if the potential benefit justifies the potential risk to the embryo, fetus, or neonate. Collaboration with the patient's obstetrician is indicated.

Women who are breast-feeding: Safety and efficacy of buprenorphine pharmacotherapy for women who are breast-feeding and their neonates and infants have not been established. The amount of buprenorphine that is excreted in breast milk is unknown. Avoid prescribing buprenorphine pharmacotherapy to women who are breast-feeding. If buprenorphine pharmacotherapy is required, breast-feeding probably should be discontinued. If desired, lactation may be maintained and breast-feeding resumed following the discontinuation of short-term buprenorphine pharmacotherapy. Collaboration with the patient's pediatrician may be required.

Elderly, frail, or debilitated patients: Initially, 0.15 mg intramuscularly or intravenously every six hours, as needed. Inject intramuscularly into a large healthy muscle site (e.g., dorsogluteal). Slowly inject intravenously over at least two minutes. Repeat the 0.15-mg dose, if needed, 20 to 60 minutes after the initial dose. Note that this recommended dosage is half of the usual adult dosage. Generally prescribe lower dosages for elderly, frail, or debilitated patients. These patients may be more sensitive to the pharmacologic actions of buprenorphine pharmacotherapy than are younger or healthier adult patients.

Children 2 to 12 years of age: 2 to 6 μg/kg (0.002 to 0.006 mg/kg) intramuscularly or intravenously every four to eight hours, as needed. Inject intramuscularly into a large healthy muscle site (e.g., dorsogluteal site, vastus lateralis site). Inject intravenously slowly over at least two minutes. Extreme caution is required with intravenous injection, particularly with the initial dose, until the child's response to intravenous buprenorphine pharmacotherapy is known.

Adolescents 13 years of age and older: 0.3 mg intramuscularly or intravenously every six hours, as needed. Repeat the 0.3-mg dose, if needed, 30 to 60 minutes after the initial dose. Note that this recommended dosage is the same as the usual adult dosage. Inject intramuscularly into a large healthy muscle site (e.g., dorsogluteal site). Slowly inject intravenously over at least two minutes. Extreme caution is required with intravenous injection, particularly with the initial dose, until the adolescent's response to intravenous buprenorphine pharmacotherapy is known.

Notes, Pain Disorders: Moderate to Severe Pain

The analgesic and respiratory depressant actions of 0.3 mg of buprenorphine (Buprenex®) are approximately equivalent to those produced by 10 mg of morphine.

Buprenorphine injectable pharmacotherapy: Inject intramuscularly, deeply into healthy muscle sites. Rotate intramuscular injection sites if more than one injection is required to avoid, or minimize, muscle damage.

Buprenorphine intravenous pharmacotherapy: Extreme caution is required with intravenous injection, particularly with the initial dose, until the patient's response to intravenous buprenorphine pharmacotherapy is known.

AVAILABLE DOSAGE FORMS, STORAGE, AND COMPATIBILITY

Injectable, intramuscular or intravenous: 0.3 mg/ml (glass ampule)

Notes

Protect injectables from prolonged exposure to light or to temperatures exceeding 40 °C (104 °F). Injectable formulations that are discolored or contain particulate matter should be returned to the dispensing pharmacy or manufacturer for safe and appropriate disposal. Buprenorphine injectable is *not* compatible with injectable formulations of diazepam or lorazepam. Do not mix these injectables in the same syringe.

General instructions for patients: Instruct patients who are receiving buprenorphine pharmacotherapy to

- obtain an available patient information sheet regarding buprenorphine pharmacotherapy from their pharmacist at the time that their prescription is dispensed. Encourage patients to clarify any questions that they may have regarding buprenorphine pharmacotherapy with their pharmacist or, if needed, to consult their prescribing psychologist.

PROPOSED MECHANISM OF ACTION

Buprenorphine's exact mechanism of action has not been fully determined. However, it probably exerts its analgesic action by binding to mu-opiate receptors, for which it has high affinity. Although it may be classified as a partial agonist, under conditions of recommended use, it acts much like a classical mu agonist, such as morphine. However, unlike other opiate agonists or agonists/antagonists, buprenorphine appears to dissociate from its receptor sites. This unusual dissociation from receptor sites may account for its longer duration of action when compared to morphine, its unpredictable reversal by opiate antagonists, and its apparently lower addiction potential.

See also "Opiate Analgesics, General Monograph."

PHARMACOKINETICS/PHARMACODYNAMICS

Buprenorphine is rapidly, but variably (i.e., 40% to 90%), absorbed following intramuscular injection. Pharmacologic actions after intramuscular injection occur within ~15 minutes. Peak effects are achieved within 1 hour, with analgesic action persisting for 6 hours or longer. Onset and peak actions are shortened with intravenous injection. It is highly (96%) plasma protein bound, primarily to α and β globulins, with little binding to plasma albumin. Buprenorphine's apparent volume of distribution is ~200 liters. Buprenorphine is virtually completely metabolized in the liver. It has a mean half-life of elimination of ~3 hours (range: 1 to 8 hours) and a total body clearance of 1.3 liters/minute. Buprenorphine is metabolized to an active metabolite, norbuprenorphine, which has a mean half-life of elimination of ~35 hours (range: 1 to 66 hours). Additional data are not available.

RELATIVE CONTRAINDICATIONS

Hypersensitivity to buprenorphine

CAUTIONS AND COMMENTS

Buprenorphine may cause addiction and habituation similar to that associated with morphine, probably because of its opiate-like euphoric action. However, a buprenorphine withdrawal syndrome has not been demonstrated.

Prescribe buprenorphine pharmacotherapy cautiously to patients who

- have acute alcoholism or delirium tremens.
- have adrenal cortical insufficiency (Addison's disease).
- are elderly, frail, or debilitated. These patients may be more sensitive to buprenorphine's respiratory and CNS depressant actions.
- have biliary tract dysfunction. Buprenorphine may increase intracholeductal pressure much like other opiate analgesics.
- have CNS depression or coma. These clinical conditions may be exacerbated by buprenorphine's CNS depressant actions.
- have head injuries, intracranial lesions, and other medical disorders associated with increased cerebrospinal fluid pressure. Buprenorphine may elevate cerebrospinal fluid pressure. Among these patients, the dosage should be reduced by one-half. Note that buprenorphine can produce abnormal contraction of the pupils (i.e., miosis) and changes in the patient's level of consciousness. These actions may interfere with the monitoring of the patient's clinical condition.
- have histories of problematic patterns of abusable psychotropic use. Addiction and habituation may occur with buprenorphine pharmacotherapy. Buprenorphine also may induce the opiate withdrawal syndrome among patients who are currently addicted to opiate analgesics because of its partial action as an opiate antagonist.
- have hypothyroidism (myxedema).
- have lateral curvature and convex prominence of the spine (kyphoscoliosis). This condition may compromise respiratory function.
- have respiratory dysfunction. Buprenorphine pharmacotherapy may increase respiratory depression among patients who have medical disorders that compromise respiratory function (e.g., chronic obstructive lung disease). As with other potent opiate analgesics, clinically significant respiratory depression may occur among patients who are receiving usual recommended dosages of buprenorphine. Particular caution is advised when patients also are receiving concurrent pharmacotherapy with other drugs that have CNS and respiratory depressant actions. The dosage of buprenorphine should be reduced by approximately one-half for these patients. It is important to note that naloxone (Narcan®) may *not* adequately reverse the respiratory depression produced by buprenorphine.
- have severe liver or kidney dysfunction.
- have toxic psychoses.

Caution patients who are receiving buprenorphine pharmacotherapy against

- drinking alcohol or using other drugs that produce CNS depression. Buprenorphine may produce drowsiness and other effects that can be potentiated by these drugs. Advise patients to avoid or limit their use of alcohol while receiving buprenorphine pharmacotherapy. They also should be advised not to use other drugs (prescription or nonprescription) that produce CNS depression without first checking with their prescribing psychologist

and to notify their other prescribers that they are receiving buprenorphine pharmacotherapy.
- performing activities that require alertness, judgment, or physical coordination (e.g., driving an automobile, operating dangerous equipment, supervising children). Buprenorphine may impair these mental and physical functions by its direct depressant action on the CNS.

In addition to these general precautions, caution patients who are receiving buprenorphine pharmacotherapy to

- understand that buprenorphine is addicting and habituating. Advise patients not to exceed the prescribed dosage or to use buprenorphine more frequently than prescribed without first checking with their prescribing psychologist.

CLINICALLY SIGNIFICANT DRUG INTERACTIONS

Concurrent buprenorphine pharmacotherapy and the following may result in clinically significant drug interactions:

Alcohol Use

Concurrent alcohol use may increase the CNS depressant action of buprenorphine. Advise patients to avoid, or limit, their use of alcohol while receiving buprenorphine pharmacotherapy.

Pharmacotherapy With Drugs That Affect Hepatic Metabolism

Concurrent buprenorphine pharmacotherapy with drugs known to affect hepatic metabolism (e.g., barbiturates, SSRIs) may result in increased or prolonged buprenorphine action. Buprenorphine is metabolized in the liver.

Pharmacotherapy With CNS Depressants and Other Drugs That Produce CNS Depression

Concurrent buprenorphine pharmacotherapy and pharmacotherapy with opiate analgesics, sedative-hypnotics, or other drugs that produce CNS depression (e.g., antihistamines, phenothiazines, TCAs) may result in additive CNS depression. When concurrent pharmacotherapy is required, dose reductions are indicated.

See also "Opiate Analgesics, General Monograph."

ADVERSE DRUG REACTIONS

Buprenorphine pharmacotherapy has been associated with the following ADRs, listed according to body system:

Cardiovascular: decreased pulse rate and blood pressure (rarely, may be increased)
CNS: dizziness, drowsiness, headache, and sedation
Cutaneous: sweating (excessive)
GI: nausea and vomiting
Ocular: abnormal contraction of the pupils (miosis)
Respiratory: hypoventilation. Buprenorphine produces dose-related respiratory depression similar to morphine. At therapeutic doses, buprenorphine (i.e., 0.3 mg) can decrease the respiratory rate similar to that produced by an analgesic dose of morphine (i.e., 10 mg).

See also "Opiate Analgesics, General Monograph."

OVERDOSAGE

Clinical experience with buprenorphine overdosage is limited. Buprenorphine's antagonist action may be observed at dosages somewhat above the usual recommended dosage. Dosages within the therapeutic range may produce clinically significant respiratory depression among certain patients (e.g., patients who are elderly, frail, or debilitated, and those who have respiratory disorders). Buprenorphine overdosage requires emergency symptomatic medical support of body systems with attention to maintaining respiratory and cardiovascular function. Mechanical ventilation may be required because the respiratory depression produced by buprenorphine, a partial opiate agonist/antagonist, may not be reversed effectively by the opiate antagonist, naloxone (Narcan®).

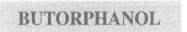

BUTORPHANOL

(byoo tore′ fan ol)

TRADE NAMES

Stadol®
Stadol NS®

CLASSIFICATION

Opiate analgesic agonist/antagonist

See also "Opiate Analgesics, General Monograph"

APPROVED INDICATIONS FOR NEUROPSYCHOLOGICAL DISORDERS

Adjunctive pharmacotherapy for the symptomatic management of:

• pain disorders: acute pain

USUAL DOSAGE AND ADMINISTRATION

Acute Pain

Adults: 1 mg intravenously every three or four hours, as needed; *or* 2 mg intramuscularly every three or four hours, as needed; *or* 1 mg intranasal spray (1 spray in *one* nostril). If adequate pain relief is not achieved within 60 to 90 minutes following the initial intranasal spray, an additional 1 mg intranasal spray (1 spray in *one* nostril) may be administered. This initial two-dose intranasal spray sequence may be repeated in three or four hours, as needed. Adherence to this intranasal spray dosage reduces the incidence of dizziness and drowsiness. However, for severe pain, an initial intranasal spray of 2 mg (1 spray in *each* nostril) may be prescribed for patients who are able to remain lying down in the event of associated dizziness or drowsiness. For these patients, do *not* prescribe additional 2 mg intranasal sprays for three or four hours.

MAXIMUM: The safety and efficacy of intramuscular doses of butorphanol exceeding 4 mg have not been established.

Women who are, or who may become, pregnant: FDA Pregnancy Category C. Safety and efficacy of butorphanol pharmacotherapy for women who are pregnant have not been established. There are no adequate and well-controlled studies of butorphanol use among pregnant women before 37 weeks of gestation. Avoid prescribing butorphanol pharmacotherapy to

For details and discussion regarding related basic principles of clinical pharmacology, readers are referred to the first text in this series, *The Pharmacologic Basis of Psychotherapeutics: An Introduction for Psychologists.*

women who are pregnant. If butorphanol pharmacotherapy is required, advise patients of potential benefits and possible risks to themselves and the embryo, fetus, or neonate (see also "Opiate Analgesics, General Monograph"). Collaboration with the patient's obstetrician is indicated.

Women who are breast-feeding: Safety and efficacy of butorphanol pharmacotherapy for women who are breast-feeding and their neonates and infants have not been established. Butorphanol has been detected in breast milk. However, the amount that a neonate or an infant would receive from breast-feeding is probably clinically insignificant (estimated as 4 μg/liter of breast milk for a mother receiving 2 mg intramuscularly four times a day). Although there are no data regarding the use of the nasal spray among women who are breast-feeding, butorphanol probably is excreted in breast milk in similar amounts following intranasal use. Avoid prescribing butorphanol pharmacotherapy to women who are breast-feeding. If butorphanol pharmacotherapy is required, monitor breast-fed neonates and infants for associated pharmacologic effects (e.g., drowsiness, lethargy). If noted, breast-feeding probably should be discontinued. If desired, lactation may be maintained and breast-feeding resumed following the discontinuation of short-term butorphanol pharmacotherapy. Collaboration with the patient's pediatrician may be required.

Elderly, frail, or debilitated patients and those who have kidney or liver dysfunction: Generally, prescribe lower dosages of butorphanol and increase the dosing interval for elderly, frail, or debilitated patients. Determine the dosage and dosing interval according to the method of administration and individual patient response.

INJECTABLE PHARMACOTHERAPY: Initially, 0.5 to 1 mg intravenously or 1 mg intramuscularly every six to eight hours, as needed. Note that the initial injectable dose recommended for these patients is half the usual adult dose at twice the usual dosing interval. Prescribe subsequent doses and dosing intervals according to individual patient response.

INTRANASAL PHARMACOTHERAPY: Initially, 1 mg intranasal spray (1 spray in *one* nostril). Allow 90 to 120 minutes to elapse before deciding whether an additional 1 mg intranasal spray (1 spray in *one* nostril) is needed. The mean half-life of butorphanol is increased by 25% (to over 6 hours) among patients who are older than 65 years of age because of age-related changes in the elimination of butorphanol. Elderly patients may be more sensitive to the ADRs associated with the intranasal spray formulation (Stadol NS®), particularly dizziness, than are younger or healthier adult patients. Patients who have kidney or liver dysfunction also require lower dosages and increased dosing intervals (see "Cautions and Comments").

Children and adolescents younger than 18 years of age: Safety and efficacy of butorphanol pharmacotherapy for children and adolescents have not been established. Butorphanol pharmacotherapy is *not* recommended for this age group.

Notes, Acute Pain

Butorphanol is not prescribed widely. The injectable and intranasal spray are indicated for the symptomatic management of pain when the use of an opiate analgesic is appropriate. Approximate equivalent analgesic action has been reported to be: 2 mg butorphanol, 10 mg morphine, 40 mg pentazocine, and 80 mg meperidine. Factors for consideration when determining the butorphanol dosage include age, body weight, general health, presenting clinical condition, and other concurrent pharmacotherapy. Patients who are receiving butorphanol intramuscular or intravenous pharmacotherapy should remain lying down during and following their injection in the event of associated dizziness or drowsiness.

Butorphanol pharmacotherapy is *not* recommended for patients who are addicted or habituated to opiate analgesics. Butorphanol has precipitated the opiate analgesic withdrawal syndrome among patients who were receiving long-term opiate analgesic agonist pharmacotherapy. Signs and symptoms of the opiate analgesic withdrawal syndrome include: agitation, anxiety, diarrhea, dysphoria, hallucinations, mood changes, and weakness. Only prescribe butorphanol pharmacotherapy for these patients when they have had an adequate period of detoxification from their long-term opiate analgesic pharmacotherapy, or regular personal use.

AVAILABLE DOSAGE FORMS, STORAGE, AND COMPATIBILITY

Injectable, intramuscular or intravenous: 1, 2 mg/ml multidose vials
Intranasal spray, metered: 10 mg/ml (14 or 15 doses, 1 mg/spray); 2.5-ml bottle

Notes

Butorphanol injectable formulation: Stadol® injectable is supplied in sealed delivery systems that have a low risk for accidental exposure of butorphanol to health care workers by inadvertent aerosol inhalation. However, care should be taken to avoid aerosol inhalation when preparing a syringe for injection. In the event of inadvertent skin contact, rinse well with cool water. Stadol® injectable has been associated with contact dermatitis.

Store butorphanol injectables safely at room temperature below 30 °C (86 °F). Discard cloudy solutions appropriately.

Butorphanol intranasal formulation: Stadol NS® is supplied in a child-resistant prescription vial containing a metered-dose spray pump with a protective tip and dust cover, a bottle of intranasal spray solution, and patient instructions for use. The intranasal spray is administered as a metered spray to the nasal mucosa. The pump reservoir must be fully primed prior to initial use. The patient's pharmacist will assemble the Stadol NS® prior to dispensing to the patient. On average, one 2.5-ml bottle will deliver 14 or 15 doses if no repriming is required.

After initial priming, each metered spray delivers an average of 1 mg of butorphanol. The unit must be *reprimed* if not used for 48 hours or longer. With intermittent use requiring repriming before each dose, the 2.5-ml bottle will deliver an average of 8 to 10 doses depending on the number of times repriming is required.

Stadol NS® is an open delivery system that may pose increased risk of exposure to health care workers and other people (or pets) who are in the immediate environment (e.g., hospital or home) when the metered-spray pump is initially primed or reprimed. A certain amount of butorphanol may be aerosolized during the priming process. Therefore, the pump sprayer should be aimed away from the face and away from the patient, other people, or pets. The unit should be disposed of by unscrewing the cap, rinsing the bottle, and placing the parts in an appropriate waste container.

General instructions for patients: Instruct patients who are receiving butorphanol pharmacotherapy to

- safely store the butorphanol intranasal spray out of the reach of children at controlled room temperature (15° to 30°C; 59° to 86°F).
- obtain an available patient information sheet regarding butorphanol pharmacotherapy from their pharmacist at the time that their prescription is dispensed. Encourage patients to clarify any questions that they may have regarding butorphanol with their pharmacist or, if needed, to consult their prescribing psychologist.

PROPOSED MECHANISM OF ACTION

Butorphanol is a synthetically derived opiate agonist/antagonist analgesic. Its major metabolites are agonists at kappa-opiate receptors and mixed agonists/antagonists at mu-opiate receptors. The interaction of butorphanol with these receptors in the CNS apparently mediates most of its pharmacologic actions, including abnormal contraction of the pupils (miosis), analgesia, depression of spontaneous respirations and cough, stimulation of the emetic (vomiting) center, and sedation. Other actions possibly mediated by non-CNS mechanisms include alteration in cardiovascular resistance and capacitance, bronchomotor tone, GI secretion and motility, and bladder sphincter activity.

Although butorphanol appears to elicit its analgesic and CNS and respiratory depressant actions primarily by binding to the endorphin receptors in the CNS, the exact mechanism of action has not yet been fully determined. The partial antagonist activity associated with butorphanol is probably due to competitive inhibition at the receptor sites. See "Opiate Analgesics, General Monograph."

PHARMACOKINETICS/PHARMACODYNAMICS

Butorphanol is absorbed rapidly following intramuscular injection and obtains peak blood concentrations within 20 to 40 minutes. After a 1-mg intranasal dose, mean peak blood concentrations occur within 30 to 60 minutes. The absolute bioavailability of the intranasal formulation is 60% to 70%. Bioavailability is unchanged among patients who have allergic rhinitis. Among patients using a nasal vasoconstrictor (e.g., oxymetazoline [Dristan® Long Lasting Nasal Spray]), the fraction of the dose absorbed is reportedly unchanged, but the rate of absorption is slowed. The peak blood concentrations are approximately half those achieved in the absence of the vasoconstrictor. Following its initial absorption/distribution phase, the single-dose pharmacokinetics of butorphanol by intravenous, intramuscular, or intranasal administration have been found to be similar.

Plasma protein binding (~80%) is independent of blood concentration over the range achieved in clinical practice. The apparent volume of distribution of butorphanol ranges from 4 to 13 liters/kg. Butorphanol is transported across the blood–brain and placental barriers. It also is excreted in breast milk. Butorphanol is extensively metabolized in the liver, with less than 5% excreted in unchanged form in the urine. A small amount is excreted in the feces. The mean half-life of elimination is ~5 hours (range: 2 to 9 hours).

The analgesic action of butorphanol is influenced by its method of administration. Onset of analgesia is within a few minutes of intravenous injection (i.e., when used as a preanesthetic). Peak analgesic activity occurs within 30 to 60 minutes following intramuscular injection and within 1 to 2 hours following the administration of the intranasal spray. The duration of analgesia varies depending on the severity of pain and method of administration, but is generally 3 to 4 hours with intramuscular or intravenous injection. When compared to the injectable formulation and other opiate analgesics or agonists/antagonists, butorphanol intranasal spray has a longer duration of action (4 to 5 hours).

RELATIVE CONTRAINDICATIONS

Hypersensitivity to butorphanol or the preservative benzethonian chloride found in some formulations (i.e., Stadol® injectable multidose vial and Stadol NS®)

CAUTIONS AND COMMENTS

Butorphanol appears to have a low abuse potential. However, it may precipitate the opiate analgesic withdrawal syndrome among patients who are addicted to opiate agonist analgesics. Although the mixed agonist/antagonist opiate analgesics, as a class, have lower abuse potential than morphine, problematic patterns of use, including addiction and habituation, have been associated with these drugs. The discontinuation of long-term injectable butorphanol use has been associated with a mild withdrawal syndrome.

The regular use of Stadol NS® for 2 months or longer has been associated with problematic patterns of use. Upon abrupt discontinuation of use of 16 mg or more daily for longer than 3 months, signs and symptoms of anxiety, agitation, and diarrhea have been observed. These signs and symptoms suggest the opiate analgesic withdrawal syndrome.

Prescribe butorphanol pharmacotherapy cautiously to patients who

- are elderly or have kidney and liver dysfunction. These patients may have a diminished ability to metabolize and eliminate butorphanol. For these patients, increase the initial dosage interval for the injectable and intranasal spray to 6 to 8 hours until their response to butorphanol pharmacotherapy is known. Subsequent doses should be determined by individual patient response rather than fixed dosing intervals.
- have cardiovascular dysfunction. Butorphanol may increase the work load of the heart, especially the pulmonary circuit. The use of butorphanol among patients who have acute myocardial infarction, ventricular dysfunction, or coronary insufficiency should be limited to those situations where the benefits clearly outweigh the risks. Collaboration with the patient's cardiologist is indicated.
- have head injuries or other conditions associated with increased intracranial pressure. Butorphanol pharmacotherapy (and other opiate analgesic pharmacotherapy) may be associated with carbon dioxide retention and a secondary increase in cerebrospinal fluid pressure; drug-induced constriction of the pupils (miosis); and alterations in mental function that may obscure the interpretation of the patient's clinical course. Among these patients, butorphanol should be prescribed only if the benefits clearly outweigh the potential risks. Collaboration with the patient's family physician or a specialist (e.g., neurologist) is indicated.
- have histories of addiction and habituation to opiate analgesics or other abusable psychotropics. Carefully evaluate the need for butorphanol pharmacotherapy and assure that these patients have undergone adequate detoxification.
- have recently received repeated doses of opiate agonist analgesics. It is difficult to assess opiate analgesic tolerance among these patients.
- have respiratory dysfunction. Butorphanol can produce respiratory depression, especially among patients who are concurrently receiving pharmacotherapy with other drugs that produce CNS depression or who have medical disorders (e.g., sleep apnea) that affect CNS or respiratory function.

CLINICALLY SIGNIFICANT DRUG INTERACTIONS

Concurrent butorphanol pharmacotherapy and the following may result in clinically significant drug interactions:

Pharmacotherapy With Drugs That Affect Hepatic Metabolism

It is unknown whether butorphanol pharmacotherapy is altered by concurrent pharmacotherapy with drugs known to affect hepatic metabolism (e.g., barbiturates, cimetidine [Tagamet®], erythromycin [E-Mycin®], theophylline [Theo-Dur®]). However, prescribing psychologists should be alert to the possibility that a lower initial dosage and longer dosing intervals may be needed for patients who are receiving concurrent pharmacotherapy with drugs that affect hepatic metabolism.

Pharmacotherapy With CNS Depressants and Other Drugs That Produce CNS Depression

Concurrent butorphanol pharmacotherapy and pharmacotherapy with CNS depressants (e.g., sedative-hypnotics) or other drugs that produce CNS depression (e.g., antihistamines, phenothiazines, TCAs) may result in additive CNS depression. When concurrent pharmacotherapy is required, the dose of butorphanol should be the lowest effective dose and the frequency of dosing (i.e., the dosing interval) should be extended as much as possible.

Pharmacotherapy With Nasal Vasoconstrictors

The fraction of Stadol NS® absorbed is unaffected by the concomitant use of a nasal vasoconstrictor (oxymetazoline). However, the rate of absorption is decreased. Therefore, a slower onset of action can be anticipated if Stadol NS® is administered with, or immediately following, a nasal vasoconstrictor.

See also "Opiate Analgesics, General Monograph."

ADVERSE DRUG REACTIONS

The ADRs associated with butorphanol pharmacotherapy, either the injectable or the intranasal spray, are similar to those commonly associated with other mixed opiate analgesic agonists/antagonists. These ADRs include dizziness, drowsiness, nausea, sedation, somnolence, and vomiting. Butorphanol, like pentazocine (Talwin®) and other mixed agonists/antagonists that have a high affinity for the kappa-opiate receptor, may produce unpleasant psychotomimetic reactions among susceptible patients. Intranasal administration has been associated with dizziness, drowsiness, insomnia, and nasal congestion.

Severe hypertension rarely has been associated with butorphanol pharmacotherapy. In such cases, immediately discontinue butorphanol pharmacotherapy. Collaboration with the patient's family physician or a specialist (e.g., cardiologist) is indicated for the appropriate medical management of the associated hypertension, which may require antihypertensive pharmacotherapy.

See also "Opiate Analgesics, General Monograph."

OVERDOSAGE

Signs and symptoms of butorphanol overdosage are similar to those associated with other opiate analgesic overdosage. The most serious signs and symptoms are hypoventilation, cardiovascular insufficiency, and coma. Overdosage has involved accidental ingestion among young children who gained access to the drug in the home and intentional overdosage by suicidal patients. Although butorphanol is more potent than morphine, it appears to have a ceiling effect in terms of respiratory depression. This ceiling effect is a theoretical advantage because an overdosage involving a large amount of butorphanol should not produce a correspondingly excessive respiratory depression. However, suspected or actual butorphanol overdosage requires emergency symptomatic medical support of body systems with attention to increasing butorphanol elimination. The use of the opiate analgesic antagonist naloxone (Narcan®) may be required. Repeated dosing with naloxone is usually required, because the duration of butorphanol action usually exceeds that of naloxone.

CARBAMAZEPINE

(kar ba maz′ e peen)

TRADE NAMES

Atretol®
Mazepine®
Novo-Carbamaz®
Tegretol®

CLASSIFICATION

Anticonvulsant (iminostilbene derivative)

APPROVED INDICATIONS FOR NEUROPSYCHOLOGICAL DISORDERS

Adjunctive pharmacotherapy for the management of:

- pain disorders: pain associated with trigeminal neuralgia. Although carbamazepine pharmacotherapy is indicated for the symptomatic management of the pain associated with trigeminal neuralgia, it is *not* indicated for the symptomatic management of any other pain disorder.
- seizure disorders. Carbamazepine pharmacotherapy is indicated alone or in combination with other anticonvulsants for the prophylactic and symptomatic management of partial seizures with complex symptomatology; generalized tonic-clonic seizures; mixed seizure patterns; and psychomotor or temporal lobe seizures.

USUAL DOSAGE AND ADMINISTRATION

Pain Disorders: Trigeminal Neuralgia Pain

Adults: 200 mg daily orally in two to four divided doses. Gradually increase the daily dosage by 200 mg, as needed, according to individual patient response. (See "Available Dosage Forms, Storage, and Compatibility," "Notes.")

MAXIMUM: 1200 mg daily orally

Women who are, or who may become, pregnant: FDA Pregnancy Category C. Safety and efficacy of carbamazepine pharmacotherapy for women who are pregnant have not been established. However, the preponderance of available data suggests that carbamazepine is a human teratogen that can cause a variety of congenital malformations (i.e., birth defects) including

---

For details and discussion regarding related basic principles of clinical pharmacology, readers are referred to the first text in this series, *The Pharmacologic Basis of Psychotherapeutics: An Introduction for Psychologists.*

cleft lip, depressed nasal bridge, hypoplastic nails, mental retardation, and spina bifida. Carbamazepine pharmacotherapy also may cause or aggravate folic acid deficiency during pregnancy. Folic acid deficiencies may contribute to the increased incidence of teratogenic effects. Prenatal folic acid supplements are, therefore, generally recommended. Avoid prescribing carbamazepine pharmacotherapy to women who are pregnant. If carbamazepine pharmacotherapy is required, advise patients of potential benefits and possible risks to themselves and the embryo, fetus, or neonate. Concurrent carbamazepine and other anticonvulsant pharmacotherapy has been associated with significant teratogenic risk. Collaboration with the patient's obstetrician is indicated.

Women who are breast-feeding: Safety and efficacy of carbamazepine pharmacotherapy for women who are breast-feeding and their neonates and infants have not been established. Carbamazepine and its active metabolite, carbamazepine-epoxide, are excreted in breast milk in concentrations equal to ~50% of the maternal blood concentration. Lethargy, poor sucking, or sedation may occur among breast-fed neonates and infants. A severe hypersensitivity skin reaction involving a breast-fed infant also has been reported. Avoid prescribing carbamazepine pharmacotherapy to women who are breast-feeding. If carbamazepine pharmacotherapy is required, breast-feeding should be discontinued. Collaboration with the patient's pediatrician is indicated.

Elderly, frail, or debilitated patients: Generally prescribe lower dosages for elderly, frail, or debilitated patients. Gradually increase the dosage, if needed, according to individual patient response. These patients may be more sensitive to the pharmacologic actions of carbamazepine than are younger or healthier adult patients.

Children: Safety and efficacy of carbamazepine pharmacotherapy for the symptomatic management of trigeminal neuralgia pain among children have not been established. Carbamazepine pharmacotherapy is *not* recommended for this indication for this age group.

Notes, Pain Disorders: Trigeminal Neuralgia Pain

Pharmacologically, carbamazepine is *not* an analgesic. Thus, carbamazepine should *not* be prescribed for the symptomatic management of any pain disorder other than trigeminal neuralgia. The ingestion of carbamazepine with meals may decrease associated gastric irritation.

Initiating carbamazepine pharmacotherapy: Before initiating carbamazepine pharmacotherapy, obtain baseline blood counts, including platelets, and evaluate kidney and liver function. Carbamazepine pharmacotherapy has been associated with bone marrow depression and serious blood disorders, including aplastic anemia and, rarely, agranulocytosis. It also has been associated with kidney and liver dysfunction. Collaboration with the patient's family physician or a specialist (e.g., hematologist, internist, nephrologist) may be indicated.

Maintaining carbamazepine pharmacotherapy: Prescribe the lowest effective dosage. TDM of carbamazepine blood levels is generally of assistance for guiding pharmacotherapy. Regularly monitor patients for signs and symptoms of blood disorders, kidney dysfunction, and liver dysfunction. Discontinue carbamazepine pharmacotherapy immediately if any signs and symptoms suggesting these conditions are noted. Carbamazepine pharmacotherapy also has been associated with severe skin reactions, such as Stevens–Johnson syndrome and Lyell's syndrome. Discontinue carbamazepine pharmacotherapy immediately if signs and symptoms suggesting a severe skin reaction are noted. The management of carbamazepine pharmacotherapy generally requires collaboration with the patient's family physician or other specialists (e.g., dermatologist, hematologist, internist, nephrologist) because of the possible occurrence of these potentially serious ADRs.

Discontinuing carbamazepine pharmacotherapy: Discontinue carbamazepine pharmacotherapy gradually. Abrupt discontinuation of carbamazepine pharmacotherapy may result in seizures, including status epilepticus.

Seizure Disorders

Adults: Initially, 400 mg daily orally in two to four divided doses. Gradually increase the daily dosage by 200 mg at weekly intervals, according to individual patient response. Monitor patients for the achievement of therapeutic benefit or dose-limiting ADRs.

MAXIMUM: 1600 mg daily orally

Women who are, or who may become, pregnant: FDA Pregnancy Category C. Safety and efficacy of carbamazepine pharmacotherapy for women who are pregnant have not been established. However, the preponderance of available data suggests that carbamazepine is a human teratogen that can cause a variety of malformations including cleft lip, depressed nasal bridge, hypoplastic nails, mental retardation, and spina bifida. Carbamazepine pharmacotherapy also may cause or aggravate folic acid deficiency during pregnancy. Folic acid deficiencies also may contribute to the increased occurrence of teratogenic effects. Prenatal folic acid supplements are, therefore, generally recommended. Avoid prescribing carbamazepine pharmacotherapy to women who are pregnant. If carbamazepine pharmacotherapy is required, advise patients of potential benefits and possible risks to themselves and the embryo, fetus, or neonate. Teratogenic risk and incidence appear to increase significantly if concurrent carbamazepine pharmacotherapy is prescribed with other anticonvulsant pharmacotherapy. Collaboration with the patient's obstetrician is indicated.

Women who are breast-feeding: Safety and efficacy of carbamazepine pharmacotherapy for women who are breast-feeding and their neonates and infants have not been established. Carbamazepine and its active metabolite, carbamazepine-epoxide, are excreted in breast milk in concentrations equal to ~50% of the maternal blood concentration. Lethargy, poor sucking, or sedation may occur among breast-fed neonates and infants. A severe hypersensitivity skin reaction involving a breast-fed infant also has been reported. Avoid prescribing carbamazepine pharmacotherapy to women who are breast-feeding. If carbamazepine pharmacotherapy is required, breast-feeding should be discontinued. Collaboration with the patient's pediatrician is indicated.

Elderly, frail, or debilitated patients: Generally prescribe lower dosages for elderly, frail, or debilitated patients. Gradually increase the dosage, if needed, according to individual patient response. These patients may be more sensitive to the pharmacologic actions of carbamazepine than are younger or healthier adult patients.

Children younger than 6 years of age: Initially, 10 to 20 mg/kg daily orally in two to four divided doses. Increase the dosage according to individual patient response at weekly intervals, as needed to obtain optimal clinical response.

MAXIMUM: 35 mg/kg daily orally

Children 6 to 12 years of age: 200 mg daily orally in two to four divided doses. Gradually increase the daily dosage by 100 mg at weekly intervals, according to individual patient response, until therapeutic benefit is achieved or dose-limiting ADRs are observed.

MAXIMUM: 1000 mg daily orally

Notes, Seizure Disorders

See "Notes, Pain Disorders: Trigeminal Pain."
See "Available Dosage Forms, Storage, and Compatibility, Notes"

AVAILABLE DOSAGE FORMS, STORAGE, AND COMPATIBILITY

Suspension, oral: 100 mg/5 ml (citrus-vanilla flavored)
Tablets, oral: 200 mg
Tablets, oral chewable: 100, 200 mg
Tablets, oral extended-release: 100, 200, 400 mg

Notes

Carbamazepine oral extended-release tablets provide a lower average maximal blood concentration without a reduction in the average minimal concentration. Thus, carbamazepine pharmacotherapy with extended-release tablets helps to ensure that the blood concentrations remain relatively stable throughout the day and allows twice-daily dosing. It also results in a lower incidence of intermittent concentration-dependent ADRs. Carbamazepine pharmacotherapy with extended-release tablets is *not* indicated for children younger than 6 years of age.

Carbamazepine oral suspension produces higher peak carbamazepine blood concentrations than does an equivalent dose of the oral tablets. Therefore, when switching a patient from carbamazepine oral tablets to the oral suspension, the same total daily dosage should be divided into more frequent and smaller doses (i.e., tablets in two divided daily doses and suspension in three or four divided daily doses).

General instructions for patients: Instruct patients who are receiving carbamazepine pharmacotherapy to

- shake the carbamazepine oral suspension well before measuring each dose to help to assure that an accurate dose is measured and ingested.
- ingest each dose of the carbamazepine oral dosage forms with food to decrease associated gastric irritation.
- Thoroughly chew each dose of the carbamazepine oral chewable tablets or allow them to completely dissolve in the mouth before swallowing.
- safely store carbamazepine oral dosage forms out of the reach of children in tightly closed, child- and light-resistant containers at controlled room temperature (15° to 30°C; 59° to 86°F).

- obtain an available patient information sheet regarding carbamazepine pharmacotherapy from their pharmacist at the time that their prescription is dispensed. Encourage patients to clarify any questions that they may have regarding carbamazepine pharmacotherapy with their pharmacist or, if needed, to consult their prescribing psychologist.

PROPOSED MECHANISM OF ACTION

The exact mechanism of carbamazepine's anticonvulsant action has not been fully determined. It appears to be related to decreased neurochemical activity in the nucleus ventralis of the thalamus and decreased summation of temporal stimulation leading to neuronal discharge. More specifically, carbamazepine appears to limit seizure propagation by reducing the post-tetanic potentiation of synaptic neurotransmission. Its action in regard to the symptomatic management of trigeminal neuralgia pain appears to be related to a reduction of synaptic transmission within the trigeminal nucleus.

PHARMACOKINETICS/PHARMACODYNAMICS

Carbamazepine is slowly but well absorbed (over 70%) following oral ingestion. Generally, peak blood concentrations are obtained within 4 to 12 hours. There are no clinically significant differences in bioavailability among oral dosage forms. In addition, the ingestion of food has no significant effect on either the rate or extent of carbamazepine absorption, regardless of oral dosage form. Plasma protein binding is moderate ($\sim$75%) and carbamazepine is widely distributed in the body with an apparent volume of distribution of 1 to 2 liters/kg. Carbamazepine is distributed into the cerebrospinal fluid and saliva in concentrations of $\sim$20% of the blood concentration (i.e., representative of the nonprotein-bound portion of carbamazepine) and is excreted in breast milk in concentrations of $\sim$50% of the maternal blood concentration. Carbamazepine is extensively metabolized, primarily in the liver, with less than 3% eliminated in unchanged form in the urine. Mean total body clearance is 100 ml/minute (range: 50 to 125 ml/minute). The mean half-life of elimination is $\sim$36 hours (range: 25 to 65 hours) following a single oral dose. However, repeated doses over 2 to 4 weeks result in autoinduction of hepatic enzymes and a reduction in the half-life of elimination to 16 to 24 hours.

Therapeutic Drug Monitoring

Dosage must be determined by individual patient response and not carbamazepine blood concentrations. However, blood concentrations may be useful for monitoring the patient's ability to manage carbamazepine pharmacotherapy or possible overdosage. For TDM, it is generally recommended to sample from trough concentrations just prior to the next dose. However, in cases of suspected overdosages, sampling may be done at any time. The therapeutic blood concentration range for the management of both *seizure disorders* and *trigeminal neuralgia* is generally estimated as 17 to 43 μmol/liter (4 to 10 μg/ml). Generally pain relief from trigeminal neuralgia is achieved within 48 hours of the initiation of carbamazepine pharmacotherapy.

RELATIVE CONTRAINDICATIONS

Atrioventricular block
Blood disorders, severe

Bone marrow depression, current *or* history of

Hypersensitivity to carbamazepine or to TCAs (e.g., amitriptyline, imipramine, trimipramine) or their analogues or metabolites. Carbamazepine has a similar tricyclic chemical structure to these drugs and their analogues or metabolites.

Liver dysfunction

MAOI pharmacotherapy, concurrent or within 14 days. Do *not* prescribe carbamazepine pharmacotherapy immediately before, concurrently with, or immediately after MAOI pharmacotherapy. When carbamazepine pharmacotherapy is required for these patients, assure a drug-free interval for as long as clinically possible before initiating carbamazepine pharmacotherapy. In no case should this interval be less than 14 days. Initially prescribe a lower dosage of carbamazepine and gradually increase the dosage according to individual patient response.

Porphyria, acute intermittent

CAUTIONS AND COMMENTS

Prescribe carbamazepine pharmacotherapy cautiously to patients who

- have histories of adverse hematological reactions to other pharmacotherapy. Baseline and periodic monitoring for signs and symptoms of bone marrow depression is required for these patients. Discontinue carbamazepine pharmacotherapy immediately if such signs and symptoms are identified.
- have histories of interrupted courses of pharmacotherapy with carbamazepine.
- have histories of kidney dysfunction. Baseline and periodic monitoring of kidney function is required. Discontinue carbamazepine pharmacotherapy immediately if signs and symptoms of kidney dysfunction are identified.
- have histories of liver dysfunction. Baseline and periodic monitoring of liver function is required, particularly for elderly, frail, or debilitated patients and those who have histories of liver disease, including alcoholic cirrhosis. Discontinue carbamazepine pharmacotherapy immediately if signs and symptoms of aggravated liver dysfunction or active liver disease are identified.
- have histories of partial seizures with complex symptomatology. Some children who have mixed seizure disorders, particularly those who have a generalized absence or atypical absence component, have experienced a carbamazepine associated increase in seizure activity. Prolonged video-EEG monitoring of these children prior to the initiation of carbamazepine pharmacotherapy may assist in the identification of the children who are most at risk for this ADR.

Caution patients who are receiving carbamazepine pharmacotherapy against

- performing activities that require alertness, judgment, or physical coordination (e.g., driving an automobile, operating dangerous equipment, supervising children) until their response to carbamazepine pharmacotherapy is known. Carbamazepine may adversely affect these mental and physical functions.

In addition to this general precaution, caution patients to

- immediately report early signs and symptoms of potentially serious ADRs, particularly dermatologic, hematologic, hepatic, and renal reactions. The onset of such potentially serious reactions may be rapid. Advise patients to inform their prescribing psychologist immediately if they develop such early signs and symptoms of these ADRs as a fever, sore throat, rash, ulcers in the mouth, or easy bruising.

CLINICALLY SIGNIFICANT DRUG INTERACTIONS

Concurrent carbamazepine pharmacotherapy and the following may result in clinically significant drug interactions:

Felbamate (Febatol®) Pharmacotherapy

Concurrent felbamate and carbamazepine pharmacotherapy may result in an increased felbamate total body clearance and decreased carbamazepine blood concentrations. However, blood concentrations of carbamazepine epoxide, an active metabolite of carbamazepine, may be increased. Both blood concentrations and patient response should be closely monitored. If required, adjust the dosage of felbamate and carbamazepine accordingly.

Pharmacotherapy With Drugs and Beverages That Are Hepatic Microsomal Enzyme Inhibitors

The hepatic metabolism of carbamazepine may be inhibited and its actions increased by concurrent cimetidine (Tagamet®), diltiazem (Cardizem®), erythromycin (E-Mycin®), fluoxetine (Prozac®), isoniazid (INH®), propoxyphene (Darvon®), troleandomycin (TAO®), or verapamil (Calan®) pharmacotherapy. Grapefruit juice also inhibits hepatic microsomal enzyme metabolism, particularly isoenzyme CYP3A4, and can result in a significant increase in carbamazepine blood concentrations.

Pharmacotherapy With Drugs That Are Primarily Metabolized by the Liver

Carbamazepine, a hepatic microsomal enzyme inducer, may increase the hepatic metabolism of benzodiazepines (i.e., alprazolam, clonazepam), corticosteroids, ethosuximide (Zarontin®), haloperidol (Haldol®), imipramine (Tofranil®), methadone (Methadose®), oral anticoagulants (e.g., warfarin [Coumadin®]), oral contraceptives (the efficacy of oral contraceptives may be affected by carbamazepine adversely), theophylline (Theo-Dur®), thyroid hormones, valproic acid (Depakene®), and other drugs that are primarily metabolized by the liver. Collaboration with other prescribers may be required to help to assure optimal pharmacotherapy.

ADVERSE DRUG REACTIONS

Carbamazepine has moderate anticholinergic actions. Tolerance may develop to these actions after a few months of pharmacotherapy. Carbamazepine pharmacotherapy has been commonly associated with: dizziness (vertigo), double vision (diplopia), drowsiness, headache, nausea, and vomiting. Carbamazepine pharmacotherapy also has been associated with the following ADRs, listed according to body system:

> **Cardiovascular:** congestive heart failure, edema, fainting (syncope), hypotension, and suppression of ventricular automaticity (due to its membrane-depressant action associated with suppression of phase-4 depolarization of heart muscle fiber, similar to the action of the antidysrhythmics, quinidine and procainamide). This ADR is associated with suppression of phase-4 depolarization of the heart muscle fiber. (Cardiovascular ADRs are

potentially fatal for patients who have existing serious cardiovascular dysfunction. Collaboration with the patient's cardiologist is indicated.)

CNS: activation of psychosis, aggressive behavior, agitation, confusion, dizziness, drowsiness, fatigue, hallucinations (rare), headache, impaired taste, incoordination (ataxia), irritability, and somnolence

Cutaneous: pigmentary changes, rash, sensitivity to light (photosensitivity), Stevens–Johnson syndrome (rare), and toxic epidermal necrolysis (Lyell's syndrome; rare)

Genitourinary: impotence, kidney failure (rare), and urinary retention

GI: abdominal pain, constipation, dry mouth, and loss of appetite (anorexia)

Hematologic: blood disorders (potentially fatal aplastic anemia, but relatively rare), also agranulocytosis, eosinophilia, leukopenia, purpura, and thrombocytopenia

Hepatic: hepatocellular and cholestatic jaundice and hepatitis. (Generally, hepatic ADRs are associated with long-term carbamazepine pharmacotherapy.)

Ocular: blurred vision and conjunctivitis

Renal: albumin in the urine (albuminuria), glucose in the urine (glycosuria), and syndrome of inappropriate antidiuretic hormone secretion (SIAHS)

OVERDOSAGE

Signs and symptoms of carbamazepine overdosage include agitation, ataxia, blurred vision, coma, convulsions, dilation of the pupils (mydriasis), disorientation, dizziness, drowsiness, flushing, impaired consciousness, involuntary cyclical rapid movement of the eyeball (nystagmus), irregular breathing, neuromuscular disturbances, tachycardia, tremor, urinary retention, and vomiting. Carbamazepine overdosage requires emergency symptomatic medical support of body systems with attention to increasing carbamazepine elimination. There is no known antidote.

CHLORDIAZEPOXIDE

(klor dye az e pox′ ide)

TRADE NAMES

Librium®
Novo-Poxide®

CLASSIFICATION

Sedative-hypnotic (benzodiazepine) (C-IV)

See also "Benzodiazepines, General Monograph."

APPROVED INDICATIONS FOR NEUROPSYCHOLOGICAL DISORDERS

Adjunctive pharmacotherapy for the short-term prophylactic and symptomatic management of:

- seizure disorders. Chlordiazepoxide pharmacotherapy is indicated for the prophylactic and symptomatic management of seizures associated with the acute alcohol withdrawal syndrome.

USUAL DOSAGE AND ADMINISTRATION

Seizure Disorders: Seizures Associated With the Acute Alcohol Withdrawal Syndrome

Adults: Initially, 50 to 100 mg intramuscularly, intravenously, or orally. Repeat every two to four hours, as needed, to a maximum of 300 mg daily. Usually, injectable pharmacotherapy is required initially for the management of acute signs and symptoms.

MAXIMUM: 300 mg daily intramuscularly, intravenously, or orally

Women who are, or who may become, pregnant: FDA Pregnancy Category D. Safety and efficacy of chlordiazepoxide pharmacotherapy for women who are pregnant have not been established. Collaboration with the patient's obstetrician is indicated.

Women who are breast-feeding: Safety and efficacy of chlordiazepoxide pharmacotherapy for women who are breast-feeding and their neonates and infants have not been established. Chlordiazepoxide is excreted into breast milk. Breast-fed neonates and infants may display

For details and discussion regarding related basic principles of clinical pharmacology, readers are referred to the first text in this series, *The Pharmacologic Basis of Psychotherapeutics: An Introduction for Psychologists.*

drowsiness or lethargy. They also may become addicted. Avoid prescribing chlordiazepoxide pharmacotherapy to women who are breast-feeding. If chlordiazepoxide pharmacotherapy is required, breast-feeding probably should be discontinued. If desired, lactation may be maintained and breast-feeding resumed following the discontinuation of short-term chlordiazepoxide pharmacotherapy. Collaboration with the patient's pediatrician is indicated.

Elderly, frail, or debilitated patients and those who have liver dysfunction: 25 to 50 mg intramuscularly, intravenously, or orally. Repeat every two to four hours, as needed, to a maximum of 150 mg daily. Initially prescribe lower dosages according to individual patient response. Elderly, frail, or debilitated patients and those who have liver dysfunction usually require half the recommended adult dosage because they may be more sensitive to chlordiazepoxide's CNS depressant action.

MAXIMUM: 150 mg daily intramuscularly, intravenously, or orally

Children 12 years of age and younger: Safety and efficacy of chlordiazepoxide pharmacotherapy for the symptomatic management of alcohol or other drug withdrawal syndromes for children 12 years of age and younger have not been established. Chlordiazepoxide pharmacotherapy for this indication is not recommended for this age group.

Adolescents 13 years of age and older: Initially, 25 to 50 mg intramuscularly, intravenously, or orally. Repeat every two to four hours, as needed, to a maximum of 150 mg daily. Initially prescribe lower dosages for adolescents. Gradually increase the dosage according to individual patient response. Adolescents usually require half the recommended adult dosage.

MAXIMUM: 150 mg daily intramuscularly, intravenously, or orally

Notes, Seizures Associated With the Acute Alcohol Withdrawal Syndrome

The optimal chlordiazepoxide dosage varies in relation to the signs and symptoms of the alcohol withdrawal syndrome and individual patient response. Prescribe the lowest effective dosage adjusted to individual patient response.

Injectable pharmacotherapy: Maximum recommended injectable dose is 300 mg daily in divided doses. Generally, the acute signs and symptoms of the alcohol withdrawal syndrome may be rapidly controlled by intramuscular or intravenous chlordiazepoxide pharmacotherapy. Replace injectable pharmacotherapy with oral pharmacotherapy as soon as possible.

Occasionally, injectable pharmacotherapy has produced mild transitory fluctuations in blood pressure. This effect generally has not been clinically problematic and emergency supportive medical management has not been required. Some patients may become drowsy or unsteady following the injection. Thus, patients should lie down for injectable chlordiazepoxide pharmacotherapy and remain lying down for 30 to 60 minutes following the injection.

INTRAMUSCULAR INJECTION: For intramuscular injection, reconstitute the injectable formulation immediately before injection. Add the diluent solution supplied with the injectable formulation for intramuscular use only according to manufacturer's directions. Do not use the diluent solution if it is cloudy. Agitate gently until a clear solution is obtained. Inject the dose intramuscularly into a healthy muscle site (e.g., dorsogluteal or ventrogluteal site). Do *not* inject the dose intravenously because air bubbles are formed when the injectable is reconstituted for intramuscular use. Intravenous injection may result in air embolism. Discard any unused drug appropriately.

INTRAVENOUS INJECTION: Intravenous pharmacotherapy is indicated for the management of acute agitation and hyperactivity associated with the acute alcohol withdrawal syndrome when rapid action is required and oral ingestion or intramuscular injection is not feasible. For intravenous injection, dilute 100 mg with 5 ml sterile water for injection or isotonic sodium chloride (i.e., normal saline) for injection. Agitate gently. Do not add to intravenous solutions or mix with any other drugs. Do not dilute further. Slowly (over 1 minute) inject intravenously into a large lumen vein. Use caution when injecting patients for whom a drop in blood pressure may lead to cardiac complications. Dosage may need to be reduced for patients who have liver dysfunction. Do *not* inject intramuscularly because the intravenous solution diluted with normal saline or sterile water causes significant pain upon intramuscular injection. Discard any unused drug appropriately.

AVAILABLE DOSAGE FORMS, STORAGE, AND COMPATIBILITY

Capsules, oral: 5, 10, 25 mg
Injectable, intramuscular or intravenous duplex pack: 100 mg. The duplex pack consists of one ampule of dry drug and one 2-ml ampule of special diluent for intramuscular use. The dry drug also can be reconstituted with 5 ml of normal saline or sterile water for intravenous injection.
Tablets, oral: 5, 10, 25 mg

Notes

Store the duplex pack diluent at 2° to 8°C (36° to 46°F). Do not use if cloudy. Return to dispensing pharmacy or manufacturer for safe and appropriate disposal. Dry drug may be stored at 15° to 30°C (59° to 86°F). Refrigerate injectable after reconstitution. Do not freeze.

PROPOSED MECHANISM OF ACTION

Chlordiazepoxide has sedative, hypnotic, and muscle relaxant actions. The exact mechanism of chlordiazepoxide's actions has not been fully determined. However, they appear to be mediated by the actions of the inhibitory neurotransmitter, GABA. Chlordiazepoxide acts selectively on polysynaptic neuronal pathways and may inhibit, or augment, neuronal transmission, depending on the endogenous function of GABA. See also "Benzodiazepines, General Monograph."

PHARMACOKINETICS/PHARMACODYNAMICS

Chlordiazepoxide is absorbed completely (100%) following oral ingestion. Generally, intramuscular absorption is slow and erratic. Following oral ingestion, chlordiazepoxide appears in the blood stream in 30 to 60 minutes. Peak blood concentrations occur in 2 to 4 hours. After intramuscular injection, effects appear within 15 to 30 minutes, and following intravenous injection, effects appear within 3 to 30 minutes. Chlordiazepoxide is highly plasma protein bound (95%

to 98%), and it has an apparent volume of distribution of ~0.3 liters/kg. Chlordiazepoxide is metabolized extensively, primarily in the liver. Less than 2% is excreted in unchanged form in the urine. Chlordiazepoxide has several active metabolites, including desmethyldiazepam and oxazepam. The mean half-life of elimination is ~10 hours (range: 5 to 30 hours). The mean total body clearance is ~35 ml/minute.

RELATIVE CONTRAINDICATIONS

Coma
Glaucoma, acute narrow-angle (See "Benzodiazepines, General Monograph")
Hypersensitivity to chlordiazepoxide or other benzodiazepines
Myasthenia gravis
Shock, acute

CAUTIONS AND COMMENTS

Addiction and habituation rarely have been associated with the use of recommended dosages of chlordiazepoxide. (See "Benzodiazepines, General Monograph.")
    Prescribe chlordiazepoxide pharmacotherapy cautiously to patients who

- are elderly, frail, or debilitated. Initially, prescribe the lowest effective dosage that does not cause incoordination (ataxia) or over-sedation. Gradually increase the dosage, as needed, according to individual patient response.
- have histories of problematic patterns of other abusable psychotropic use in addition to their problematic patterns of alcohol use. These patients may be at risk for developing problematic patterns of chlordiazepoxide use.
- have severe liver or kidney dysfunction.

Caution patients who are receiving chlordiazepoxide pharmacotherapy against

- performing activities that require alertness, judgment, and physical coordination (e.g., smoking tobacco cigarettes) until their response to chlordiazepoxide pharmacotherapy is known. Chlordiazepoxide's CNS depressant actions may adversely affect these mental and physical functions.

CLINICALLY SIGNIFICANT DRUG INTERACTIONS

Concurrent chlordiazepoxide pharmacotherapy and the following may result in clinically significant drug interactions:

Alcohol Use

Concurrent alcohol use may increase the CNS depressant action of chlordiazepoxide.

Pharmacotherapy With CNS Depressants and Other Drugs That Produce CNS Depression

Concurrent chlordiazepoxide pharmacotherapy and pharmacotherapy with opiate analgesics, other sedative-hypnotics, or other drugs that produce CNS depression (e.g., antihistamines, phenothiazines, TCAs) may result in additive CNS depression.

See also "Benzodiazepines, General Monograph."

ADVERSE DRUG REACTIONS

Chlordiazepoxide pharmacotherapy has been associated with the following ADRs, listed according to body system. Most ADRs occur infrequently and generally can be managed by reducing the dosage.

Cardiovascular: fainting (syncope)
CNS: confusion; drowsiness; extrapyramidal reactions; EEG pattern alterations (e.g., low voltage, fast activity), which may appear during or after chlordiazepoxide pharmacotherapy; incoordination (ataxia); and paradoxical reactions (e.g., elevation of mood, rage, unusual excitement), particularly among patients who have histories of psychoses or children who are hyperactive and aggressive. Monitor patients for these reactions, particularly during initial pharmacotherapy.
Cutaneous: edema and skin eruptions
Genitourinary: rarely, changes in sex drive (increase or decrease)
GI: constipation, nausea
Hematologic: blood disorders, including leukopenia and agranulocytosis (rare)
Hepatic: jaundice, liver dysfunction (occasional)

See also "Benzodiazepines, General Monograph."

OVERDOSAGE

Signs and symptoms of chlordiazepoxide overdosage include confusion, diminished reflexes, drowsiness, incoordination (ataxia), and coma. Depression of the cardiovascular and respiratory centers may occur. Chlordiazepoxide overdosage requires emergency symptomatic medical support of body systems with attention to increasing chlordiazepoxide elimination. Flumazenil (Anexate®, Romazicon®), the benzodiazepine antagonist, may be required. Note that patients whose seizure disorders have been managed with benzodiazepine pharmacotherapy may be at increased risk for the occurence of seizures when their benzodiazepine overdosage is treated with flumazenil pharmacotherapy.

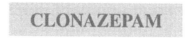

CLONAZEPAM

(kloe na′ ze pam)

TRADE NAMES

Klonopin®
Rivotril®

CLASSIFICATION

Anticonvulsant (benzodiazepine) (C-IV)

See also "Benzodiazepines, General Monograph."

APPROVED INDICATIONS FOR NEUROPSYCHOLOGICAL DISORDERS

Pharmacotherapy for the prophylactic and symptomatic management of:

- seizure disorders: akinetic and myoclonic seizures, Lennox–Gastaut syndrome (petit mal variant epilepsy), and absence (petit mal) seizures that are refractory to succinimides (e.g., ethosuximide [Zarontin®], methsuximide [Celontin®]). Clonazepam is prescribed alone or as adjunctive pharmacotherapy to other anticonvulsant pharmacotherapy for the prophylactic and symptomatic management of seizure disorders.

USUAL DOSAGE AND ADMINISTRATION

Seizure Disorders

Adults: Initially, 1.5 mg daily orally in three divided doses. Gradually increase the daily dosage by 0.5 to 1 mg every third day, according to individual patient response, until therapeutic benefit or dose-limiting ADRs are observed. Usual maintenance dosage is 8 to 10 mg daily orally in three divided doses.

MAXIMUM: 20 mg daily orally

Women who are, or who may become, pregnant: FDA Pregnancy Category "not established." Safety and efficacy of clonazepam pharmacotherapy for women who are pregnant have not been established (see also "Benzodiazepines, General Monograph"). Avoid prescribing clonazepam pharmacotherapy to women who are pregnant. If clonazepam pharmacotherapy is required, advise patients of potential benefits and possible risks to themselves and the embryo, fetus, or neonate. Collaboration with the patient's obstetrician is indicated.

For details and discussion regarding related basic principles of clinical pharmacology, readers are referred to the first text in this series, *The Pharmacologic Basis of Psychotherapeutics: An Introduction for Psychologists.*

Women who are breast-feeding: Safety and efficacy of clonazepam pharmacotherapy for women who are breast-feeding and their neonates and infants have not been established. Although maximal intake of clonazepam by breast-feeding infants may be low (~2.5% of maternal dosage), avoid prescribing clonazepam pharmacotherapy to women who are breast-feeding. If clonazepam pharmacotherapy is required, breast-feeding probably should be discontinued.

Elderly, frail, or debilitated patients: Generally prescribe lower dosages for elderly, frail, or debilitated patients. These patients may be more sensitive to the pharmacologic actions of clonazepam than are younger or healthier adult patients.

Children younger than 10 years of age or weighing less than 30 kg: Initially, 10 to 30 μg/kg/day orally in three divided doses. Gradually increase the daily dosage by 250 to 500 μg every third day, according to individual patient response, until therapeutic benefit or dose-limiting ADRs are observed. Usual maintenance dosage is 100 to 200 μg/kg/day orally in three divided doses. Note that the dosage is in *micrograms*.

Notes, Seizure Disorders

Up to one-third of treated patients may develop tolerance or refractoriness to the anticonvulsant action of clonazepam within three months of the initiation of pharmacotherapy. Dosage adjustment may reestablish efficacy in some cases, but not in most cases.

Abrupt discontinuation of clonazepam pharmacotherapy, particularly long-term or high-dosage pharmacotherapy, may result in status epilepticus. Therefore, do *not* discontinue clonazepam pharmacotherapy abruptly. Gradually reduce the dosage according to individual patient response.

See also "Benzodiazepines, General Monograph."

AVAILABLE DOSAGE FORMS, STORAGE, AND COMPATIBILITY

Tablets, oral: 0.5, 1, 2 mg

Notes

General instructions for patients: Instruct patients who are receiving clonazepam pharmacotherapy to

- safely store tablets out of the reach of children in tightly closed, light- and child-resistant containers at controlled room temperature (15° to 30°C; 59° to 86°F).
- obtain an available patient information sheet regarding clonazepam pharmacotherapy from their pharmacist at the time that their prescription is dispensed. Encourage patients to clarify any questions that they may have regarding clonazepam pharmacotherapy with their pharmacist or, if needed, to consult their prescribing psychologist.

PROPOSED MECHANISM OF ACTION

The exact mechanism of the anticonvulsant action of clonazepam has not yet been fully determined. Clonazepam appears to augment presynaptic inhibition and thus suppresses, but does not abolish, seizure activity. See also "Benzodiazepines, General Monograph."

PHARMACOKINETICS/PHARMACODYNAMICS

Clonazepam is generally well absorbed from the GI tract following oral ingestion ($F = 0.9$). Onset of action is within 1 hour and peak blood concentrations are achieved within 2 hours. Clonazepam is highly protein bound (~86%) with a mean apparent volume of distribution of 3.2 liters/kg. Clonazepam is extensively metabolized in the liver with only small amounts (<1%) eliminated in unchanged form in the urine. Its mean half-life of elimination is 23 hours and its mean total body clearance is ~90 ml/hour/kg. The half-life of elimination ranges from 19 to 50 hours. Duration of action ranges from 6 to 12 hours. Additional data are not available.

Therapeutic Drug Monitoring

Therapeutic blood concentrations for the anticonvulsant action of clonazepam have not yet been clearly established. Available data indicate that most patients experience seizure control at blood concentrations between 20 and 80 ng/ml.

RELATIVE CONTRAINDICATIONS

Glaucoma, acute angle-closure (See "Benzodiazepines, General Monograph.")
Hypersensitivity to clonazepam or other benzodiazepines
Liver dysfunction, significant

CAUTIONS AND COMMENTS

Rarely, clonazepam pharmacotherapy may increase seizure activity among some patients. In addition, when used to treat seizure activity among patients in whom several different types of seizures coexist, clonazepam pharmacotherapy may increase the incidence, or precipitate the onset, of generalized tonic-clonic (grand mal) seizures.

Prescribe clonazepam pharmacotherapy cautiously to patients who

• have histories of alcohol or other substance use disorders.
• have histories of chronic respiratory disorders (e.g., chronic obstructive lung disease).

Caution patients who are receiving clonazepam pharmacotherapy against

• performing activities that require alertness, judgment, or physical coordination (e.g., driving an automobile, operating dangerous equipment, supervising children) until their response to clonazepam pharmacotherapy is known. Clonazepam may affect these mental and physical functions adversely.

In addition to this general precaution, caution patients to

- inform their prescribing psychologist if they begin or discontinue any other pharmacotherapy while receiving clonazepam pharmacotherapy.

CLINICALLY SIGNIFICANT DRUG INTERACTIONS

Concurrent clonazepam pharmacotherapy and the following may result in clinically significant drug interactions:

Alcohol Use

Concurrent alcohol use may increase the CNS depressant action of clonazepam. Advise patients to avoid, or limit, their use of alcohol while receiving clonazepam pharmacotherapy.

Pharmacotherapy With CNS Depressants and Other Drugs That Produce CNS Depression

Concurrent clonazepam pharmacotherapy and pharmacotherapy with opiate analgesics, sedative-hypnotics, or other drugs that produce CNS depression (e.g., antihistamines, phenothiazines, TCAs) may result in additive CNS depression.

See also "Benzodiazepines, General Monograph."

ADVERSE DRUG REACTIONS

Clonazepam pharmacotherapy commonly has been associated with: drowsiness, hypotonia, incoordination (ataxia), and sedation. Clonazepam pharmacotherapy also has been associated with the following ADRs, listed according to body system:

Cardiovascular: palpitations
CNS: agitation, aggression, antisocial behavior (particularly among children), confusion, depression, dizziness, drowsiness, fatigue, headache, hyperactivity, insomnia, irritability, mental confusion, nervousness, psychosis, and slurred speech. Behavioral ADRs (e.g., aggressiveness, hyperactivity) are noted primarily among children or adults who have pre-existing brain damage or mental retardation. These ADRs have been reported to occur in up to 25% of patients receiving clonazepam pharmacotherapy.
Cutaneous: abnormal hair growth (hirsutism), dehydration, edema (ankle and facial), and hair loss (alopecia)
Genitourinary: difficult or painful urination (dysuria), excessive urination during the night (nocturia), involuntary urination (enuresis), and urinary retention
GI: abnormal thirst, dry mouth, dyspepsia, inflammation of the stomach (gastritis), and nausea
Hematologic: anemia, eosinophilia, leukopenia, and thrombocytopenia
Hepatic: abnormal liver function tests and enlargement of the liver (hepatomegaly)
Musculoskeletal: muscle weakness and low back pain
Ophthalmic: blurred vision, double vision (diplopia), and involuntary rapid cyclic movement of the eyeballs (nystagmus)
Respiratory: chest congestion, hypersecretion in the upper respiratory passages, respiratory depression, and shortness of breath
Miscellaneous: fever and lymphadenopathy

See also "Benzodiazepines, General Monograph."

OVERDOSAGE

Signs and symptoms of clonazepam overdosage include coma, confusion, diminished reflexes, incoordination (ataxia), and somnolence. Clonazepam overdosage requires emergency symptomatic medical support of body systems with attention to increasing clonazepam elimination. The benzodiazepine antagonist, flumazenil (Anexate®; Romazicon®), may be required. Note that patients whose seizure disorders have been managed with benzodiazepine pharmacotherapy may be at increased risk for the occurrence of seizures when their benzodiazepine overdosage is treated with flumazenil pharmacotherapy.

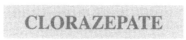

CLORAZEPATE

(klor az′ e pate)

TRADE NAMES

Gen-XENE®
Novo-Clopate®
Tranxene®
Tranxene-SD®

CLASSIFICATION

Anticonvulsant (sedative-hypnotic) (benzodiazepine prodrug) (C-IV)

See also "Benzodiazepines, General Monograph."

APPROVED INDICATIONS FOR NEUROPSYCHOLOGICAL DISORDERS

Adjunctive pharmacotherapy for the symptomatic management of:

- seizure disorders: partial seizures and those associated with the acute alcohol withdrawal syndrome. Clorazepate pharmacotherapy has been found to be of benefit for the symptomatic management of the agitation, delirium tremens (impending or acute), hallucinations, tremor, and seizures associated with the acute alcohol withdrawal syndrome.

USUAL DOSAGE AND ADMINISTRATION

Seizure Disorders: Partial Seizures

Adults: Initially, 22.5 mg daily orally in three divided doses. Gradually increase the dosage by no more than 7.5 mg per week according to individual patient response.

MAXIMUM: 90 mg daily orally

Women who are, or who may become, pregnant: FDA Pregnancy Category C. An increased risk for congenital malformations (i.e., birth defects) has been associated with the use of benzodiazepines, such as chlordiazepoxide (Librium®) and diazepam (Valium®), during the first trimester of pregnancy. Clorazepate, a benzodiazepine derivative, has not been clearly associated with an increased risk. However, clorazepate may be teratogenic if prescribed during the first trimester of pregnancy. Avoid prescribing clorazepate pharmacotherapy to women who are pregnant because of its similarity to these and other benzodiazepines. If clorazepate pharmacotherapy

For details and discussion regarding related basic principles of clinical pharmacology, readers are referred to the first text in this series, *The Pharmacologic Basis of Psychotherapeutics: An Introduction for Psychologists.*

is required, advise patients of potential benefits and possible risks to themselves and the embryo, fetus, or neonate. Collaboration with the patient's obstetrician is indicated.

Women who are breast-feeding: Safety and efficacy of clorazepate pharmacotherapy for women who are breast-feeding and their neonates and infants have not been established. The active metabolite of clorazepate, nordiazepam, is excreted in breast milk. Drowsiness and lethargy may occur among breast-fed neonates and infants, who also may become addicted. Avoid prescribing clorazepate to women who are breast-feeding. If clorazepate pharmacotherapy is required, breast-feeding probably should be discontinued. If desired, lactation may be maintained and breast-feeding resumed following the discontinuation of short-term clorazepate pharmacotherapy. Collaboration with the patient's pediatrician is indicated.

Elderly, frail, or debilitated patients and those who have kidney or liver dysfunction: Initially, 7.5 to 15 mg daily orally in two to four divided doses. Gradually increase the dosage by no more than 7.5 mg per week, according to individual patient response. Generally prescribe lower dosages initially for elderly, frail, or debilitated patients. Increase the dosage more gradually in order to avoid associated incoordination (ataxia) or excessive sedation among these patients. Also prescribe lower dosages for patients who have kidney or liver dysfunction.

MAXIMUM: 60 mg daily orally

Children younger than 9 years of age: Safety and efficacy of clorazepate pharmacotherapy for the management of seizure disorders among children younger than 9 years of age have not been established. Clorazepate pharmacotherapy for this indication is *not* recommended for this age group.

Children 9 to 12 years of age: Initially, 15 mg daily orally in two divided doses. Gradually increase the dosage by no more than 7.5 mg per week according to individual patient response.

MAXIMUM: 60 mg daily orally

Notes, Seizure Disorders

Initiating and maintaining clorazepate pharmacotherapy: Drowsiness may occur upon the initiation of clorazepate pharmacotherapy and with incremental increases in dosage. Periodically monitor blood counts and liver function tests for patients who require long-term clorazepate pharmacotherapy. Collaboration with the patient's family physician or a specialist (e.g., hematologist) may be indicated.

Discontinuing clorazepate pharmacotherapy: Long-term clorazepate pharmacotherapy, or regular personal use, may lead to addiction and habituation. Abrupt discontinuation of long-term clorazepate pharmacotherapy, or of regular personal use, may result in the clorazepate withdrawal syndrome. This syndrome may include seizures. Discontinue clorazepate pharmacotherapy, or regular personal use, gradually.

Seizures and Other Symptoms Associated With the Acute Alcohol Withdrawal Syndrome

Adults: The following daily schedule is recommended for the prophylactic and symptomatic management of the acute alcohol withdrawal syndrome:

Day 1 (first 24 hours): Initially, 30 mg orally, then an additional 30 to 60 mg orally in two to four divided doses
Day 2 (second 24 hours): 45 to 90 mg orally in two to four divided doses
Day 3 (third 24 hours): 22.5 to 45 mg orally in two to four divided doses
Day 4 (fourth 24 hours): 15 to 30 mg orally in two to four divided doses
Day 5 (fifth 24 hours) and thereafter: Gradually reduce the previous daily dosage to 7.5 to 15 mg. Completely discontinue clorazepate pharmacotherapy as soon as the patient's condition stabilizes.

MAXIMUM: 90 mg daily orally

Notes, Alcohol Withdrawal Syndrome, Acute

Avoid excessive reductions in the total daily dosage prescribed on successive days, 1 through 4, to adequately manage the signs and symptoms of the acute alcohol withdrawal syndrome.

AVAILABLE DOSAGE FORMS, STORAGE, AND COMPATIBILITY

Capsules, oral: 3.75, 7.5, 15 mg
Tablets, oral: 3.75, 7.5, 11.25, 15 mg
Tablets, oral extended-release: 11.25, 22.5 mg (not generally prescribed for the prophylactic or symptomatic management of the acute alcohol withdrawal syndrome)

Notes

General instructions for patients: Instruct patients who are receiving clorazepate pharmacotherapy to

- swallow each dose of clorazepate oral capsules or extended-release tablets whole without breaking, chewing, or crushing, with adequate liquid chaser (e.g., 60 to 120 ml of water).

PROPOSED MECHANISM OF ACTION

Clorazepate has the chemical characteristics of the benzodiazepines and produces similar depressant actions on the CNS. The exact mechanism of action of clorazepate has not yet been fully determined. However, it appears to be mediated by or to work in concert with the inhibitory neurotransmitter, GABA.

See also the "Benzodiazepines, General Monograph."

PHARMACOKINETICS/PHARMACODYNAMICS

Clorazepate, a *prodrug*, is rapidly metabolized in the liver to its active major metabolite, nordiazepam (desmethyldiazepam). There is virtually no circulating parent drug in the blood. Nordiazepam is highly plasma protein bound (~98%). It is further extensively metabolized in the liver, and its metabolites are primarily excreted in the urine (i.e., less than 1% of nordiazepam is excreted in unchanged form in the urine). The mean half-life of elimination for nordiazepam is approximately 2 to 3 days. The mean total body clearance is ~1 ml/minute.

RELATIVE CONTRAINDICATIONS

Glaucoma, acute narrow-angle (See "Benzodiazepines, General Monograph.")
Hypersensitivity to clorazepate or other benzodiazepines
Myasthenia gravis
Pain, severe uncontrolled

CAUTIONS AND COMMENTS

Clorazepate is addicting and habituating. A clorazepate withdrawal syndrome similar to the alcohol and barbiturate withdrawal syndromes has occurred following the abrupt discontinuation of long-term, high-dosage clorazepate pharmacotherapy, or of regular personal use. Signs and symptoms of the clorazepate withdrawal syndrome include diarrhea, hallucinations, insomnia, irritability, memory impairment, muscle aches, nervousness, and tremor. Monitor all patients for whom clorazepate pharmacotherapy is discontinued for signs and symptoms of withdrawal because abrupt discontinuation of other benzodiazepine pharmacotherapy, even prescribed therapeutic dosages over several months, has resulted in a benzodiazepine withdrawal syndrome.

Prescribe clorazepate pharmacotherapy cautiously to patients who

- have depression accompanied with anxiety and for whom suicide tendencies may be present. Prescribe the least amount of clorazepate feasible for dispensing to these patients. Other suicide precautions may be indicated.
- have histories of problematic patterns of alcohol or other abusable psychotropic use. Clorazepate is addicting and habituating. These patients may be more likely to develop problematic patterns of clorazepate use, including addiction and habituation.
- have kidney or liver dysfunction.

Caution patients who are receiving clorazepate pharmacotherapy against

- drinking alcohol or using other drugs that cause CNS depression (e.g., antihistamines, barbiturates, opiate analgesics, phenothiazines). Excessive CNS depression may result.
- performing activities that require alertness, judgment, or physical coordination (e.g., driving an automobile, operating dangerous equipment, supervising children) until their response to clorazepate pharmacotherapy is known. Clorazepate pharmacotherapy may affect these mental and physical functions adversely, particularly during the first few days of pharmacotherapy, because of its sedative action.

In addition to these general precautions for patients, caution women who are receiving clorazepate pharmacotherapy to

- inform their prescribing psychologist if they become or intend to become pregnant while receiving clorazepate pharmacotherapy so that their pharmacotherapy can be discontinued safely.

CLINICALLY SIGNIFICANT DRUG INTERACTIONS

Concurrent clorazepate pharmacotherapy and the following may result in clinically significant drug interactions:

Alcohol Use

Concurrent alcohol use may significantly increase the CNS depressant action of clorazepate. Advise patients to avoid, or limit, their use of alcohol while receiving clorazepate pharmacotherapy.

Cimetidine Pharmacotherapy

Cimetidine (Tagamet®), a hepatic microsomal enzyme inhibitor, may decrease the hepatic clearance of clorazepate. This interaction may result in clorazepate toxicity.

Pharmacotherapy With CNS Depressants and Other Drugs That Produce CNS Depression

Concurrent clorazepate pharmacotherapy and pharmacotherapy with opiate analgesics, other sedative-hypnotics, or other drugs that cause CNS depression (e.g., MAOIs, phenothiazines, TCAs) may result in additive CNS depression.

See also "Benzodiazepines, General Monograph."

ADVERSE DRUG REACTIONS

Clorazepate pharmacotherapy commonly has been associated with drowsiness. Clorazepate pharmacotherapy also has been associated with the following ADRs, listed according to body system:

Cardiovascular: rarely, decreased systolic blood pressure
CNS: confusion, depression, dizziness, drowsiness, fatigue, headache, insomnia, irritability, mental confusion, nervousness, and slurred speech
Cutaneous: transient skin rashes
Genitourinary: genitourinary complaints
GI: dry mouth and other GI complaints
Hematologic: rarely, decreased hematocrit
Hepatic: abnormal liver function tests
Musculoskeletal: incoordination (ataxia) and tremor
Ocular: blurred vision and double vision (diplopia)
Renal: rarely, abnormal kidney function tests

See also "Benzodiazepines, General Monograph."

OVERDOSAGE

Signs and symptoms of clorazepate overdosage correspond to varying degrees of CNS depression ranging from slight sedation to coma. Clorazepate overdosage requires emergency symptomatic medical support of body systems with attention to increasing clorazepate elimination. The benzodiazepine antagonist, flumazenil (Anexate®, Romazicon®), may be required. Note that patients whose seizure disorders have been managed with benzodiazepine pharmacotherapy may be at increased risk for the occurrence of seizures when their benzodiazepine overdosage is treated with flumazenil pharmacotherapy.

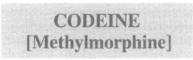

CODEINE
[Methylmorphine]

(koe′ deen)

TRADE NAMES

Codeine Contin®
Paveral®

CLASSIFICATION

Opiate analgesic (agonist) (C-II)

See also "Opiate Analgesics, General Monograph."

APPROVED INDICATIONS FOR NEUROPSYCHOLOGICAL DISORDERS

Adjunctive pharmacotherapy for the short-term symptomatic management of:

- pain disorders: mild to moderate pain. The codeine extended-release formulation (Codeine Contin®) is indicated for the long-term symptomatic management of moderate cancer pain.

USUAL DOSAGE AND ADMINISTRATION

Pain, Mild to Moderate

Adults: 0.5 to 2 mg/kg intramuscularly, orally, or subcutaneously every four to six hours

MAXIMUM: 60 mg/dose; 300 mg daily

Women who are, or who may become, pregnant: FDA Pregnancy Category C. Safety and efficacy of codeine pharmacotherapy for women who are pregnant have not been established. Generally, codeine pharmacotherapy is not recommended for women who are pregnant because codeine crosses the placenta. However, it is unlikely that codeine is a teratogen. If it is, its potency and incidence as a teratogen are extremely low. Codeine is widely used during pregnancy, particularly in combination analgesic and cough and cold products. Only a few cases of possible teratogenic effects (e.g., cleft lip and palate) have been reported in the published literature. Maternal use near term may result in neonatal depression, which is associated with the expected actions

For details and discussion regarding related basic principles of clinical pharmacology, readers are referred to the first text in this series, *The Pharmacologic Basis of Psychotherapeutics: An Introduction for Psychologists.*

of an opiate analgesic. Long-term maternal pharmacotherapy, or regular personal use, may result in the neonatal opiate withdrawal syndrome. Avoid prescribing codeine pharmacotherapy to women who are pregnant. If codeine pharmacotherapy is required, advise patients of potential benefits and possible risks to themselves and the embryo, fetus, or neonate. Collaboration with the patient's obstetrician is indicated.

Women who are breast-feeding: Safety and efficacy of codeine pharmacotherapy for women who are breast-feeding and their neonates and infants have not been established. The active metabolites of codeine (e.g., morphine) are excreted in low concentrations in breast milk. Neonatal respiratory depression following several days (4 or 5 days) of breast-feeding has been reported among neonates. Drowsiness and lethargy may occur among breast-fed neonates and infants. These neonates and infants also may become addicted. Avoid prescribing codeine to women who are breast-feeding. If codeine pharmacotherapy is required, breast-feeding probably should be discontinued. If desired, lactation may be maintained and breast-feeding resumed following the discontinuation of short-term codeine pharmacotherapy. Collaboration with the patient's pediatrician may be indicated.

Elderly, frail, or debilitated patients and those who have kidney or liver dysfunction: Initially prescribe lower dosages for elderly, frail, or debilitated patients. Gradually increase the dosage, as needed, according to individual patient response. These patients may be more sensitive to the CNS or respiratory depressant actions of codeine than are younger or healthier adult patients. Also prescribe lower dosages for patients who have severe kidney or liver dysfunction.

Children: 0.5 to 1 mg/kg intramuscularly, orally, or subcutaneously every four to six hours, according to individual signs and symptoms of pain and clinical response

MAXIMUM: 1.5 mg/kg/dose to a maximum of 60 mg

Notes, Cancer Pain, Moderate

In terms of analgesic action, orally administered codeine is ~60% as potent as intramuscularly administered codeine. Orally administered codeine phosphate is approximately one-tenth as potent as orally administered morphine sulfate (i.e., 10 mg codeine ≈1 mg morphine). Oral doses may be only two-thirds as effective as equal injectable doses because of differences in bioavailability. Avoid intravenous injection because of the associated release of histamine.

Injectable formulation: The injectable formulation of some manufacturers contains sodium bisulfite or sodium metabisulfite. Sulfites have been associated with hypersensitivity reactions, including anaphylactic reactions, among susceptible patients. Although relatively uncommon, these reactions appear to occur with a higher incidence among patients who have asthma.

Oral formulations: The oral extended-release tablets contain two codeine salts, codeine monohydrate and codeine sulfate trihydrate. However, the formulation is labeled and dosed in terms of anhydrous codeine. For example, the 100-mg extended-release tablet contains 53 mg of codeine monohydrate and 62.7 mg of codeine sulfate trihydrate. Each salt form is equivalent to 50 mg of anhydrous codeine. The oral extended-release tablets are scored and can be split (e.g., halved) for dosage adjustment.

Extended-release tablets are *not* recommended for patients whose pain is adequately managed with 90 mg daily or less of codeine phosphate. See the table "Approximate Oral Opiate Analgesic Equivalents."

*Approximate oral opiate analgesic equivalents.**

Opiate analgesic	Oral dose (mg)	Duration of action (hours)
Codeine	**200**	**3 to 4**
Anileridine	75	2 to 3
Heroin	20	3 to 4
Hydromorphone	7.5	2 to 4
Levorphanol	4	4 to 8
Meperidine	300	1 to 3
Morphine	30	3 to 4
Oxycodone	30	2 to 4
Pentazocine	180	3 to 4
Propoxyphene	100	2 to 4

* The sensations of pain and analgesia are the result of a complex interaction between both physiological and psychological variables. Thus, significant variation is noted among patients.

Extended-release codeine tablets are only recommended for cancer patients who have moderate pain and require long-term analgesic pharmacotherapy. The "Approximate Oral Opiate Analgesic Equivalents" table provides a general guide for oral dosage equivalents and duration of analgesic action for several commonly prescribed opiate analgesics. (See also "Opiate Analgesics, General Monograph.") This table and a knowledge of the patient's current opiate analgesic requirements provide a useful guide for estimating a patient's total daily codeine dosage requirements. Prescribe an ~25% *lower* daily dosage. Dose half of the daily dosage every 12 hours. If breakthrough pain occurs toward the end of the dosing interval, gradually increase the dosage, as needed, according to individual patient response. Once pain relief has been achieved, gradually reduce the dosage to the lowest effective dosage. At regular intervals, reevaluate the patient's need for a further decrease or increase in dosage.

MAXIMUM, EXTENDED-RELEASE TABLET: 600 mg daily orally in two equally divided doses at 12-hour intervals

AVAILABLE DOSAGE FORMS, STORAGE, AND COMPATIBILITY

Elixir, oral: 10 mg/5 ml (contains 7% alcohol)
Injectables, intramuscular or subcutaneous: 15, 30, 60 mg/ml
Solution, oral: 15 mg/5 ml
Syrup, oral: 25 mg/5 ml
Tablets, oral: 15, 30, 60 mg
Tablets, oral extended-release: 100, 150, 200 mg

Notes

The injectable formulations contain sodium metabisulfite. Sulfites have been associated with hypersensitivity reactions, including anaphylactic reactions, among susceptible patients. Although relatively uncommon, these reactions appear to occur with a higher incidence among patients who have asthma.

The injectable formulations are chemically and/or physically *incompatible* with (i.e., should *not* be mixed with): aminophylline, amobarbital (Amytal®), chlorothiazide (Diuril®), heparin, methicillin (Staphcillin®), nitrofurantoin (Furadantin®), pentobarbital (Nembutal®), phenobarbital (Luminal®), and thiopental (Pentothal®).

General instructions for patients: Instruct patients who are receiving codeine pharmacotherapy to

- safely store codeine oral tablets out of the reach of children in tightly closed, child- and light-resistant containers at controlled room temperature (15° to 30°C; 59° to 86°F).
- swallow each dose of the codeine oral extended-release tablets whole, with adequate liquid chaser (60 to 120 ml), without breaking, chewing, or crushing. These tablets are scored and can be split (e.g., halved) for dosage adjustment.
- obtain an available patient information sheet regarding codeine pharmacotherapy from their pharmacist at the time that their prescription is dispensed. Encourage patients to clarify any questions that they may have regarding their codeine pharmacotherapy with their pharmacist or, if needed, to consult their prescribing psychologist.

PROPOSED MECHANISM OF ACTION

Codeine appears to elicit its analgesic action primarily by binding to the endorphin receptors in the CNS. This binding to receptors is thought to result in the inhibition of neurotransmission in the ascending pain pathways and in diminished pain perception. However, the exact mechanism of action has not yet been fully determined.

Similar to other opiate analgesics, codeine produces other actions in addition to analgesia. These actions are mediated by both central and peripheral mechanisms of action and include: cough reduction associated with suppression of the central cough center; constipation associated with decreased GI motility; nausea and vomiting associated with stimulation of the chemoreceptor trigger zone (CTZ) in the medulla; and respiratory depression associated with decreased responsiveness of the central respiratory center to stimulation by carbon dioxide (CO_2).

PHARMACOKINETICS/PHARMACODYNAMICS

The oral availability of codeine is variable (i.e., 40% to 70%; mean = 53%). It is only slightly (7%) bound to plasma protein and has an apparent volume of distribution of 2 to 3 liters/kg. The onset of action is generally within 30 minutes after oral ingestion or intramuscular or subcutaneous injection. The duration of action is 4 to 6 hours and is extended to ∼12 hours for the extended-release formulation. Codeine is metabolized in the liver to several active metabolites, including morphine, ∼10% (see the morphine monograph). Less than 5% is excreted in unchanged form in the urine. The mean half-life of elimination is ∼3 hours. The total body clearance is ∼800 ml/minute.

RELATIVE CONTRAINDICATIONS

Alcoholism, acute
CNS depression, severe
Cor pulmonale
Hypersensitivity to codeine or other opiate analgesics
Liver dysfunction, severe
Respiratory depression, severe

CAUTIONS AND COMMENTS

Long-term, high-dosage pharmacotherapy, or regular personal use, may lead to the development of addiction and habituation.

Prescribe codeine pharmacotherapy cautiously to patients who

- are children. The respiratory center of young children is particularly sensitive to the CNS depressant action of codeine.
- have obstructive airway disorders, such as sleep apnea. Codeine's depressant action on respiratory drive may significantly exacerbate these conditions and may produce apnea.
- have respiratory dysfunction, including asthma and emphysema. Codeine's drying action on airway secretions and its depressant action on the cough reflex may aggravate these conditions.
- have traumatic head injury, brain tumors, or other conditions associated with increased intracranial fluid pressure. Codeine pharmacotherapy may exacerbate these clinical conditions because of its ability to increase cerebrospinal fluid pressure. It also may mask the clinical course of these patients.

Caution patients who are receiving codeine pharmacotherapy against

- performing activities that require alertness, judgment, or physical coordination (e.g., driving an automobile, operating dangerous equipment, supervising children) until their response to codeine pharmacotherapy is known. Codeine may cause marked sedation and affect these mental and physical functions adversely.

CLINICALLY SIGNIFICANT DRUG INTERACTIONS

Concurrent codeine pharmacotherapy and the following may result in clinically significant drug interactions:

Alcohol Use

Concurrent alcohol use may increase the CNS depressant action of codeine. Advise patients to avoid, or limit, their use of alcohol while receiving codeine pharmacotherapy. (See "Relative Contraindications.")

Pharmacotherapy With CNS Depressants and Other Drugs That Produce CNS Depression

Concurrent codeine pharmacotherapy and pharmacotherapy with other opiate analgesics, sedative-hypnotics, or other drugs that produce CNS depression (e.g., antihistamines, phenothiazines, TCAs) may result in additive CNS depression. It also is important to note that codeine is one of the most common opiates found in prescription and nonprescription cough products. Concurrent use of these products should be avoided.

See also "Opiate Analgesics, General Monograph."

ADVERSE DRUG REACTIONS

Codeine pharmacotherapy commonly has been associated with constipation, dizziness, light-headedness, nausea, sedation, sweating (excessive), and vomiting. Codeine pharmacotherapy also has been associated with the following ADRs, listed according to body system:

CNS: depression, drowsiness, and headache
Cutaneous: flushing
Genitourinary: urinary retention
GI: cramps, dry mouth, and loss of appetite (anorexia)
Ocular: abnormal contraction of the pupils (miosis); blurred vision; constant, involuntary cyclical movement of the eyeball (nystagmus); and double vision (diplopia)
Respiratory: bronchospasm and laryngospasm (generally related to hypersensitivity reactions)
Miscellaneous: chills

See also "Opiate Analgesics, General Monograph."

OVERDOSAGE

See "Opiate Analgesics, General Monograph."

DEXTROAMPHETAMINE
[Dexamphetamine]

(dex troe am fet′ a meen)

TRADE NAME

Dexedrine®

CLASSIFICATION

CNS stimulant (sympathomimetic) (amphetamine) (C-II)

See also "Amphetamines, General Monograph."

APPROVED INDICATIONS FOR NEUROPSYCHOLOGICAL DISORDERS

Adjunctive pharmacotherapy for the symptomatic management of:

* sleep disorders: narcolepsy

USUAL DOSAGE AND ADMINISTRATION

Sleep Disorders: Narcolepsy

Adults: 5 to 60 mg daily orally in a single dose or two or three divided doses

Women who are, or who may become, pregnant: FDA Pregnancy Category C. Safety and efficacy of dextroamphetamine pharmacotherapy for women who are pregnant have not been established. Studies published to date on the use of dextroamphetamine during the first trimester of pregnancy have provided mixed results in relation to congenital malformations (i.e., birth defects) and, thus, are inconclusive. Neonates born to mothers who are addicted to amphetamines have an increased risk for premature delivery and low birth weight. During the neonatal period they also may display signs and symptoms of the amphetamine withdrawal syndrome. These signs and symptoms include agitation and lassitude. Avoid prescribing dextroamphetamine pharmacotherapy to women who are pregnant. If dextroamphetamine pharmacotherapy is required, advise patients of potential benefits and possible risks to themselves and the embryo, fetus, or neonate. Collaboration with the patient's obstetrician is indicated.

For details and discussion regarding related basic principles of clinical pharmacology, readers are referred to the first text in this series, *The Pharmacologic Basis of Psychotherapeutics: An Introduction for Psychologists.*

Women who are breast-feeding: Safety and efficacy of dextroamphetamine pharmacotherapy for women who are breast-feeding and their neonates and infants have not been established. Amphetamines are excreted in breast milk. Expected pharmacologic actions may be observed among breast-fed neonates and infants, who also may become addicted. Avoid prescribing dextroamphetamine pharmacotherapy to women who are breast-feeding. If dextroamphetamine pharmacotherapy is required, breast-feeding probably should be discontinued. Collaboration with the patient's pediatrician may be indicated.

Elderly, frail, or debilitated patients: Generally prescribe lower dosages for elderly, frail, or debilitated patients. Gradually increase the dosage, if needed, according to individual patient response. These patients may be more sensitive to the pharmacologic actions of dextroamphetamine than are younger or healthier patients.

Children 6 to 12 years of age: Initially, 5 mg daily orally in a single dose upon awakening in the morning. Increase the daily dosage by 5 mg weekly until optimal therapeutic response is achieved. Note that narcolepsy seldom occurs among children who are younger than 12 years of age.

MAXIMUM: 60 mg daily orally

Children 12 years of age and older: Initially, 10 mg daily orally in a single dose upon awakening in the morning. Increase the daily dosage by 10 mg weekly until optimal therapeutic response is achieved.

MAXIMUM: 60 mg daily orally

Notes, Narcolepsy

Prescribe the lowest effective dosage. Adjust the dosage according to individual patient response. Late evening doses should be avoided because of associated insomnia. Dexedrine® capsules (Spansules®) are designed to provide extended drug release into the GI tract and sustained therapeutic action for 10 to 12 hours. Prescribe these capsules for once-daily dosing, when appropriate.

AVAILABLE DOSAGE FORMS, STORAGE, AND COMPATIBILITY

Capsules, oral extended-release: 5, 10, 15 mg
Tablets, oral: 5, 10 mg

Notes

Some oral dosage forms (e.g., Dexedrine® capsules and tablets) contain tartrazine (FD & C Yellow No. 5). Tartrazine has been associated with hypersensitivity reactions (e.g., bronchial asthma) among susceptible patients, particularly those who have a hypersensitivity to aspirin.

General instructions for patients: Instruct patients who are receiving dextroamphetamine pharmacotherapy, or their parents or legal guardians as appropriate, to

- safely store dextroamphetamine capsules and tablets out of the reach of children in tightly closed, child- and light-resistant containers at controlled room temperature (15° to 30°C; 59°to 86°F).
- obtain an available patient information sheet regarding dextroamphetamine pharmacotherapy from their pharmacist at the time that their prescription is dispensed. Encourage patients, or their parents or legal guardians as appropriate, to clarify any questions that they may have regarding dextroamphetamine pharmacotherapy with their pharmacist or, if needed, to consult their prescribing psychologist.

PROPOSED MECHANISM OF ACTION

Dextroamphetamine is a member of the amphetamine group of sympathomimetic amines that have CNS stimulant action. Peripheral actions include elevation of systolic and diastolic blood pressures and weak bronchodilator and respiratory stimulant actions. Dextroamphetamine appears to elicit its stimulant action primarily by increasing the release of norepinephrine from presynaptic storage vesicles in adrenergic neurons. A direct effect on α- and β-adrenergic receptors, inhibition of the enzyme amine oxidase, and the release of dopamine also may be involved. However, the exact mechanism of action has not yet been fully determined.

PHARMACOKINETICS/PHARMACODYNAMICS

Dextroamphetamine appears to be fairly well absorbed following oral ingestion. Peak blood concentrations occur within ~2 hours. The mean half-life of elimination is 10 hours. Additional data are not available.

RELATIVE CONTRAINDICATIONS

Addiction and habituation to amphetamines or other abusable psychotropics, history of
Agitation
Arteriosclerosis, advanced
Glaucoma
Heart disease, symptomatic
Hypersensitivity to amphetamines or sympathomimetic amines
Hypertension, moderate to severe
Hyperthyroidism
MAOI pharmacotherapy, concurrent or within 14 days. Hypertensive crisis may result.

CAUTIONS AND COMMENTS

Amphetamines have a high potential for addiction and habituation. Thus, they should be prescribed cautiously as adjunctive pharmacotherapy for the symptomatic management of narcolepsy. Long-term amphetamine pharmacotherapy, or regular personal use, may lead to addiction and habituation. Thus, attention must be given to the possibility that some patients may become addicted or habituated to dextroamphetamine as a result of their pharmacotherapy. Attention also must be given to the possibility that some patients may seek dextroamphetamine prescriptions to support their addiction or habituation (i.e., regular personal use). Prescribe small quantities of dextroamphetamine and monitor pharmacotherapy closely. Limit prescriptions to the least amount that is feasible for dispensing at one time in order to minimize the possible development of problematic patterns of use.

Prescribe dextroamphetamine pharmacotherapy cautiously to patients who

- have cardiovascular disorders, including mild hypertension. Amphetamine pharmacotherapy has been associated with cardiac dysrhythmias and hypertension among these patients.
- have histories of schizophrenia or other psychotic disorders. Amphetamine pharmacotherapy for children, adolescents, and adults who have psychotic disorders may exacerbate the signs and symptoms of the psychotic disorder. Reportedly, amphetamines exacerbate motor and phonic tics and Tourette's disorder (Gilles de la Tourette's syndrome). Clinical assessment of patients for tics and Tourette's syndrome should precede the prescription of dextroamphetamine pharmacotherapy.

Caution patients who are receiving dextroamphetamine pharmacotherapy against

- performing activities that require alertness, judgment, and physical coordination (e.g., driving an automobile, operating dangerous equipment, supervising children) until their response to dextroamphetamine pharmacotherapy is known. The CNS stimulant action of dextroamphetamine may affect these mental and physical functions adversely.

See also "Amphetamines, General Monograph."

CLINICALLY SIGNIFICANT DRUG INTERACTIONS

Concurrent dextroamphetamine pharmacotherapy and the following may result in clinically significant drug interactions:

Antipsychotic Pharmacotherapy

Chlorpromazine (Largactil®, Thorazine®), haloperidol (Haldol®), and, presumably, other antipsychotics, antagonize the CNS stimulatory actions of the amphetamines. Thus, this combination of pharmacotherapy is contraindicated except in situations of dextroamphetamine overdosage. (See "Overdosage.")

Guanethidine Pharmacotherapy

Dextroamphetamine pharmacotherapy may decrease the neuronal uptake of guanethidine (Ismelin®) and, thus, decrease its antihypertensive action. An adjustment to the guanethidine dosage may be required. Collaboration with the prescriber of the guanethidine is indicated.

Insulin Pharmacotherapy

Dextroamphetamine pharmacotherapy for patients who have insulin-dependent diabetes mellitus may result in alterations in insulin requirements. A change in the insulin dosage may be required. Collaboration with the prescriber of the insulin is indicated.

MAOI Pharmacotherapy

Dextroamphetamine may interact with MAOIs (e.g., phenelzine [Nardil®]) and cause the release of large amounts of catecholamines and the hypertensive crisis. The hypertensive crisis is characterized by a severe headache and hypertension. Thus, dextroamphetamine pharmacotherapy, concurrent or within 14 days of MAOI pharmacotherapy, is ***contraindicated***.

Pharmacotherapy With Drugs That Acidify the Urine

Drugs that acidify the urine (e.g., ammonium chloride) increase the urinary excretion of dextroamphetamine.

Pharmacotherapy With Drugs That Alkalinize the Urine

Drugs that alkalinize the urine (e.g., acetazolamide, sodium bicarbonate) decrease the urinary excretion of dextroamphetamine.

TCA Pharmacotherapy

Concurrent dextroamphetamine and TCA pharmacotherapy (as with other amphetamine or sympathomimetic pharmacotherapy) may result in additive CNS stimulant actions. Monitor patients closely and adjust the dosage of both drugs carefully when concurrent pharmacotherapy is required. Each drug tends to enhance the pharmacologic actions of the other.

See also "Amphetamines, General Monograph."

ADVERSE DRUG REACTIONS

Dextroamphetamine pharmacotherapy has been associated with the following ADRs, listed according to body system:

Cardiovascular: increased blood pressure (hypertension), increased heart rate (tachycardia), and palpitations

CNS: dizziness, dysphoria, euphoria, headache, insomnia, and overstimulation. Psychotic episodes and Tourette's disorder (Gilles de la Tourette's syndrome) rarely have been reported at recommended dosages.

Cutaneous: hives (urticaria)

Genitourinary: changes in sex drive and impotence

GI: constipation, diarrhea, dry mouth, gastrointestinal complaints, loss of appetite (anorexia), weight loss, and unpleasant taste

Musculoskeletal: restlessness and tremor. Suppression of growth also has been reported among children who have received long-term dextroamphetamine pharmacotherapy.

See also "Amphetamines, General Monograph."

OVERDOSAGE

Signs and symptoms of acute dextroamphetamine overdosage include acute, sometimes fatal, destruction of skeletal muscle (rhabdomyolysis), assaultiveness, cardiovascular reactions (e.g., dysrhythmias, hypertension or hypotension, and circulatory collapse), confusion, elevated body temperature (hyperpyrexia), GI complaints (e.g., abdominal cramps, diarrhea, nausea, and vomiting), dilated and reactive pupils, hallucinations, increased action of the reflexes (hyperreflexia), panic, rapid respirations, restlessness, and tremor. Depression and fatigue usually follow the central stimulation. Fatal overdosage usually terminates in convulsions and coma.

Dextroamphetamine overdosage requires emergency symptomatic medical support of body systems with attention to increasing dextroamphetamine elimination. There is no known antidote. However, the antipsychotics, chlorpromazine (Largactil®, Thorazine®) and haloperidol (Haldol®), block dopamine and norepinephrine re-uptake and, thus, inhibit the central stimulant actions of dextroamphetamine.

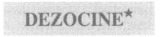

DEZOCINE*

(dez′ oh seen)

TRADE NAME

Dalgan®

CLASSIFICATION

Opiate analgesic (mixed agonist/antagonist)

See also "Opiate Analgesics, General Monograph."

APPROVED INDICATIONS FOR NEUROPSYCHOLOGICAL DISORDERS

Adjunctive pharmacotherapy for the symptomatic management of:

- pain disorders: acute or chronic pain, moderate to severe.

USUAL DOSAGE AND ADMINISTRATION

Acute or Chronic Pain, Moderate to Severe

Adults: 5 to 20 mg intramuscularly every three to six hours; *or* 2.5 to 10 mg intravenously every two to four hours.

MAXIMUM: 20 mg/dose intramuscularly; 120 mg daily intramuscularly

Women who are, or who may become, pregnant: FDA Pregnancy Category C. Safety and efficacy of dezocine pharmacotherapy for women who are pregnant have not been established. Avoid prescribing dezocine pharmacotherapy to women who are pregnant. If dezocine pharmacotherapy is required, advise patients of potential benefits and possible risks to themselves and the embryo, fetus, or neonate. Collaboration with the patient's obstetrician is indicated.

Women who are breast-feeding: Safety and efficacy of dezocine pharmacotherapy for women who are breast-feeding and their neonates and infants have not been established. Avoid prescribing dezocine pharmacotherapy to women who are breast-feeding. If dezocine pharmacotherapy is required, breast-feeding probably should be discontinued. If desired, lactation may be maintained and breast-feeding resumed following the discontinuation of short-term dezocine pharmacotherapy.

For details and discussion regarding related basic principles of clinical pharmacology, readers are referred to the first text in this series, *The Pharmacologic Basis of Psychotherapeutics: An Introduction for Psychologists.*

Elderly, frail, or debilitated patients: Generally prescribe lower dosages for elderly, frail, or debilitated patients. Gradually increase the dosage, if needed, according to individual patient response. These patients may be more sensitive to the pharmacologic actions of dezocine than are younger or healthier adult patients.

Children and adolescents younger than 18 years of age: Safety and efficacy of dezocine pharmacotherapy for children and adolescents have not been established. Dezocine pharmacotherapy is *not* recommended for this age group.

Notes, Acute or Chronic Pain, Moderate to Severe

Note differences in recommended intramuscular and intravenous dosages. Subcutaneous injection is irritating and should be avoided.

AVAILABLE DOSAGE FORMS, STORAGE, AND COMPATIBILITY

Injectable, intramuscular or intravenous: 5, 10, 15 mg/ml

Notes

The injectable formulation contains sodium metabisulfite. Sulfites have been associated with hypersensitivity reactions, including anaphylactic reactions, among susceptible patients. Although relatively uncommon, these reactions appear to occur with a higher incidence among patients who have asthma.

Inspect injectable formulations for precipitate prior to use. Do not use the formulation if a precipitate is noted. Return the formulation to the dispensing pharmacy or manufacturer for safe and appropriate disposal.

Safely store dezocine injectable, protected from light, at room temperature below 30 °C (86 °F).

PROPOSED MECHANISM OF ACTION

Dezocine elicits its analgesic, CNS depressant, and respiratory depressant actions primarily by binding to the endorphin receptors in the CNS. However, the exact mechanism of action has not yet been fully determined. See also "Opiate Analgesics, General Monograph."

PHARMACOKINETICS/PHARMACODYNAMICS

Dezocine is rapidly and completely absorbed following intramuscular injection ($F = 1$). Dezocine is highly plasma protein bound (~92%) and has an apparent volume of distribution of 6 to 10 liters/kg. Dezocine is extensively metabolized in the liver with less than 1% excreted in unchanged form in the urine. The mean half-life of elimination is 4 hours (range: 1 to 7 hours) and the mean total body clearance is ~1.5 liters/kg/hour.

RELATIVE CONTRAINDICATIONS

Hypersensitivity to dezocine

CAUTIONS AND COMMENTS

Dezocine is addicting and habituating. Long-term dezocine pharmacotherapy, or regular personal use, may result in addiction and habituation. Abrupt discontinuation after long-term dezocine pharmacotherapy, or regular personal use, may result in a reportedly mild form of the opiate withdrawal syndrome.

Prescribe dezocine pharmacotherapy cautiously for patients who

- have acute cholecystitis or pancreatitis or will be undergoing surgery of the biliary tract. Opiate analgesics generally increase biliary tract pressure. Although dezocine reportedly causes little or no elevation of biliary pressure, caution is advised.
- are receiving long-term opiate analgesic pharmacotherapy with pure opiate agonists (e.g., morphine). Dezocine pharmacotherapy may cause the opiate withdrawal syndrome among these patients because it has mixed opiate agonist/antagonist properties.
- have head injuries, intracranial lesions, or other medical disorders associated with increased intracranial pressure. The respiratory depressant action associated with dezocine and its potential for elevating cerebrospinal fluid pressure may markedly exaggerate intracranial pressure among these patients. Dezocine's analgesic and sedative actions also may obscure the clinical course of these patients.
- have histories of opiate agonist analgesic addiction. Patients who are addicted to opiate agonist analgesics may experience signs and symptoms of the opiate withdrawal syndrome. Dezocine, a mixed agonist/antagonist, has weak opiate antagonist action.
- have liver dysfunction. Serious liver dysfunction appears to predispose patients to a higher incidence of ADRs (e.g., anxiety, dizziness, drowsiness, marked apprehension) even when usual recommended dosages are prescribed. These ADRs may be the result of decreased dezocine metabolism by the liver and resultant accumulation and toxicity.
- have respiratory depression, limited respiratory function (e.g., severely limited respiratory reserve, severe bronchial asthma, or other obstructive respiratory conditions, such as sleep apnea), or cyanosis. The respiratory depressant action of dezocine may further compromise the respiratory function of these patients.

Caution patients who are receiving dezocine pharmacotherapy against

- performing activities that require alertness, judgment, and physical coordination (e.g., driving an automobile, operating dangerous equipment, supervising children) until their response to dezocine pharmacotherapy is known. The CNS depressant action of dezocine may affect these mental and physical functions adversely.

CLINICALLY SIGNIFICANT DRUG INTERACTIONS

Concurrent dezocine pharmacotherapy and the following may result in clinically significant drug *interactions:*

Alcohol Use

Concurrent alcohol use may increase the CNS depressant action of dezocine. Advise patients to avoid, or limit, their use of alcohol while receiving dezocine pharmacotherapy.

Pharmacotherapy With CNS Depressants and Other Drugs That Produce CNS Depression

Concurrent dezocine pharmacotherapy and pharmacotherapy with other opiate analgesics, sedative-hypnotics, or other drugs that produce CNS depression (e.g., antihistamines, phenothiazines, TCAs) may result in additive CNS depression.

See also "Opiate Analgesics, General Monograph."

ADVERSE DRUG REACTIONS

Dezocine pharmacotherapy has been commonly associated with nausea, sedation, and vomiting. Dezocine pharmacotherapy also has been associated with the following ADRs, listed according to body systems:

Cardiovascular: hypotension
CNS: anxiety, confusion, depression, dizziness, and headache
Cutaneous: edema, itching, local irritation at the injection site, rash, and redness of the skin
GI: constipation and dry mouth
Hematologic: low hemoglobin
Musculoskeletal: cramps and muscle pain
Ocular: blurred vision and double vision
Otic: congestion in the ears and ringing in the ears (tinnitus)
Respiratory: respiratory depression

See also "Opiate Analgesics, General Monograph."

OVERDOSAGE

Signs and symptoms of dezocine overdosage are similar to the signs and symptoms associated with other opiate analgesic overdosage (e.g., acute respiratory depression, cardiovascular compromise, and delirium). Dezocine overdosage requires emergency symptomatic medical support of body systems with attention to increasing dezocine elimination. Naloxone (Narcan®) is a specific and effective antidote.

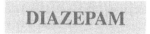

DIAZEPAM

(dye az′ e pam)

TRADE NAMES

Diazemuls®
Dizac®
Novo-Dipam®
Valium®
Vivol®

CLASSIFICATION

Anticonvulsant (sedative-hypnotic) (benzodiazepine) (C-IV)

See also "Benzodiazepines, General Monograph."

APPROVED INDICATIONS FOR NEUROPSYCHOLOGICAL DISORDERS

Pharmacotherapy for the prophylactic and symptomatic management of:

- seizure disorders: status epilepticus (acute repetitive seizures). Diazepam pharmacotherapy also is indicated for the prophylactic and symptomatic management of seizures associated with the acute alcohol withdrawal syndrome. Diazepam pharmacotherapy has been found to be of benefit for the management of the agitation, delirium tremens (impending or acute), hallucinations, tremor, and seizures associated with the acute alcohol withdrawal syndrome.
- skeletal muscle spasticity. Diazepam pharmacotherapy is indicated for the symptomatic management of skeletal muscle spasticity when it is associated with athetosis, stiff-man syndrome, tetanus, and upper motor neuron disorders (e.g., cerebral palsy, paraplegia).

USUAL DOSAGE AND ADMINISTRATION

Seizure Disorders: Status Epilepticus

Adults: 5 to 10 mg intravenously. Repeat dose at 10- to 15-minute intervals, if needed, to a maximum total dosage of 30 mg. The initial dose may be repeated in two to four hours, if needed. If preferred, rectal pharmacotherapy may be prescribed for use in either the home or hospital setting. See the "Notes, Seizure Disorders" and table "Diazepam Rectal Gel Dosing Guidelines."

MAXIMUM: 30 mg intravenously or 40 mg rectally per total episode of status epilepticus

For details and discussion regarding related basic principles of clinical pharmacology, readers are referred to the first text in this series, *The Pharmacologic Basis of Psychotherapeutics: An Introduction for Psychologists.*

Elderly, frail, or debilitated patients: 2 to 5 mg intravenously. Generally prescribe lower dosages for elderly, frail, or debilitated patients. Gradually increase the dosage, if needed, according to individual patient response. These patients may be more sensitive to the pharmacologic actions of diazepam than are younger or healthier adult patients. Intravenous injections of diazepam must be administered with extreme care among these patients and those who have cardiovascular or respiratory dysfunction. These patients are at particular risk for apnea and cardiac arrest associated with diazepam intravenous pharmacotherapy. Resuscitative equipment and emergency personnel should be readily available when intravenous diazepam pharmacotherapy is administered.

Children: Initially, 0.25 mg/kg intravenously. Slowly inject diazepam intravenously over a three-minute period. Do *not* exceed 0.25 mg/kg. After an interval of 15 to 30 minutes, the initial dose can be safely repeated, if needed. The initial dose may be repeated in two to four hours, if needed. These recommendations for injectable diazepam pharmacotherapy will help to assure maximal therapeutic benefit with the minimal dose of drug and will help to reduce the risk for serious ADRs (e.g., apnea or prolonged periods of somnolence). If the signs and symptoms are not managed after a third injection, other adjunctive therapy appropriate for the symptomatic management of status epilepticus is recommended. If preferred, rectal pharmacotherapy may be prescribed for use in either the home or hospital setting. See "Notes, Seizure Disorders" and the table "Diazepam Rectal Gel Dosing Guidelines."

MAXIMUM: 10 mg intravenously total dosage per episode of status epilepticus

Notes, Seizure Disorders

Adjust the diazepam dosage according to individual patient response for optimal therapeutic benefit. While most patients will benefit from usual recommended dosages, some patients may require higher dosages. Once seizures (i.e., status epilepticus) have been terminated, appropriate supportive measures should be implemented. Maintenance anticonvulsant pharmacotherapy should be initiated immediately.

Diazepam injectable pharmacotherapy: Patients should be lying down for injectable pharmacotherapy. Monitor patients carefully following injectable diazepam pharmacotherapy until complete alertness and psychomotor functions are restored. Do not mix or dilute the injectable formulation with other drugs or solutions in the syringe or intravenous solution. Injectable diazepam is contraindicated for patients who are in shock or coma, are acutely intoxicated with alcohol, or have cardiovascular and respiratory depression. Once acute signs and symptoms have been appropriately managed with injectable diazepam pharmacotherapy, replace the injectable pharmacotherapy with oral diazepam pharmacotherapy, if further pharmacotherapy is required.

INTRAMUSCULAR PHARMACOTHERAPY: Inject diazepam deeply intramuscularly into healthy muscle sites. Rotate injection sites carefully if more than one injection is required.

INTRAVENOUS PHARMACOTHERAPY: Facilities and personnel for emergency medical support of respiratory function should be readily available when intravenous pharmacotherapy is initiated. To reduce possible venous thrombosis, phlebitis, local irritation, and swelling associated with intravenous injection and, rarely, vascular impairment, slowly inject intravenously, taking at least one minute for each 5 mg (1 ml) injected. Avoid injecting the small veins on the back of the hand or near the wrist. Assure correct placement of the needle or catheter in the vein before injection and use extreme care to avoid extravasation or intra-arterial injection. Diazepam may be slowly injected intravenously through the tubing of a patent continuous intravenous infusion at an intravenous port as close as possible to the vein insertion site.

Diazepam rectal pharmacotherapy: Diazepam pharmacotherapy with the rectal gel formulation (Diastat®) is indicated for the symptomatic management of acute repetitive seizures among selected refractory patients who have seizure disorders and are generally stabilized on other anticonvulsant pharmacotherapy. These patients may require intermittent diazepam rectal gel pharmacotherapy to control acute episodes of seizure activity. Diazepam rectal gel pharmacotherapy may be administered in the home setting by a family member or other caregiver during an acute repetitive seizure to stop the seizure. It is generally recommended that diazepam rectal gel be used only once in any five-day period for the treatment of acute repetitive seizures and for no more than five such episodes per month.

Doses of the diazepam rectal gel for children range from 0.3 to 0.5 mg/kg. Doses for adults are generally 0.2 mg/kg. The initial dose may be repeated in four to twelve hours, if needed. See the table "Diazepam Rectal Gel Dosing Guidelines," for additional information.

Diazepam rectal gel dosing guidelines. *

Children				Adolescents and adults	
2 to 5 years of age (0.5 mg/kg)		6 to 11 years of age (0.3 mg/kg)		12+ years of age (0.2 mg/kg)	
Weight (kg)	Dose (mg)	Weight (kg)	Dose (mg)	Weight (kg)	Dose (mg)
6 to 11	5	10 to 18	5	14 to 27	5
12 to 22	10	19 to 37	10	28 to 50	10
23 to 33	15	38 to 55	15	51 to 75	15
34 to 44	20	56 to 74	20	76 to 111	20

* **Note that because the diazepam rectal gel is only available in fixed, unit-doses of 5, 10, 15, and 20 mg, the prescribed dosage is obtained by rounding upward to the next available dosage.**

Diazepam rectal gel should *only* be administered by family members or others involved with the patient's care who are, in the opinion of the prescribing psychologist, able to meet the following criteria: 1) they are able to distinguish the distinct cluster of seizures (and/or the events presumed to herald their onset) from the patient's usual seizure activity; 2) they have received adequate instruction concerning the administration of diazepam rectal gel; 3) they are evaluated as being competent to safely administer the diazepam rectal gel; 4) they explicitly understand the indication for the administration of diazepam rectal gel (i.e., they can differentiate the types of seizure activity that should and should not be treated with diazepam rectal gel); 5) they are able to appropriately monitor the patient's clinical response to diazepam rectal gel pharmacotherapy; and 6) they are competent to evaluate the patient's response and determine when therapeutic response may be sufficiently inadequate or inappropriate so as to warrant action to secure immediate supportive medical intervention (e.g., calling for emergency assistance and/or an ambulance for transporting the patient to a hospital emergency department).

Skeletal Muscle Spasticity

Adults: 5 to 10 mg intravenously. Repeat the dose in three or four hours, if needed, according to individual patient response.

Women who are, or who may become, pregnant: FDA Pregnancy Category D. An increased risk for congenital malformations (e.g., cleft lip and palate, limb and digit malformations) has been associated with diazepam pharmacotherapy during the first trimester of pregnancy. However, data are inconclusive. Maternal use near term has been associated with expected pharmacologic actions among neonates, including: hypotonia, low Apgar scores, poor feeding, and signs and symptoms of the neonatal benzodiazepine withdrawal syndrome. Avoid prescribing diazepam pharmacotherapy to women who are pregnant. If diazepam pharmacotherapy is required, advise patients of potential benefits and possible risks to themselves and the embryo, fetus, or neonate. Collaboration with the patient's obstetrician is indicated.

Women who are breast-feeding: Safety and efficacy of diazepam pharmacotherapy for women who are breast-feeding and their neonates and infants have not been established. Diazepam is excreted in breast milk in sufficient quantities to cause sedation and addiction among breast-fed neonates and infants. Avoid prescribing diazepam pharmacotherapy to women who are breast-feeding. If diazepam pharmacotherapy is required, breast-feeding probably should be discontinued. If desired, lactation may be maintained and breast-feeding resumed following the discontinuation of short-term diazepam pharmacotherapy. Collaboration with the patient's pediatrician is indicated.

Notes, Skeletal Muscle Spasticity

See "Notes, Seizure Disorders."

Seizures and Other Symptoms Associated With the Acute Alcohol Withdrawal Syndrome

Adults: Initially, 30 to 40 mg orally during the first 24 hours in three or four divided doses. Depending on the severity of the patient's signs and symptoms, reduce the dosage to 15 to 20 mg daily orally in three or four divided doses, as needed. Some patients may require initially, 10 mg intramuscularly or intravenously. This dose may be followed by an additional dose of 5 to 10 mg intramuscularly or intravenously in three or four hours, if needed.

Women who are, or who may become, pregnant: See the "Skeletal Muscle Spasticity" subsection of "Usual Dosage and Administration," above.

Women who are breast-feeding: See the "Skeletal Muscle Spasticity" subsection of "Usual Dosage and Administration," above.

Elderly, frail, or debilitated patients: Initially, 15 mg daily orally in three divided doses. Gradually increase the dosage, if needed, according to individual patient response. Generally prescribe lower dosages for elderly, frail, or debilitated patients. These patients may be more sensitive to the pharmacologic actions of diazepam than are younger or healthier adult patients.

Children: Safety and efficacy of diazepam pharmacotherapy for the symptomatic manage-ment of the acute alcohol withdrawal syndrome for children have not been established. Diazepam pharmacotherapy is *not* recommended for this indication for this age group.

Notes, Alcohol Withdrawal Syndrome

See "Notes, Seizure Disorders."

AVAILABLE DOSAGE FORMS, STORAGE, AND COMPATIBILITY

Capsules, oral extended-release (Valrelease®): 15 mg
Gel, rectal (Diastat®): 2.5, 5, 10, 15, 20 mg (see Notes)
Injectable, intramuscular or intravenous (Diazemuls®): 5 mg/ml (oil/water emulsion)
Injectable, intravenous (Dizac®, Zetran®): 5 mg/ml
Injectable, Tel-E-Ject® disposable syringe: 5 mg/ml
Solution, oral: 1 mg/ml
Solution, oral concentrate (Diazepam Intensol®): 5 mg/ml (contains 19% alcohol)
Tablets, oral: 2, 5, 10 mg

Notes

Diazepam injectable formulations: Diazepam injectable emulsion (Diazemuls®) is for intramuscular and intravenous use. Diazemuls® is incompatible with morphine and glycopyr-rolate (Robinul®). For intravenous injection, do *not* administer with intravenous infusion sets containing polyvinyl chloride. Only use glass, polyethylene, or polyethylene/polypropylene sy-ringes and infusion sets for intravenous diazepam pharmacotherapy.

Diazepam injectable (Dizac®, Valium®, Zetran®) contains benzyl alcohol, ethanol, and propylene glycol and is for intravenous injection *only*. Safely store the diazepam injectable, pro-tected from light at room temperature below 25 °C (77 °F). Avoid freezing. Diazepam injectable is incompatible with morphine and glycopyrrolate (Robinul®). It generally is recommended to *avoid* mixing injectable diazepam in the same syringe with other drugs or intravenous fluids.

Diazepam oral formulations: Do not confuse the regular diazepam oral solution with the concentrated oral solution. Serious overdosage may result.

Diazepam rectal formulation: The diazepam rectal gel is formulated as a non-sterile gel with benzyl alcohol, ethanol (10%), and propylene glycol. It is available in a pre-filled, unit-dose rectal delivery system. The rectal delivery system includes a plastic applicator with a flexi-ble, molded tip available in two lengths. These lengths are specifically designated as "pediatric" (4.4 cm) and "adult" (6 cm).

General instructions for patients: Instruct patients who are receiving diazepam pharma-cotherapy to

- safely store diazepam oral and rectal dosage forms out of the reach of children in tightly closed, child- and light-resistant containers at controlled room temperature (15° to 30 °C; 59° to 86 °F).

- obtain an available patient information sheet regarding diazepam pharmacotherapy from their pharmacist at the time that their prescription is dispensed. Encourage patients to clarify any questions that they may have regarding diazepam pharmacotherapy with their pharmacist or, if needed, to consult their prescribing psychologist.

PROPOSED MECHANISM OF ACTION

The exact mechanism of action of diazepam has not yet been fully determined. However, it appears to be primarily mediated by, or to work in concert with, the inhibitory neurotransmitter, GABA. Thus, diazepam appears to act by binding to the benzodiazepine receptors within the GABA complex.

See also "Benzodiazepines, General Monograph."

PHARMACOKINETICS/PHARMACODYNAMICS

Diazepam is virtually completely absorbed following oral ingestion ($F \approx 1$) and rectal insertion ($F = 0.9$). Peak blood concentrations are achieved within 1 to 2 hours following either oral ingestion or rectal insertion. Following intravenous injection, peak blood concentrations are achieved within 15 minutes. Although absorption following intramuscular injection may be erratic depending upon blood flow to intramuscular sites, peak absorption usually occurs within 2 hours. Diazepam is highly plasma protein bound (~98%) and has an apparent volume of distribution of ~1 liter/kg. It is extensively metabolized in the liver to both active (e.g., desmethyldiazepam, oxazepam) and inactive metabolites. Less than 1% is excreted in unchanged form in the urine. The mean half-life of elimination is 43 hours and the mean total body clearance is 28 ml/minute.

Therapeutic Drug Monitoring

Therapeutic and toxic blood concentrations for diazepam have *not* been established. However, it has been reported that anxiolytic actions occur at blood concentrations in the range of 300 to 400 ng/ml. Anticonvulsant actions generally occur at blood concentrations in excess of 600 ng/ml.

RELATIVE CONTRAINDICATIONS

Glaucoma, acute narrow-angle. Diazepam pharmacotherapy may be prescribed to patients who have open-angle glaucoma and who are receiving appropriate pharmacotherapy. Collaboration with the patient's ophthalmologist is indicated. See "Benzodiazepines, General Monograph."
Hypersensitivity to diazepam or other benzodiazepines

CAUTIONS AND COMMENTS

Diazepam pharmacotherapy may result in addiction and habituation. Abrupt discontinuation of long-term, high-dosage pharmacotherapy, or regular personal use, has been associated with the benzodiazepine withdrawal syndrome, which is similar to the alcohol or barbiturate withdrawal syndromes. Signs and symptoms of the diazepam withdrawal syndrome include abdominal and muscle cramps, convulsions, tremor, vomiting, and sweating. Milder withdrawal signs and symptoms, such as dysphoria and insomnia, have been associated with the abrupt discontinuation of benzodiazepine pharmacotherapy among patients who were receiving recommended dosages over several months. Avoid discontinuing diazepam pharmacotherapy abruptly, particularly when pharmacotherapy has been extended over several months. In this clinical situation, a gradual reduction of dosage is recommended for discontinuing diazepam pharmacotherapy.

Prescribe diazepam pharmacotherapy cautiously to patients who

- have depression, severe or latent.
- have kidney or liver dysfunction.
- have histories of problematic patterns of alcohol or other abusable psychotropic use. Diazepam can produce addiction and habituation. Monitor patients closely for signs and symptoms of problematic patterns of use.

Caution patients who are receiving diazepam pharmacotherapy against

- drinking alcohol or using other drugs that produce CNS depression while receiving diazepam pharmacotherapy. The depressant actions of these drugs may be additive.
- increasing their prescribed dosages, using their diazepam more frequently than prescribed, or abruptly discontinuing their pharmacotherapy without first consulting with their prescribing psychologist. Diazepam may produce addiction and habituation. A withdrawal syndrome has been associated with abrupt discontinuation.
- performing activities that require alertness, judgment, or physical coordination (e.g., driving an automobile, operating dangerous equipment, supervising children) until their response to diazepam pharmacotherapy is known. Diazepam's associated CNS depressant action may affect these mental and physical functions adversely.

In addition to these general precautions for patients, caution women who are receiving diazepam pharmacotherapy to

- inform their prescribing psychologist if they become or intend to become pregnant while receiving diazepam pharmacotherapy so that their pharmacotherapy can be discontinued safely.

CLINICALLY SIGNIFICANT DRUG INTERACTIONS

Concurrent diazepam pharmacotherapy and the following may result in clinically significant drug interactions:

Alcohol Use

Concurrent alcohol use may increase the CNS depressant action of diazepam. Advise patients to avoid, or limit, their use of alcohol while receiving diazepam pharmacotherapy.

Cimetidine Pharmacotherapy

Concurrent diazepam and cimetidine (Tagamet®) pharmacotherapy may result in the delayed or decreased elimination of diazepam. The clinical significance of this interaction is unclear.

Pharmacotherapy With CNS Depressants and Other Drugs That Produce CNS Depression

Concurrent diazepam pharmacotherapy with opiate analgesics, other sedative-hypnotics, or other drugs that produce CNS depression (e.g., antihistamines, phenothiazines, TCAs) may result in additive CNS depression.

See also "Benzodiazepines, General Monograph."

ADVERSE DRUG REACTIONS

Diazepam pharmacotherapy commonly has been associated with drowsiness, fatigue, and incoordination (ataxia). Hypotension and muscle weakness have been associated with injectable diazepam pharmacotherapy, particularly among patients who were using alcohol or who were concurrently receiving barbiturate or opiate analgesic pharmacotherapy. The intravenous injection of diazepam has been associated with phlebitis and venous thrombosis at the injection site. Other ADRs associated with diazepam pharmacotherapy, listed according to body system, include:

Cardiovascular: bradycardia, cardiovascular collapse, fainting (syncope), and hypotension
CNS: confusion, depression, headache, hypoactivity, slurred speech, tremor, and vertigo. Paradoxical reactions, including anxiety (acute), hyperexcited states, hallucinations, insomnia, rage, sleep disturbances, and over-stimulation have been reported. If these ADRs are observed, discontinue diazepam pharmacotherapy. Minor changes in EEG pattern, usually low-voltage, fast activity, also have been observed among patients during and following diazepam pharmacotherapy. These changes are of no known clinical significance.
Cutaneous: hives (urticaria) and skin rash
Genitourinary: urinary incontinence and urinary retention
GI: changes in salivation, constipation, fecal incontinence, hiccups, and nausea
Hematologic: decreased neutrophils (neutropenia)
Hepatic: jaundice
Musculoskeletal: difficult and defective speech due to impairment of the tongue or other muscles essential to speech (dysarthria), muscle spasms, and tremor
Ocular: blurred vision; constant, involuntary, cyclical movement of the eyeball (nystagmus); and double vision (diplopia)
Miscellaneous: changes in sex drive

See also "Benzodiazepines, General Monograph."

OVERDOSAGE

Signs and symptoms of diazepam overdosage include confusion, somnolence, coma, and diminished reflexes. Diazepam overdosage requires emergency symptomatic medical support of body systems with attention to increasing diazepam elimination. Flumazenil (Anexate®, Romazicon®), the benzodiazepine antagonist, may be required. See flumazenil monograph.

DIHYDROERGOTAMINE

(dye hye droe er got′ a meen)

TRADE NAMES

DHE-45®
Migranol®

CLASSIFICATION

Antimigraine (ergot alkaloid)

APPROVED INDICATIONS FOR NEUROPSYCHOLOGICAL DISORDERS

Adjunctive pharmacotherapy for the symptomatic management of:

- vascular headache: migraine headache. Dihydroergotamine pharmacotherapy is indicated for the symptomatic management of acute migraine headache with or without aura (see "Relative Contraindications").
- vascular headache: cluster and other vascular headaches. Dihydroergotamine pharmacotherapy is indicated for the symptomatic management of cluster and other vascular headaches when rapid relief is desired.

USUAL DOSAGE AND ADMINISTRATION

Vascular Headache

Adults: Dosage is prescribed according to injectable or intranasal dihydroergotamine pharmacotherapy.

INJECTABLE PHARMACOTHERAPY: 1 mg intramuscularly, intravenously (slowly), or subcutaneously at the first sign of headache. Dosage may be repeated, if required, after 60 minutes.
Maximum 3 mg intramuscularly or subcutaneously per attack or per day; *or* 2 mg intravenously (slowly) per attack or per day. The total *weekly* injectable dosage should not exceed 6 mg.

INTRANASAL PHARMACOTHERAPY: Initially, 0.5 mg intranasal spray in each nostril. Repeat 0.5 mg intranasal spray in each nostril after 15 minutes.
Maximum Intranasal pharmacotherapy, 2 mg daily intranasally

For details and discussion regarding related basic principles of clinical pharmacology, readers are referred to the first text in this series, *The Pharmacologic Basis of Psychotherapeutics: An Introduction for Psychologists.*

Women who are, or who may become, pregnant: FDA Pregnancy Category "not established." Dihydroergotamine pharmacotherapy is contraindicated during pregnancy because it has been associated with teratogenic effects (i.e., congenital or birth defects) in animal studies (see "Relative Contraindications"). In addition, dihydroergotamine possesses oxytoxic actions.

Women who are breast-feeding: Safety and efficacy of dihydroergotamine pharmacotherapy for women who are breast-feeding and their neonates and infants have not been established. Avoid prescribing dihydroergotamine pharmacotherapy to women who are breast-feeding. If dihydroergotamine pharmacotherapy is required, breast-feeding probably should be discontinued. If desired, lactation may be maintained and breast-feeding resumed following the discontinuation of short-term dihydroergotamine pharmacotherapy.

Elderly, frail, or debilitated patients: Initially, generally prescribe lower dosages of dihydroergotamine for elderly, frail, or debilitated patients. These patients may be more sensitive to the pharmacologic actions of dihydroergotamine than are younger or healthier adult patients.

Children and adolescents younger than 18 years of age: Safety and efficacy of dihydroergotamine pharmacotherapy for children and adolescents who are younger than 18 years of age have not been established. Dihydroergotamine pharmacotherapy is *not* recommended for this age group.

Notes, Vascular Headaches

Following the initial dose of dihydroergotamine, instruct patients to lie down in a quiet, cool, darkened room for maximal effect.

AVAILABLE DOSAGE FORMS, STORAGE, AND COMPATIBILITY

Spray, intranasal: 4 mg (in 1-ml glass ampule) (see "Notes").
Injectables, intramuscular, intravenous, subcutaneous: 1 mg/ml (contains ~5% alcohol)

Notes

Dihydroergotamine injectable formulation: Dihydroergotamine decomposes upon exposure to air. Therefore, the injectable should be prepared immediately prior to use. The unused contents of opened ampules should be appropriately discarded within 8 hours after opening. Also discard in a safe and appropriate manner injectable solutions that have become discolored. Slowly inject intravenously in order to reduce the risk of severe vasospasm. Pretreatment with an antiemetic may be considered to prevent vomiting occasionally associated with intravenous dihydroergotamine pharmacotherapy (not migraine related vomiting).

Dihydroergotamine intranasal formulation: The dihydroergotamine intranasal spray is provided as a kit containing four unit dose trays, an assembly case, a patient instruction booklet, and a patient information sheet. Each tray contains 4 mg of dihydroergotamine in a 1-ml glass ampule, a nasal spray applicator, and an ampule breaker cap that is attached to the ampule. Prior to administration, prime the pump of the nasal spray applicator by squeezing four times.

General instructions for patients: Instruct patients who are receiving dihydroergotamine pharmacotherapy to

- safely store dihydroergotamine intranasal spray kits and injectables out of the reach of children in light- and child-resistant containers at controlled room temperature (15° to 25 °C; 59° to 77 °F).
- safely and appropriately discard, within 8 hours, any dihydroergotamine remaining in the opened ampule together with the nasal spray applicator.
- obtain an available patient information sheet regarding dihydroergotamine pharmacotherapy from their pharmacist at the time that their prescription is dispensed. Encourage patients to clarify any questions that they may have regarding dihydroergotamine pharmacotherapy with their pharmacist or, if needed, to consult their prescribing psychologist.

PROPOSED MECHANISM OF ACTION

Dihydroergotamine is an ergot alkaloid that has potent vasoconstricting actions. It is a catecholamine-, dopamine-, and serotonin-receptor agonist. Dihydroergotamine also displays blocking action at alpha-adrenergic receptors and has a direct stimulating effect upon the smooth muscle of peripheral blood vessels. The exact mechanism of its antimigraine action has not yet been fully determined. However, it appears to relieve migraine headache pain by means of serotonin (i.e., 5-HT$_{1D}$) receptor-mediated vasoconstriction. It may also act by preventing the release of inflammatory peptides from sensory nerve endings in the trigeminal system.

PHARMACOKINETICS/PHARMACODYNAMICS

Dihydroergotamine has limited oral bioavailability. Thus, dihydroergotamine pharmacotherapy is prescribed for intramuscular, intravenous, or subcutaneous injection or intranasal insufflation. Dihydroergotamine is ~93% protein bound and has an apparent volume of distribution of 30 liters/kg. The total body clearance is ~1.5 liters/minute. Clearance is predominantly by hepatic clearance (i.e., >90%). The major route of elimination is by way of the bile in the feces. Less than 10% is excreted in unchanged form in the urine. The half-life of elimination is ~15 hours.

RELATIVE CONTRAINDICATIONS

Arteriosclerosis, severe
Basilar migraine
Breast-feeding
Coronary artery spasm
Ergot pharmacotherapy, within the previous 24 hours
Hemiplegic migraine
Hepatic dysfunction, severe
Hypersensitivity to dihydroergotamine or other ergot alkaloids
Hypertension, uncontrolled
Ischemic heart disease
Peptic ulcer
Peripheral artery disease
Prinzmetal angina

Pregnancy
Pruritus, severe
Raynaud's disease
Renal dysfunction, severe
Sepsis
Shock
Thrombophlebitis
Vascular surgery, recent
Vasoconstrictor pharmacotherapy, concurrent
Vasospastic angina

CAUTIONS AND COMMENTS

Intra-arterial injection of dihydroergotamine may result in severe arterial spasm and must be avoided. Should inadvertent intra-arterial injection occur, an alpha-blocker, such as phentolamine (Regitine®, Rogitine®), should be administered immediately and the patient monitored appropriately.

CLINICALLY SIGNIFICANT DRUG INTERACTIONS

Dihydroergotamine pharmacotherapy and the following may result in clinically significant drug interactions:

Clarithromycin, Erythromycin, and Troleandomycin Antibiotic Pharmacotherapy

Clarithromycin (Biaxin®), erythromycin (E-mycin®), and troleandomycin (TAO®) may inhibit the hepatic metabolism of dihydroergotamine. Presumably, the mechanism of this interaction is by means of inhibition of the hepatic isoenzyme CYP450–3A4. Severe vasospastic reactions have occurred as a result of this interaction.

Sympathomimetic and Vasoconstrictor Pharmacotherapy

Concurrent sympathomimetic (e.g., phenylpropanolamine) or vasoconstrictor (e.g., epinephrine) pharmacotherapy and dihydroergotamine pharmacotherapy may result in hypertension.

ADVERSE DRUG REACTIONS

Dihydroergotamine pharmacotherapy has been commonly associated with altered taste perception (bitter or unusual taste) and nose or throat irritation. Dihydroergotamine pharmacotherapy also has been associated with the following ADRs, listed according to body system:

Cardiovascular: bradycardia or tachycardia (transient) and vasospasm (potentially severe, particularly with the intravenous injection of high dosages)
CNS: dizziness
Cutaneous: itching and localized edema

GI: nausea and vomiting
Musculoskeletal: muscle pain and a sensation of leg weakness
Respiratory: runny nose (rhinitis)
Miscellaneous: numbness or tingling sensation in the fingers and toes

OVERDOSAGE

Signs and symptoms of dihydroergotamine overdosage include coma, confusion, dizziness, drowsiness, increased heart rate over 100 beats per minute (tachycardia), nausea, and vomiting. Numbness, tingling, and pain in the extremities also may occur due to associated ischemia. Acute dihydroergotamine overdosage requires emergency symptomatic medical support of body systems with attention to the elimination of dihydroergotamine. Measures aimed at the prevention of tissue damage (e.g., local application of warmth) also are required. There is no known antidote. However, in cases of severe vasospasm, the use of potent vasodilators, such as sodium nitroprusside (Nipride®), may be indicated.

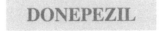

DONEPEZIL

(doe nep′ ih zil)

TRADE NAME

Aricept®

CLASSIFICATION

Nootropic (cholinesterase inhibitor)

APPROVED INDICATIONS FOR NEUROPSYCHOLOGICAL DISORDERS

Adjunctive pharmacotherapy for the symptomatic management of:

- dementia of the Alzheimer's type, mild to moderate

USUAL DOSAGE AND ADMINISTRATION

Dementia of the Alzheimer's Type, Mild to Moderate

Adults: Initially, 5 mg daily orally in a single evening dose 30 minutes before retiring for bed in the evening. Once steady state has been achieved (after ∼ two weeks), increase the dosage to 10 mg, according to individual patient response. Although the daily dosage may be increased at this time, it is generally recommended that the 5-mg daily oral dosage be continued for four to six weeks before increasing the dosage (see "Notes").

MAXIMUM: 10 mg daily orally

Women who are, or who may become, pregnant: FDA Pregnancy Category C. Safety and efficacy of donepezil pharmacotherapy for women who are pregnant have not been established. Avoid prescribing donepezil pharmacotherapy to women who are pregnant.

Women who are breast-feeding: Safety and efficacy of donepezil pharmacotherapy for women who are breast-feeding and their neonates and infants have not been established. Avoid prescribing donepezil pharmacotherapy to women who are breast-feeding.

Elderly, frail, or debilitated patients: Adjustment of the usual recommended adult dosage generally is not required when prescribing donepezil pharmacotherapy for elderly patients. Donepezil was developed primarily for use among this population group. However, a

For details and discussion regarding related basic principles of clinical pharmacology, readers are referred to the first text in this series, *The Pharmacologic Basis of Psychotherapeutics: An Introduction for Psychologists.*

significantly increased incidence of ADRs has been noted among older elderly (i.e., those elderly who are 85 years of age or older) who generally have low body weight. It is generally recommended that the donepezil dosage *not* exceed 5 mg daily orally for these patients.

Children and adolescents younger than 18 years of age: Safety and efficacy of donepezil pharmacotherapy for children and adolescents who are younger than 18 years of age have not been established. Donepezil pharmacotherapy is *not* recommended for this age group.

Notes, Dementia of the Alzheimer's Type, Mild to Moderate

Gradually increasing the dosage of donepezil from 5 mg daily to 10 mg daily over a six-week period has been associated with a significant decrease in the incidence of ADRs.

AVAILABLE DOSAGE FORMS, STORAGE, AND COMPATIBILITY

Tablets, oral: 5, 10 mg

Notes

General instructions for patients: Instruct patients who are receiving donepezil pharmacotherapy, or those assisting with their pharmacotherapy, to

- safely store donepezil oral tablets out of the reach of children in tightly closed, child-resistant containers at controlled room temperature (15° to 30°C; 59° to 86°F).
- obtain an available patient information sheet regarding donepezil pharmacotherapy from their pharmacist at the time that their prescription is dispensed. Encourage patients, or those assisting them with their pharmacotherapy, to clarify any questions that they may have regarding donepezil pharmacotherapy with their pharmacist or, if needed, to consult their prescribing psychologist.

PROPOSED MECHANISM OF ACTION

It has been hypothesized that the predominant clinical manifestations of Alzheimer's disease are caused by the degeneration of cholinergic neuronal pathways within the CNS. Donepezil is a piperidine-based, reversible inhibitor of acetylcholinesterase. Thus, donepezil appears to enhance cholinergic function among patients who have this disease by inhibiting the metabolic degradation of the neurotransmitter, acetylcholine. This inhibition of acetylcholine degradation, in turn, increases the concentration of acetylcholine at its sites of action along the cholinergic neuronal pathways. Although donepezil pharmacotherapy may be of benefit to patients who have Alzheimer's dementia, unfortunately it does not alter the underlying pathology or clinical course of this disease.

PHARMACOKINETICS/PHARMACODYNAMICS

Donepezil is completely absorbed from the GI tract following oral ingestion ($F = 1$). Peak blood concentrations are achieved within 3 to 4 hours. Neither food nor time of dose (i.e., morning or evening) affect donepezil's oral bioavailability. Donepezil is highly plasma protein bound ($\sim$12 liters/kg). Approximately 17% of donepezil is eliminated in unchanged form in the urine. The remainder is extensively metabolized in the liver, principally by CYP450 isoenzymes 2D6 and 3A4. The half-life of elimination is $\sim$70 hours. The total body clearance is $\sim$0.13 liters/hour/kg.

RELATIVE CONTRAINDICATIONS

Hypersensitivity to donepezil or to piperidine derivatives

CAUTIONS AND COMMENTS

Prescribe donepezil pharmacotherapy cautiously to patients who

- are 85 years of age or older. The incidence of ADRs associated with donepezil pharmacotherapy increases significantly in this age group. Women who are 85 years of age or older and who also have low body weight are at particular risk for experiencing ADRs associated with donepezil pharmacotherapy.
- are receiving succinylcholine (Anectine®) or related neuromuscular blocker pharmacotherapy. Donepezil decreases the metabolism of succinylcholine by inhibiting plasma cholinesterase. This action may enhance neuromuscular blockade and associated respiratory paralysis significantly.

CLINICALLY SIGNIFICANT DRUG INTERACTIONS

Donepezil pharmacotherapy has not been demonstrated to significantly interact with other drugs. However, because of its mechanism of action as a cholinesterase inhibitor, donepezil is expected to have the potential to significantly interact with anticholinergic (e.g., atropine and benztropine [Cogentin®]) and cholinergic (e.g., bethanechol [Urecholine®]) agonists. When concurrent pharmacotherapy is required, collaboration with the prescriber of the anticholinergic or cholinergic agonists is indicated. (See also "Cautions and Comments.")

ADVERSE DRUG REACTIONS

Donepezil pharmacotherapy has been commonly associated with diarrhea, nausea, and vomiting. Donepezil pharmacotherapy also has been associated with the following ADRs, listed according to body systems:

CNS: abnormal dreams, dizziness, headache, and insomnia
GI: loss of appetite (anorexia)
Musculoskeletal: muscle cramps
Miscellaneous: fatigue

OVERDOSAGE

Signs and symptoms of donepezil overdosage are consistent with cholinergic crisis and include the following signs and symptoms: bradycardia, cardiovascular collapse, convulsions, hypotension, muscle weakness, nausea (severe), respiratory depression (which may be fatal), salivation (excessive), sweating (extreme), and vomiting. Donepezil overdosage requires emergency symptomatic medical support of body systems with attention to increasing donepezil elimination. The anticholinergic, atropine, is a specific antidote for donepezil overdosage.

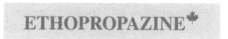

ETHOPROPAZINE⚜

(eth oh proe′ pa zeen)

TRADE NAME

Parsitan®

CLASSIFICATION

Antiparkinsonian (tertiary amine antimuscarinic, phenothiazine derivative)

APPROVED INDICATIONS FOR NEUROPSYCHOLOGICAL DISORDERS

Pharmacotherapy for the symptomatic management of:

- Parkinson's disease. Ethopropazine pharmacotherapy is indicated for the symptomatic management of the various forms of Parkinson's disease, including drug-induced Parkinson's disease.

USUAL DOSAGE AND ADMINISTRATION

Parkinson's Disease, Including Drug-Induced Parkinson's Disease

Adults: Initially, 150 mg daily orally in three divided doses. Increase the daily dosage by 50 to 100 mg at intervals of two or three days according to individual patient response. The usual effective dosage ranges from 100 to 500 mg daily.

MAXIMUM: 1000 mg daily orally

Women who are, or who may become, pregnant: FDA Pregnancy Category "not established." Safety and efficacy of ethopropazine pharmacotherapy for women who are pregnant have not been established. Avoid prescribing ethopropazine pharmacotherapy to women who are pregnant. If ethopropazine pharmacotherapy is required, advise patients of potential benefits and possible risks to themselves and the embryo, fetus, or neonate. Collaboration with the patient's obstetrician is indicated.

Women who are breast-feeding: Safety and efficacy of ethopropazine pharmacotherapy for women who are breast-feeding and their neonates and infants have not been established. Avoid prescribing ethopropazine pharmacotherapy to women who are breast-feeding. If ethopropazine pharmacotherapy is required, breast-feeding probably should be discontinued.

For details and discussion regarding related basic principles of clinical pharmacology, readers are referred to the first text in this series, *The Pharmacologic Basis of Psychotherapeutics: An Introduction for Psychologists.*

Elderly, frail, or debilitated patients: Generally prescribe lower dosages of etho-propazine for elderly, frail, or debilitated patients. These patients may be more sensitive to the pharmacologic actions of ethopropazine than are younger or healthier adult patients.

Children and adolescents younger than 18 years of age: Safety and efficacy of etho-propazine pharmacotherapy for children and adolescents who are younger than 18 years of age have not been established. Ethopropazine pharmacotherapy is *not* recommended for this age group.

AVAILABLE DOSAGE FORMS, STORAGE, AND COMPATIBILITY

Tablets, oral: 50 mg

Notes

General instructions for patients: Instruct patients who are receiving ethopropazine pharmacotherapy to

- safely store ethopropazine oral tablets out of the reach of children in tightly closed, light- and child-resistant containers at controlled room temperature (15 ° to 30 °C; 59 ° to 86 °F).
- obtain an available patient information sheet regarding ethopropazine pharmacotherapy from their pharmacist at the time that their prescription is dispensed. Encourage patients to clarify any questions that they may have regarding ethopropazine pharmacotherapy with their pharmacist or, if needed, to consult their prescribing psychologist.

PROPOSED MECHANISM OF ACTION

The exact mechanism of the antiparkinsonian action of ethopropazine has not yet been fully determined. However, it appears to involve its anticholinergic action.

PHARMACOKINETICS/PHARMACODYNAMICS

Data are not available.

RELATIVE CONTRAINDICATIONS

Glaucoma
Hypersensitivity to ethopropazine or other phenothiazines

CAUTIONS AND COMMENTS

Prescribe ethopropazine pharmacotherapy cautiously to patients who

- have cardiac dysfunction. The significant anticholinergic action of ethopropazine may affect this clinical condition adversely.
- have prostatic hypertrophy. The significant anticholinergic action of ethopropazine may affect this clinical condition adversely.
- have pyloric obstruction. The significant anticholinergic action of ethopropazine may affect this clinical condition adversely.

Caution patients who are receiving ethopropazine pharmacotherapy against

- performing activities that require alertness, judgment, and physical coordination (e.g., driving an automobile, operating dangerous equipment, supervising children) until their response to ethopropazine pharmacotherapy is known. Ethopropazine may affect these mental and physical functions adversely.

CLINICALLY SIGNIFICANT DRUG INTERACTIONS

Concurrent ethopropazine pharmacotherapy and the following may result in clinically significant drug interactions:

Alcohol Use

Concurrent alcohol use may increase the CNS depressant action of ethopropazine. Advise patients to avoid, or limit, their use of alcohol while receiving ethopropazine pharmacotherapy.

Pharmacotherapy With Anticholinergics or Other Drugs That Produce Anticholinergic Actions

Concurrent ethopropazine pharmacotherapy and pharmacotherapy with anticholinergics (e.g., atropine) or other drugs that produce anticholinergic actions (e.g., phenothiazines, TCAs) may produce additive, and potentially toxic anticholinergic effects (e.g., slowed heart rate below 60 beats per minute [bradycardia], intestinal obstruction).

Pharmacotherapy With CNS Depressants and Other Drugs That Produce CNS Depression

Concurrent ethopropazine pharmacotherapy and pharmacotherapy with opiate analgesics, sedative-hypnotics, or other drugs that produce CNS depression (e.g., antihistamines, phenothiazines, TCAs) may result in additive CNS depression.

ADVERSE DRUG REACTIONS

Ethopropazine pharmacotherapy has commonly been associated with blurred vision, dizziness, drowsiness, dry mouth, headache, lassitude, and paresthesia. Ethopropazine pharmacotherapy also has been associated with the following ADRs, listed according to body system:

CNS: confusion and, rarely, incoordination (ataxia)

GI: rarely, epigastric distress

Miscellaneous: neuroleptic malignant syndrome. The major signs and symptoms of this syndrome include the following: altered mental status, autonomic nervous system instability (e.g., abnormal blood pressure or pulse), increased body temperature (hyperpyrexia), and muscle rigidity.

OVERDOSAGE

Clinical data concerning ethopropazine overdosage are not available. In the absence of such data, ethopropazine overdosage should be treated as a medical emergency requiring symptomatic support of body systems with attention to increasing ethopropazine elimination. There is no known antidote.

ETHOSUXIMIDE

(eth oh sux′ i mide)

TRADE NAME

Zarontin®

CLASSIFICATION

Anticonvulsant (succinimide derivative)

APPROVED INDICATIONS FOR NEUROPSYCHOLOGICAL DISORDERS

Adjunctive pharmacotherapy for the symptomatic management of:

* seizure disorders: absence (petit mal) seizures

USUAL DOSAGE AND ADMINISTRATION

Seizure Disorders: Absence (Petit Mal) Seizures

Adults: 20 mg/kg daily orally in a single dose or two divided doses

MAXIMUM: 1500 mg daily orally

Women who are, or who may become, pregnant: FDA Pregnancy Category C. Safety and efficacy of ethosuximide pharmacotherapy for women who are pregnant have not been established. However, fetal malformations, including accessory nipples and mongoloid facies, and decreased scores for gross motor index scores, have been reported among ~5% of infants who have been pre-natally exposed to ethosuximide. Thus, ethosuximide is probably a human teratogen. Avoid prescribing ethosuximide pharmacotherapy to women who are pregnant. If ethosuximide pharmacotherapy is required, advise patients of potential benefits and possible risks to themselves and the embryo, fetus, or neonate. Collaboration with the patient's obstetrician is indicated.

Women who are breast-feeding: Safety and efficacy of ethosuximide pharmacotherapy for women who are breast-feeding and their neonates and infants have not been established. However, ethosuximide is excreted in breast milk at ~80% of the maternal blood concentration. Avoid prescribing ethosuximide pharmacotherapy to women who are breast-feeding. If ethosuximide pharmacotherapy is required, breast-feeding probably should be discontinued. If desired, lactation may be maintained and breast-feeding resumed following the discontinuation of short-term ethosuximide pharmacotherapy.

For details and discussion regarding related basic principles of clinical pharmacology, readers are referred to the first text in this series, *The Pharmacologic Basis of Psychotherapeutics: An Introduction for Psychologists.*

Elderly, frail, or debilitated patients: Initially, 500 mg daily orally in divided doses. Gradually increase the dosage by 250 mg every four to seven days, if needed, according to individual patient response. Generally prescribe lower dosages of ethosuximide for elderly, frail, or debilitated patients. These patients may be more sensitive to the pharmacologic actions of ethosuximide than are younger or healthier adult patients.

Children younger than 6 years of age: Initially, 250 mg daily orally in divided doses. Gradually adjust the dosage according to individual patient response.

Children older than 6 years of age: See information for adults, earlier in this section.

Notes, Seizure Disorders: Absence (Petit Mal) Seizures

Pharmacotherapy with ethosuximide alone for the treatment of mixed seizures may increase the incidence of tonic-clonic seizures. Adjunctive phenobarbital or phenytoin (Dilantin®) pharmacotherapy may be required in this clinical situation.

Discontinuing ethosuximide pharmacotherapy: Discontinue ethosuximide pharmacotherapy gradually in order to avoid precipitating seizures, including status epilepticus. Reduce the dosage over a period of several days before completely discontinuing ethosuximide pharmacotherapy.

AVAILABLE DOSAGE FORMS, STORAGE, AND COMPATIBILITY

Capsules, oral: 250 mg
Syrup, oral: 240 mg/5 ml (contains 3% alcohol) (raspberry flavored)

Notes

General instructions for patients: Instruct patients who are receiving ethosuximide pharmacotherapy to

- safely store ethosuximide oral capsules and the oral syrup out of the reach of children in tightly closed, light- and child-resistant containers at controlled room temperature (15° to 30°C; 59° to 86°F).
- obtain an available patient information sheet regarding ethosuximide pharmacotherapy from their pharmacist at the time that their prescription is dispensed. Encourage patients to clarify any questions that they may have regarding ethosuximide pharmacotherapy with their pharmacist or, if needed, to consult their prescribing psychologist.

PROPOSED MECHANISM OF ACTION

Ethosuximide appears to elicit its anticonvulsant action by the following mechanisms: 1) elevating the seizure threshold in the basal ganglia and cerebral cortex; and 2) reducing synaptic response to low-frequency repetitive stimulation. Ethosuximide suppresses the paroxysmal spike and wave pattern observed on the EEG, which is characteristic of absence seizures.

PHARMACOKINETICS/PHARMACODYNAMICS

Ethosuximide is absorbed from the GI tract following oral ingestion. Peak blood concentrations are achieved within 4 hours. Ethosuximide is only slightly protein bound. The apparent volume of distribution is ~0.7 liters/kg. Approximately 25% is eliminated in unchanged form in the urine. Total body clearance is ~15 ml/minute. The half-life of elimination is ~60 hours among adults and ~30 hours among children. Additional data are not available.

Therapeutic Drug Monitoring

Therapeutic blood concentrations of ethosuximide reportedly range from 40 to 100 µg/ml.

RELATIVE CONTRAINDICATIONS

Hypersensitivity to ethosuximide or other succinimides.

CAUTIONS AND COMMENTS

Ethosuximide pharmacotherapy has been associated with potentially fatal blood disorders (i.e., blood dyscrasias) including agranulocytosis and aplastic anemia. Therefore, blood counts should be obtained before initiating pharmacotherapy and periodically during ethosuximide pharmacotherapy. Collaboration with the patient's advanced practice nurse or family physician may be indicated.

Prescribe ethosuximide pharmacotherapy cautiously to patients who

- have kidney dysfunction. Ethosuximide pharmacotherapy may cause microscopic hematuria. In addition, kidney dysfunction may result in a decreased rate of elimination and resultant accumulation of ethosuximide and possible toxicity. Periodic kidney function tests are recommended. Collaboration with the patient's advanced practice nurse, family physician, or other specialist (e.g., nephrologist) may be indicated.
- have liver dysfunction. Ethosuximide pharmacotherapy may cause both morphological and functional changes in the liver. In addition, liver dysfunction may result in a decreased rate of elimination with resultant accumulation of ethosuximide and possible toxicity. Periodic liver function tests are recommended. Collaboration with the patient's advanced practice nurse, family physician, or other specialists (e.g., internist) may be indicated.

Caution patients who are receiving ethosuximide pharmacotherapy against

- performing activities that require alertness, judgment, or physical coordination (e.g., driving an automobile, operating dangerous equipment, supervising children) until their response to ethosuximide pharmacotherapy is known. Ethosuximide may affect these mental and physical functions adversely.

CLINICALLY SIGNIFICANT DRUG INTERACTIONS

Concurrent ethosuximide pharmacotherapy and the following may result in clinically significant drug interactions:

Alcohol Use

Concurrent alcohol use may increase the CNS depressant action of ethosuximide. Advise patients to avoid, or limit, their use of alcohol while receiving ethosuximide pharmacotherapy.

Pharmacotherapy With CNS Depressants and Other Drugs That Produce CNS Depression

Concurrent ethosuximide pharmacotherapy and pharmacotherapy with opiate analgesics, sedative-hypnotics, or other drugs that produce CNS depression (e.g., antihistamines, phenothiazines, TCAs) may result in additive CNS depression.

ADVERSE DRUG REACTIONS

Ethosuximide pharmacotherapy has been commonly associated with abdominal pain, cramps, diarrhea, loss of appetite (anorexia), nausea, and vomiting. Ethosuximide pharmacotherapy also has been associated with the following ADRs, listed according to body system:

CNS: aggressiveness, depression, dizziness, drowsiness, fatigue, headache, incoordination (ataxia), insomnia, irritability, and paranoid psychosis (rare)

Cutaneous: hives (urticaria), itchy (pruritic) skin rashes, lupus erythematosus, and Stevens–Johnson syndrome

GI: gum hypertrophy and swelling of the tongue

Hematologic: agranulocytosis, aplastic anemia, eosinophilia, leukopenia, and pancytopenia. Periodic blood counts are recommended prior to and during ethosuximide pharmacotherapy.

Miscellaneous: increased sex drive (rare)

OVERDOSAGE

The signs and symptoms of ethosuximide overdosage include coma, nausea, respiratory depression, and vomiting. Ethosuximide overdosage requires emergency symptomatic medical support of body systems with attention to increasing ethosuximide elimination. There is no known antidote.

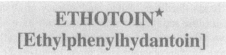

ETHOTOIN*
[Ethylphenylhydantoin]

(eth oh toyn′)

TRADE NAME

Peganone®

CLASSIFICATION

Anticonvulsant (hydantoin derivative)

APPROVED INDICATIONS FOR NEUROPSYCHOLOGICAL DISORDERS

Pharmacotherapy for the prophylactic and symptomatic management of:

- seizure disorders. Ethotoin pharmacotherapy is indicated for various seizure disorders including tonic-clonic (grand mal) seizures and partial seizures with complex symptomatology (i.e., psychomotor seizures).

USUAL DOSAGE AND ADMINISTRATION

Seizure Disorders

Adults: Initially, 1 gram daily orally in four to six divided doses. Gradually adjust the dosage over a period of several days, according to individual patient response.

MAINTENANCE: The usual daily maintenance dosage is 2 to 3 grams.

Women who are, or who may become, pregnant: FDA Pregnancy Category C. Safety and efficacy of ethotoin pharmacotherapy for women who are pregnant have not been established. However, exposure in utero has resulted in symptoms compatible with the fetal hydantoin syndrome (e.g., abnormal facies, cleft lip and palate, growth retardation). Ethotoin is probably a human teratogen. Avoid prescribing ethotoin pharmacotherapy to women who are pregnant. If ethotoin pharmacotherapy is required, advise patients of potential benefits and possible risks to themselves and the embryo, fetus, or neonate. Collaboration with the patient's obstetrician is indicated.

For details and discussion regarding related basic principles of clinical pharmacology, readers are referred to the first text in this series, *The Pharmacologic Basis of Psychotherapeutics: An Introduction for Psychologists.*

Women who are breast-feeding: Safety and efficacy of ethotoin pharmacotherapy for women who are breast-feeding and their neonates and infants have not been established. Ethotoin is excreted in breast milk. Avoid prescribing ethotoin pharmacotherapy to women who are breast-feeding. If ethotoin pharmacotherapy is required, breast-feeding should be discontinued. Collaboration with the patient's pediatrician may be indicated.

Elderly, frail, or debilitated patients: Generally prescribe lower dosages of ethotoin for elderly, frail, or debilitated patients. Gradually increase the dosage if needed, according to individual patient response. These patients may be more sensitive to the pharmacologic actions of ethotoin than are younger or healthier adult patients.

Children: 80 mg/kg daily orally in four to six divided doses

MAINTENANCE: The usual daily maintenance dosage is 0.5 to 1.5 grams.

Notes, Seizure Disorders

Generally, ethotoin is less effective, but also less toxic, than is phenytoin.

Discontinuing ethotoin pharmacotherapy: Whenever possible, discontinue ethotoin pharmacotherapy gradually in order to avoid associated seizures or status epilepticus.

AVAILABLE DOSAGE FORMS, STORAGE, AND COMPATIBILITY

Tablets, oral: 250, 500 mg

Notes

General instructions for patients: Instruct patients who are receiving ethotoin pharmacotherapy to

- safely store ethotoin oral tablets out of the reach of children in tightly closed, light- and child-resistant containers at controlled room temperature (15° to 30°C; 59° to 86°F).
- obtain an available patient information sheet regarding ethotoin pharmacotherapy from their pharmacist at the time that their prescription is dispensed. Encourage patients to clarify any questions that they may have regarding ethotoin pharmacotherapy with their pharmacist or, if needed, to consult their prescribing psychologist.

PROPOSED MECHANISM OF ACTION

The mechanism of the anticonvulsant action of ethotoin appears to be principally by means of the limitation of seizure propagation. The reduction of post-tetanic potentiation (PTP) of synaptic transmission occurs as a result of the reduction of the passive influx of sodium ions. The anticonvulsant action of ethotoin also appears to be associated with an increased efficacy of the sodium pump, which, in turn, prevents excess accumulation of intracellular sodium during tetanic stimulation.

PHARMACOKINETICS/PHARMACODYNAMICS

Ethotoin is rapidly absorbed from the GI tract following oral ingestion. However, the extent of ethotoin's absorption and bioavailability has not been determined. Ethotoin is extensively metabolized in the liver. Only a small percentage is excreted in unchanged form in the urine. Additional data are not available.

Therapeutic Drug Monitoring

A definitive therapeutic blood concentration range has not been established for ethotoin. However, a range of 15 to 50 µg/ml has been suggested.

RELATIVE CONTRAINDICATIONS

Hematologic disorders
Liver dysfunction
Phenacemide pharmacotherapy. Concurrent ethotoin and phenacemide (Phenurone®) pharmacotherapy has been associated with extreme signs and symptoms of paranoia.

CAUTIONS AND COMMENTS

Caution patients who are receiving ethotoin pharmacotherapy against

- performing activities that require alertness, judgment, or physical coordination (e.g., driving an automobile, operating dangerous equipment, supervising children) until their response to ethotoin pharmacotherapy is known. Ethotoin may affect these mental and physical functions adversely.

In addition to this general precaution, caution patients who are receiving ethotoin pharmacotherapy to

- monitor themselves for signs and symptoms associated with hematologic toxicity (e.g., easy bruising, fever, malaise, nosebleeds [epistaxis], petechiae, or sore throat). Advise patients to inform their prescribing psychologist immediately if any of these signs and symptoms are noted.

CLINICALLY SIGNIFICANT DRUG INTERACTIONS

Concurrent ethotoin pharmacotherapy and the following may result in clinically significant drug interactions:

Alcohol Use

Concurrent alcohol use may increase the CNS depressant action of ethotoin. Advise patients to avoid, or limit, their use of alcohol while receiving ethotoin pharmacotherapy.

Pharmacotherapy With CNS Depressants and Other Drugs That Produce CNS Depression

Concurrent ethotoin pharmacotherapy and pharmacotherapy with opiate analgesics, sedative-hypnotics, or other drugs that produce CNS depression (e.g., antihistamines, phenothiazines, TCAs) may result in additive CNS depression.

Phenacemide Pharmacotherapy

See "Relative Contraindications."

ADVERSE DRUG REACTIONS

Ethotoin pharmacotherapy has been associated with the following ADRs, listed according to body system:

Cardiovascular: chest pain
CNS: dizziness, fatigue, headache, incoordination (ataxia, rare), and insomnia
Cutaneous: rash
GI: diarrhea, nausea, and vomiting
Hematologic: various blood dyscrasias have been associated with ethotoin pharmacotherapy. However, the etiologic role of ethotoin in relation to the occurrence of these ADRs has not been established.
Ophthalmic: involuntary cyclical movement of the eyeball (nystagmus) and double vision (diplopia)
Miscellaneous: fever, inflammation and enlargement of the lymph nodes (lymphadenopathy), and, rarely, lupus erythematosus

OVERDOSAGE

The signs and symptoms of ethotoin overdosage include coma, dizziness, fatigue, hallucinations, hypotension, incoordination (ataxia), insomnia, motor restlessness, nausea, and vomiting. Ethotoin overdosage requires emergency symptomatic medical support of body systems with attention to increasing ethotoin elimination. There is no known antidote.

FELBAMATE*

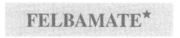

(fel′ ba mate)

TRADE NAME

Felbatol®

CLASSIFICATION

Anticonvulsant (dicarbamate)

APPROVED INDICATIONS FOR NEUROPSYCHOLOGICAL DISORDERS

Pharmacotherapy for the symptomatic management of:

- seizure disorders. Felbamate pharmacotherapy is indicated for the management of partial seizures with or without secondary generalization and for partial and generalized seizures associated with Lennox–Gastaut syndrome among children. However, felbamate pharmacotherapy is indicated *only* for patients whose seizures are refractory to safer anticonvulsant pharmacotherapy (see "Notes, Seizure Disorders").

USUAL DOSAGE AND ADMINISTRATION

Seizure Disorders

Adults: Initially, 1.2 grams daily orally in three or four divided doses. Increase the daily dosage at two-week intervals by increments of 600 mg according to individual patient response.

MAXIMUM: 3.6 grams daily orally

Women who are, or who may become, pregnant: FDA Pregnancy Category C. Safety and efficacy of felbamate pharmacotherapy for women who are pregnant have not been established. Avoid prescribing felbamate pharmacotherapy to women who are pregnant. If felbamate pharmacotherapy is required, advise patients of potential benefits and possible risks to themselves and the embryo, fetus, or neonate. Collaboration with the patient's obstetrician is indicated.

Women who are breast-feeding: Safety and efficacy of felbamate pharmacotherapy for women who are breast-feeding and their neonates and infants have not been established. Felbamate is excreted into breast milk. Avoid prescribing felbamate pharmacotherapy to women who are breast-feeding. If felbamate pharmacotherapy is required, breast-feeding probably should be discontinued. If desired, lactation may be maintained and breast-feeding resumed following the discontinuation of short-term felbamate pharmacotherapy.

For details and discussion regarding related basic principles of clinical pharmacology, readers are referred to the first text in this series, *The Pharmacologic Basis of Psychotherapeutics: An Introduction for Psychologists.*

Elderly, frail, or debilitated patients: Generally prescribe lower dosages of felbamate for elderly, frail, or debilitated patients. Gradually increase the dosage if needed, according to individual patient response. These patients may be more sensitive to the pharmacologic actions of felbamate than are younger or healthier adult patients.

Children 2 years of age and older: Felbamate pharmacotherapy is recommended *only* for the symptomatic management of partial and generalized seizures associated with Lennox–Gastaut syndrome among children 2 years of age and older. For these children, initially prescribe 15 mg/kg daily orally in three or four divided doses. Increase the daily dosage at weekly intervals by increments of 15 mg/kg, as indicated by individual patient response.

MAXIMUM: 45 mg/kg daily orally

Notes, Seizure Disorders

Felbamate pharmacotherapy is indicated only *for patients who have severe, refractory seizure disorders and for whom, in the opinion of the prescribing psychologist, the potential benefits of pharmacotherapy outweigh the potential risk for aplastic anemia and hepatic failure (see "Adverse Drug Reactions"). Felbamate pharmacotherapy should* not *be initiated until the patient, or his or her parents or legal guardian in the event the patient is a child, has been fully informed about these serious associated risks and has signed a specially developed "patient information/consent form." Collaboration with the patient's physician may be indicated.*
Additional data and copies of patient information/consent forms are available from the manufacturer, Carter-Wallace Laboratories, at 609-655-6147 or 1-800-526-3840, or from the U.S. FDA at 1-800-FDA-1088.

Discontinuing felbamate pharmacotherapy: Although not reported to date in the published clinical literature for felbamate, withdrawal seizures have been associated with the sudden discontinuation of other anticonvulsant pharmacotherapy and is a therapeutic concern in regard to discontinuing felbamate pharmacotherapy. Therefore, in order to avoid the risk for withdrawal seizures, it is generally recommended that felbamate pharmacotherapy be discontinued gradually over a period of 10 to 14 days.

AVAILABLE DOSAGE FORMS, STORAGE, AND COMPATIBILITY

Suspension, oral: 600 mg/5 ml (contains sodium saccharin)
Tablets, oral: 400, 600 mg

Notes

General instructions for patients: Instruct patients who are receiving felbamate pharmacotherapy, or their parents or legal guardians as appropriate in regard to the patient, to

- safely store the felbamate oral suspension and oral tablets out of the reach of children in tightly closed, child-resistant containers at controlled room temperature (15° to 30°C; 59° to 86°F).

- shake the oral suspension well before measuring each dose to help to assure that an accurate dose is measured and ingested.
- obtain an available patient information sheet regarding felbamate pharmacotherapy from their pharmacist at the time that their prescription is dispensed. Encourage patients, or their parents or legal guardians as appropriate, to clarify any questions that they may have regarding felbamate pharmacotherapy with their pharmacist or, if needed, to consult their prescribing psychologist.

PROPOSED MECHANISM OF ACTION

The exact mechanism of the anticonvulsant action of felbamate has not yet been determined. However, felbamate appears to increase the seizure threshold and reduce seizure spread primarily by means of the inhibition of voltage-dependent sodium ion channels.

PHARMACOKINETICS/PHARMACODYNAMICS

Felbamate is well absorbed following oral ingestion (>80%). Peak blood concentrations are obtained within 1 to 4 hours. Felbamate is ~25% bound to plasma proteins and has an apparent volume of distribution of ~0.8 liters/kg. Felbamate is metabolized in the liver and ~50% is excreted in unchanged form in the urine. The total body clearance of felbamate is ~30 ml/kg/hour. Its mean half-life of elimination is ~21 hours (range: 13 to 23 hours). Additional data are not available.

RELATIVE CONTRAINDICATIONS

Blood disorders, history of
Hypersensitivity to felbamate or other carbamates (e.g., meprobamate [Equanil®, Miltown®]).
Liver dysfunction, history of

CAUTIONS AND COMMENTS

Caution patients who are receiving felbamate pharmacotherapy against

- performing activities that require alertness, judgment, or physical coordination (e.g., driving an automobile, operating dangerous equipment, supervising children) until their response to felbamate pharmacotherapy is known. Felbamate may affect these mental and physical functions adversely.

See also "Notes, Seizure Disorders."

CLINICALLY SIGNIFICANT DRUG INTERACTIONS

Concurrent felbamate pharmacotherapy and the following may result in clinically significant drug interactions:

Alcohol Use

Concurrent alcohol use may increase the CNS depressant action of felbamate. Advise patients to avoid, or limit, their use of alcohol while receiving felbamate pharmacotherapy.

Carbamazepine Pharmacotherapy

Concurrent felbamate and carbamazepine (Tegretol®) pharmacotherapy may result in an increased total body clearance of felbamate and a decreased carbamazepine blood concentration. However, blood concentrations of carbamazepine epoxide, an active metabolite of carbamazepine, may be increased. Both blood concentrations and patient response should be monitored closely. If required, adjust the dosage of felbamate and carbamazepine accordingly.

Pharmacotherapy With CNS Depressants and Other Drugs That Produce CNS Depression

Concurrent felbamate pharmacotherapy and pharmacotherapy with opiate analgesics, sedative-hypnotics, or other drugs that produce CNS depression (e.g., antihistamines, phenothiazines, TCAs) may result in additive CNS depression.

Phenytoin Pharmacotherapy

Concurrent felbamate and phenytoin (Dilantin®) pharmacotherapy may result in an increased total body clearance of felbamate and a decreased total body clearance of phenytoin. Both blood concentrations and patient response should be monitored closely. If required, adjust the dosage of felbamate and phenytoin accordingly.

Valproic Acid Pharmacotherapy

Concurrent felbamate and valproic acid (Depakene®) pharmacotherapy may result in an increased total body clearance of felbamate and a decreased total body clearance of valproic acid. Both blood concentrations and patient response should be monitored closely. If required, adjust the dosage of felbamate and valproic acid accordingly.

ADVERSE DRUG REACTIONS

Felbamate pharmacotherapy commonly has been associated with dizziness, fatigue, headache, insomnia, loss of appetite (anorexia), nausea, somnolence, and vomiting. Felbamate pharmacotherapy also has been associated with the following ADRs, listed according to body system:

Cardiovascular: chest pain, palpitations, and tachycardia
CNS: aggressive behavior, depression, emotional lability, incoordination (ataxia), pain, paresthesia, psychosis, stupor, and tremor
Cutaneous: acne, facial edema, itching (pruritus), and rash
GI: constipation, diarrhea, dry mouth, dyspepsia, hiccups, and taste disturbances

Hematologic: aplastic anemia (occurs among ~1 in 2000 patients and is *potentially fatal*), leukopenia (~6% incidence), purpura (~13% incidence), and various other blood disorders (e.g., agranulocytosis; less than 1% incidence).

Hepatic: acute liver failure, which is *potentially fatal*

Musculoskeletal: muscle pain (myalgia)

Ophthalmic: double vision (diplopia) and reduction or dimness of vision (amblyopia)

Respiratory: cough, inflammation of the pharynx (pharyngitis), inflammation of the sinuses (sinusitis), runny nose (rhinitis), and upper respiratory tract infection

Miscellaneous: decreased body weight, fever, and low blood phosphate (hypophosphatemia)

OVERDOSAGE

Reportedly, the signs and symptoms of felbamate overdosage are mild and include gastric distress (mild), sleepiness (somnolence), and tachycardia (heart rate of ~100 beats per minute at rest). Felbamate overdosage may be managed with close monitoring of the patient and the provision of general medical supportive care, if required. There is no known antidote.

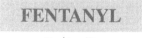
FENTANYL

(fen′ ta nil)

TRADE NAMES

Actiq®
Duragesic®
Sublimaze®

CLASSIFICATION

Opiate analgesic (C-II)

See also "Opiate Analgesics, General Monograph."

APPROVED INDICATIONS FOR NEUROPSYCHOLOGICAL DISORDERS

Adjunctive pharmacotherapy for the symptomatic management of:

- pain disorders: severe pain. Note: Fentanyl injectable pharmacotherapy is indicated primarily for patients during or immediately following surgery (e.g., to enhance anesthesia, to provide short-acting analgesia during anesthesia, and to provide analgesia immediately following surgery). It also is indicated for the symptomatic management of severe cancer pain.

USUAL DOSAGE AND ADMINISTRATION

Pain Disorders: Severe Pain

Adults: 50 to 100 µg intramuscularly for the management of post-operative pain. Repeat dose, if needed, in one or two hours according to individual patient response. Individualize dosage with attention to age, body weight, general physical health, severity of pain, degree of opiate tolerance, and concurrent pharmacotherapy. For transdermal dosage, see the transdermal fentanyl pharmacotherapy subsection of "Notes, Pain Disorders: Severe Pain."

Women who are, or who may become, pregnant: FDA Pregnancy Category C. Safety and efficacy of fentanyl pharmacotherapy for women who are pregnant have not been established (see "Opiate Analgesics, General Monograph"). Avoid prescribing fentanyl pharmacotherapy to women who are pregnant. If fentanyl pharmacotherapy is required, advise patients of potential benefits and possible risks to themselves and the embryo, fetus, or neonate. Collaboration with the patient's obstetrician is indicated.

For details and discussion regarding related basic principles of clinical pharmacology, readers are referred to the first text in this series, *The Pharmacologic Basis of Psychotherapeutics: An Introduction for Psychologists.*

Women who are breast-feeding: Safety and efficacy of fentanyl pharmacotherapy for women who are breast-feeding and their neonates and infants have not been established. Fentanyl is excreted in breast milk. Pharmacologic effects (e.g., drowsiness, lethargy) may be expected among breast-fed neonates and infants, who also may become addicted. Avoid prescribing fentanyl pharmacotherapy to women who are breast-feeding. If short-term fentanyl pharmacotherapy is required, breast-feeding probably should be discontinued, although single doses are unlikely to produce expected ADRs among breast-fed neonates and infants. If desired, lactation may be maintained and breast-feeding resumed following the discontinuation of short-term fentanyl pharmacotherapy. Collaboration with the patient's pediatrician is indicated.

Elderly, frail, or debilitated patients: Initially, prescribe lower dosages of fentanyl for elderly, frail, or debilitated patients. Dosage may be as low as one-quarter to one-third the usual recommended adult dosage. For transdermal fentanyl dosage, see the transdermal fentanyl pharmacotherapy subsection of "Notes, Pain Disorders: Severe Pain." Higher dosages are associated with a prolonged duration of action and respiratory depression, particularly among elderly patients. Consider the total dosage of all opiate analgesics comprising a patient's pharmacotherapy before prescribing fentanyl. Gradually increase the dosage according to individual patient response.

Children younger than 2 years of age: Safety and efficacy of fentanyl pharmacotherapy for children younger than 2 years of age have not been established. Injectable or transdermal fentanyl pharmacotherapy is *not* recommended for this age group.

Children 2 years of age and older and adolescents: 2 to 3 µg/kg intramuscularly or subcutaneously. The initial dose may be repeated in 30 to 60 minutes as indicated by patient response. The safety and efficacy of transdermal fentanyl pharmacotherapy for children younger than 12 years of age have not been established. Transdermal fentanyl pharmacotherapy is *not* recommended for this age group. See "Notes, Pain Disorders: Severe Pain."

Notes, Pain Disorders: Severe Pain

Concurrent fentanyl pharmacotherapy with other CNS depressant pharmacotherapy will generally necessitate a reduction in the dosage of fentanyl by 25% to 75%. Adjust the dosage cautiously, according to individual patient response. When moderate or high doses of fentanyl are required, assure that resuscitative equipment and adequately prepared medical personnel are readily available for monitoring the patient's respiratory and cardiovascular function until the patient's response to fentanyl pharmacotherapy is known. The opiate antagonist, naloxone (Narcan®), also should be immediately available. Emergency symptomatic medical support of body systems, particularly respiratory function, may be required.

Injectable fentanyl pharmacotherapy: Injectable fentanyl pharmacotherapy may be administered by intramuscular or intravenous injection. It is usually administered intravenously.

INTRAVENOUS FENTANYL PHARMACOTHERAPY: Intravenous fentanyl pharmacotherapy has been associated with muscle rigidity, particularly involving the muscles of respiration. This ADR appears to be related to the rate by which fentanyl is intravenously injected. To avoid this ADR, administer fentanyl by slow intravenous injection. Intravenous fentanyl pharmacotherapy also has been associated with abnormal contraction of the pupils (miosis), bronchospasm, bradycardia, and euphoria. Only inject fentanyl intravenously in the hospital setting, where resuscitative equipment and adequately prepared personnel are readily available for emergency symptomatic medical support of body systems, including airway maintenance (i.e., intubation) and assisted or controlled respiration. The opiate antagonist, naloxone (Narcan®), also should be readily available for emergency use if needed.

Transdermal fentanyl pharmacotherapy

INITIATING AND MAINTAINING TRANSDERMAL FENTANYL PHARMACOTHERAPY: The safety and efficacy of transdermal fentanyl pharmacotherapy for the *initial* management of chronic, moderate to severe pain have not been established. Although initial dosages have been suggested and used clinically, transdermal fentanyl pharmacotherapy generally is reserved for patients whose chronic, severe pain (e.g., terminal cancer pain), has been adequately managed with other opiate analgesics. The advantages of transdermal fentanyl pharmacotherapy for these patients include more consistent opiate blood concentrations and, therefore, analgesia; less frequent dosing; and more convenient and less painful (compared to intramuscular injection) opiate administration. See the table "Approximate Transdermal Fentanyl Dosage Equivalents for Patients Who are Receiving Oral Morphine" for approximate dosing equivalents.

Approximate transdermal fentanyl dosage equivalents for patients who are receiving oral morphine. *

Oral morphine (mg/day)	Transdermal fentanyl (μg/hour)
45 to 134	25
135 to 224	50
225 to 314	75
315 to 404	100
405 to 494	125
495 to 584	150
585 to 674	175
675 to 764	200
765 to 854	225
855 to 944	250
945 to 1034	275
1035 to 1124	300

* See "Opiate Analgesics, General Monograph" for "morphine dosage equivalents" for injectable morphine pharmacotherapy or *other* opiate analgesic pharmacotherapy.

The equivalent doses listed in the table generally are conservative. Many patients may, therefore, require dose adjustments. The maximal analgesic action of the fentanyl transdermal system generally is not apparent for at least 24 hours after its initial application. Initially prescribe supplemental doses of a different short-acting opiate analgesic (see "Opiate Analgesics, General Monograph"), based on individual patient response, to prevent breakthrough pain. After 3 days, an appropriate increase in the transdermal fentanyl dosage may be made, based upon the amount of supplemental opiate analgesia required during this transition period. For this calculation, the recommended ratio is 90 mg daily of oral morphine (or equivalent) to each 25 μg/hour increase for the fentanyl transdermal system.

Although pain may be adequately managed for most patients with the application of a fresh transdermal system every 72 hours, a small percentage of patients may require more frequent application (i.e., every 48 hours). Always prescribe the lowest effective dosage and longest effective dosing interval.

DISCONTINUING TRANSDERMAL FENTANYL PHARMACOTHERAPY: If transdermal fentanyl pharmacotherapy requires discontinuation, remove the system and monitor patient response carefully. Up to 20 hours may be required for fentanyl blood concentrations to decrease by 50%. If transdermal fentanyl pharmacotherapy is being replaced with other opiate analgesic pharmacotherapy, remove the system and titrate the dosage of the replacement opiate analgesic according to individual patient response. During this time, monitor patients for adequate pain management and signs and symptoms of toxicity.

AVAILABLE DOSAGE FORMS, STORAGE, AND COMPATIBILITY

Injectable, intramuscular or intravenous: 50 μg/ml (2- and 5-ml ampules)
Transdermal delivery systems, 72 hour: 25, 50, 75, or 100 μg/hour
Transmucosal (buccal) lozenge (Fentanyl Oralet®): 200, 300, 400 μg

Notes

Fentanyl injectable: Safely store the fentanyl injectable protected from light at controlled room temperature (15° to 30°C; 59° to 86°F).

Fentanyl transdermal systems: The 50, 75, and 100 μg/hour fentanyl transdermal systems are recommended *only* for patients who are opiate tolerant. Return the transdermal system to the manufacturer or dispensing pharmacy for appropriate disposal if the transdermal system is outdated or if the package seal has been broken.

Fentanyl transmucosal (buccal) lozenge: A buccal lozenge form of fentanyl (Fentanyl Oralet®) is available to provide fentanyl pharmacotherapy without the need for injection. However, the use of this fentanyl formulation generally is indicated for pre-operative sedation or as an adjunct to anesthesia.

General instructions for patients: Instruct patients who are receiving fentanyl pharmacotherapy to

- safely store fentanyl transdermal drug delivery systems out of the reach of children in child-resistant containers at controlled room temperature below 25°C (77°F).
- apply fentanyl transdermal drug delivery systems immediately after removal from their individual sealed packages.
- remove each used fentanyl transdermal drug delivery system from the skin and place it in its original pouch for safe disposal. The used system should be disposed of immediately to prevent inadvertent access by children or pets.
- never apply more than one transdermal system at a time. Serious toxicity may occur.
- never cut the transdermal drug delivery system to alter the dosage. Destroying the system by cutting may result in excessive drug absorption and toxicity. Instruct patients to consult their prescribing psychologist if a change in dosage is required.

- obtain an available patient information sheet regarding fentanyl pharmacotherapy from their pharmacist at the time that their prescription is dispensed. Encourage patients to clarify any questions that they may have regarding fentanyl pharmacotherapy with their pharmacist or, if needed, to consult their prescribing psychologist.

PROPOSED MECHANISM OF ACTION

Fentanyl is an opiate analgesic that has actions similar to those of morphine and meperidine. A 100-μg dose of fentanyl is approximately equivalent in analgesic action to 10 mg of morphine or 75 mg of meperidine. Fentanyl elicits its analgesic, CNS depressant, and respiratory depressant actions primarily by binding to the endorphin receptors in the CNS. The exact mechanism of action has not yet been fully determined.

See also "Opiate Analgesics, General Monograph."

PHARMACOKINETICS/PHARMACODYNAMICS

Fentanyl's onset of action is almost immediate following intravenous injection. However, its maximal analgesic and respiratory depressant actions may not occur for several minutes. The usual duration of analgesia is 30 to 60 minutes after a single intravenous dose of up to 100 μg. Following intramuscular injection, the onset of action is generally within 7 to 8 minutes and the duration of action is 1 to 2 hours. Fentanyl is ~85% plasma protein bound. Its mean apparent volume of distribution is ~4 liters/kg. Less than 10% is excreted in unchanged form in the urine. The mean half-life of elimination is ~4 hours. The mean total body clearance is ~1 liter/minute.

Similar to other opiate analgesics, the alterations in respiratory rate and alveolar ventilation associated with fentanyl may last longer than its analgesic action. As the dosage is increased, pulmonary exchange becomes decreased. Although fentanyl preserves cardiac stability and decreases stress-related hormonal changes, apnea may occur with higher dosages. Fentanyl does not display cardiovascular actions even when injected intravenously at dosages of 0.7 μg/kg. It has less emetic action than do other opiate analgesics. Fentanyl is most often used as an intravenous analgesic during surgery because of its short duration of action (i.e., 20 to 40 minutes after intravenous injection). It also may be used intramuscularly as a premedication for surgery (duration of action after intramuscular injection is 1 to 2 hours).

RELATIVE CONTRAINDICATIONS

Hypersensitivity to fentanyl or other opiate analgesics

CAUTIONS AND COMMENTS

Fentanyl is addicting and habituating. See "Opiate Analgesics, General Monograph." Prescribe fentanyl pharmacotherapy cautiously to patients who

- have a particular susceptibility to respiratory depression, such as those patients who are comatose or have brain tumors, head injuries, or other medical disorders that are associated with increased intracranial pressure. Fentanyl pharmacotherapy may exacerbate these conditions and also may obscure the clinical course of these patients.

- have cardiac bradydysrhythmias. Fentanyl may produce additional bradycardia among these patients.
- have chronic obstructive lung disease, decreased respiratory reserve, and potentially compromised respiration. Fentanyl may produce a further decrease in respiratory drive and an increase in airway resistance among these patients.
- have kidney or liver dysfunction. Kidney or liver dysfunction may affect fentanyl metabolism and excretion.

Caution patients who are receiving fentanyl pharmacotherapy against

- performing activities that require alertness, judgment, and physical coordination (e.g., driving an automobile, operating dangerous equipment, supervising children) until their response to fentanyl is known. Fentanyl's CNS depressant action may affect these mental and physical functions adversely.

In addition to this general precaution, caution patients who are receiving fentanyl pharmacotherapy to

- inform their prescribing psychologist if they begin or discontinue any other pharmacotherapy while receiving fentanyl pharmacotherapy.

CLINICALLY SIGNIFICANT DRUG INTERACTIONS

Concurrent fentanyl pharmacotherapy and the following may result in clinically significant drug interactions:

Alcohol Use

Concurrent alcohol use may increase the CNS depressant action of fentanyl. Advise patients to avoid, or limit, their use of alcohol while receiving fentanyl pharmacotherapy.

Droperidol and Other Antipsychotic Pharmacotherapy

Concurrent fentanyl pharmacotherapy and pharmacotherapy with droperidol (Inapsine®), or other antipsychotic drugs, requires the immediate availability of adequately prepared personnel and facilities for the emergency symptomatic medical support of the patient's body systems with attention to the management of hypotension. Cautiously monitor patients who are receiving concurrent fentanyl and droperidol, or other antipsychotic, pharmacotherapy for the following cardiovascular, CNS, and miscellaneous signs and symptoms:

Cardiovascular: elevated blood pressure, with or without preexisting hypertension. The hypertension may be related to unexplained alterations in sympathetic nervous system activity associated with high dosages or other factors depending on the clinical situation.
CNS: drowsiness; extrapyramidal signs and symptoms including akathisia, dystonia, and oculogyric crisis; hallucinations sometimes associated with transient periods of mental depression; and restlessness.
Miscellaneous: chills and shivering

MAOI Pharmacotherapy

The safety and efficacy of concurrent fentanyl and MAOI pharmacotherapy have not been established. Concurrent fentanyl and MAOI pharmacotherapy may result in severe and unpredictable potentiation of MAOI actions. Fentanyl and MAOI pharmacotherapy, concurrent or within 14 days, is *not* recommended.

Pharmacotherapy With CNS Depressants and Other Drugs That Produce CNS Depression

Concurrent fentanyl pharmacotherapy with other opiate analgesics, sedative-hypnotics, or other drugs that produce CNS depression (e.g., antihistamines, phenothiazines, TCAs) may result in additive CNS depression. When concurrent pharmacotherapy is required, the fentanyl dosage should be lower than usually recommended. Reduce the dosage of other CNS depressants when prescribed for patients who are receiving fentanyl pharmacotherapy. Collaboration with other prescribers (e.g., advanced practice nurse, dentist, family physician) is indicated to help to assure optimal pharmacotherapy.

See also "Opiate Analgesics, General Monograph."

ADVERSE DRUG REACTIONS

As with other opiate analgesics, the most common serious ADRs associated with fentanyl pharmacotherapy are apnea, bradycardia, respiratory depression, and skeletal and thoracic muscular rigidity. If untreated, these ADRs may result in respiratory arrest, circulatory depression, and cardiac arrest. Like other opiate analgesics, fentanyl can produce addiction and habituation. Other ADRs, listed according to body system, include:

Cardiovascular: hypotension
CNS: dizziness
GI: nausea and vomiting
Musculoskeletal: spasm of the larynx (laryngospasm)
Ocular: reduction or dimness of vision (amblyopia)
Respiratory: respiratory depression
Miscellaneous: sweating (excessive)

See also "Opiate Analgesics, General Monograph."

OVERDOSAGE

Signs and symptoms of fentanyl overdosage are variable. Generally, they are an extension of its CNS and respiratory depressant actions. Fentanyl overdosage requires emergency symptomatic medical support of body systems with attention to increasing fentanyl elimination. The opiate antagonist, naloxone (Narcan®), is usually required to manage the severe respiratory depression associated with fentanyl overdosage. The duration of respiratory depression associated with fentanyl overdosage may be longer than the duration of action for the opiate antagonist. Thus, the opiate antagonist may require periodic readministration.

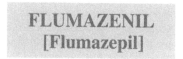

FLUMAZENIL
[Flumazepil]

(floo′ may ze nil)

TRADE NAMES

Anexate®
Romazicon®

CLASSIFICATION

Benzodiazepine receptor antagonist (imidazobenzodiazepine)

APPROVED INDICATIONS FOR NEUROPSYCHOLOGICAL DISORDERS

Pharmacotherapy for the diagnosis or symptomatic management of:

• substance-related disorders: benzodiazepine overdosage

USUAL DOSAGE AND ADMINISTRATION

Benzodiazepine Overdosage

Adults: Initially, 0.3 mg injected intravenously over 30 seconds. Repeat at 1-minute intervals until the patient clearly responds or the maximal recommended dosage of 3 mg is reached. If drowsiness recurs, repeat initial dosage at 20-minute intervals. If preferred, 0.1 to 0.4 mg/hour by continuous intravenous infusion. Adjust the rate according to individual patient response and the desired level of patient arousal.

MAXIMUM: 3 mg intravenously (total dosage)

Women who are, or who may become, pregnant: FDA Pregnancy Category C. Safety and efficacy of flumazenil pharmacotherapy for women who are pregnant have not been established. Avoid prescribing flumazenil pharmacotherapy to women who are pregnant. If flumazenil pharmacotherapy is required, advise patients (or their family members in regard to the patient, as appropriate, in the event of severe overdosage) of the importance of the use of the antidote and any possible risks to themselves and the embryo, fetus, or neonate. Collaboration with the patient's obstetrician is indicated.

For details and discussion regarding related basic principles of clinical pharmacology, readers are referred to the first text in this series, *The Pharmacologic Basis of Psychotherapeutics: An Introduction for Psychologists.*

Women who are breast-feeding: Safety and efficacy of flumazenil pharmacotherapy for women who are breast-feeding and their neonates and infants have not been established. If flumazenil pharmacotherapy is required, breast-feeding should be discontinued for at least 24 hours, lactation maintained, and breast-feeding resumed following recovery from benzodiazepine overdosage.

Elderly, frail, or debilitated patients: Generally, no special precautions or dosage modifications are required for elderly, frail, or debilitated patients. For recommended dosage, see "Adults."

Children and adolescents younger than 18 years of age: Safety and efficacy of flumazenil pharmacotherapy for children and adolescents have *not* been established. However, in cases of benzodiazepine overdosage, prescribing psychologists may consider recommending the following suggested dosages: 0.01 mg/kg/dose injected intravenously over 30 seconds. Repeat, as indicated, or follow by a continuous intravenous infusion of 0.005 to 0.01 mg/kg/hour until the patient responds or the maximal recommended dosage of 2 mg is reached. Note that limited data are available regarding flumazenil pharmacotherapy for the symptomatic management of benzodiazepine overdosage among children and adolescents.

MAXIMUM: For children and adolescents weighing 30 kg (67 lb) or less, 2 mg intravenously (total dosage). For children and adolescents weighing *over* 30 kg (67 lb), 3 mg intravenously (total dosage).

Notes, Benzodiazepine Overdosage

The manufacturer recommends that flumazenil pharmacotherapy for the symptomatic management of acute benzodiazepine overdosage be administered by a physician who has experience in anesthesiology. The manufacturer also recommends that patients have an established airway and intravenous access before intravenous flumazenil pharmacotherapy is initiated. Concurrent emergency symptomatic medical support of body systems with attention to increasing the elimination of the benzodiazepine is indicated for acute overdosage.

Flumazenil has a relatively short duration of action ($T_{1/2} = 1$ hour). Therefore, overdosages involving long-acting benzodiazepines require continued monitoring *after* initial therapeutic benefit has been achieved. If drowsiness recurs, a continuous intravenous infusion may be initiated. See "Usual Dosage and Administration."

AVAILABLE DOSAGE FORMS, STORAGE, AND COMPATIBILITY

Injectable, intravenous: 0.1 mg/ml

Notes

The flumazenil injectable formulation is compatible for 24 hours with 5% dextrose in water, lactated Ringer's, and normal saline intravenous solutions. Safely store the flumazenil injectable and diluted intravenous flumazenil admixtures at controlled room temperature (15° to 30°C; 59° to 86°F).

PROPOSED MECHANISM OF ACTION

Flumazenil is a benzodiazepine antagonist that acts at the benzodiazepine receptors to reverse, or antagonize, the actions of benzodiazepines by means of competitive inhibition (i.e., flumazenil blocks the benzodiazepines from binding to their receptors and eliciting their pharmacologic actions). The efficacy of flumazenil varies for reversing the sedation and respiratory depression associated with benzodiazepine overdosage. Efficacy is greatest for sedation, but is limited or incomplete for respiratory depression. Flumazenil also possesses weak anticonvulsant (i.e., benzodiazepine agonist) activity. However, this action does not appear to be of any therapeutic significance.

PHARMACOKINETICS/PHARMACODYNAMICS

Flumazenil is moderately bound to plasma proteins ($\sim$50%). It has a mean apparent volume of distribution of 1 liter/kg. Flumazenil is extensively metabolized by the liver with less than 1% excreted in unchanged form in the urine. The mean half-life of elimination is 1 hour and the mean total body clearance is $\sim$70 liters/hour. Generally, the onset of the reversal of the signs and symptoms of benzodiazepine overdosage occurs within 2 minutes of the intravenous injection of flumazenil.

RELATIVE CONTRAINDICATIONS

Cyclic antidepressant overdosage (see "Cautions and Comments")
Head injury (flumazenil may precipitate seizures among these patients)
Hypersensitivity to flumazenil or the benzodiazepines
Seizure disorders, including epilepsy (flumazenil may precipitate seizures among these patients)

CAUTIONS AND COMMENTS

Excessive or rapid administration of flumazenil to patients who are addicted to benzodiazepines may induce the benzodiazepine withdrawal syndrome. Signs and symptoms of the benzodiazepine withdrawal syndrome include, depending upon the severity of addiction and habituation: anxiety, dizziness, excessive sweating, seizures, and tachycardia. Cardiac dysrhythmias and seizures also have been observed, particularly among patients whose overdosage has involved the benzodiazepines and cyclic antidepressants.

Recommend cautious flumazenil pharmacotherapy for patients who

- have histories of panic disorder. Flumazenil pharmacotherapy may precipitate a panic attack among these patients.
- have histories of seizure disorders. Flumazenil pharmacotherapy may precipitate a seizure among these patients.
- have histories of severe liver dysfunction. The clearance of flumazenil may be reduced by up to two-thirds among these patients. Although a lower initial flumazenil dose is not *generally required*, subsequent dosage may need to be reduced for these patients.

CLINICALLY SIGNIFICANT DRUG INTERACTIONS

Concurrent flumazenil pharmacotherapy and the following may result in clinically significant drug interactions:

Zopiclone Pharmacotherapy

Zopiclone (Imovane®, Rhovane®), a non-benzodiazepine sedative-hypnotic, acts by binding to the benzodiazepine receptor. Thus, flumazenil blocks the action of zopiclone and also may be of benefit for the symptomatic management of zopiclone overdosage.

ADVERSE DRUG REACTIONS

Generally, flumazenil pharmacotherapy is well tolerated. Occasionally, slight pain and irritation has been noted at the injection site. Other ADRs associated with flumazenil pharmacotherapy (e.g., agitation, anxiety, crying, seizures) are most likely signs and symptoms of the benzodiazepine withdrawal syndrome.

Occasionally, flumazenil pharmacotherapy for the symptomatic management of overdosage, or following a diagnostic procedure, has resulted in seizures or cardiac dysrhythmias. Patients particularly at risk generally have histories of one or more of the following: 1) long-term benzodiazepine pharmacotherapy or regular personal use; 2) seizure disorder; or 3) TCA overdosage (see "Cautions and Comments").

OVERDOSAGE

Flumazenil overdosage has not been reported. Intravenous dosages of up to 100 mg have failed to produce signs and symptoms of overdosage among healthy volunteers (see "Adverse Drug Reactions").

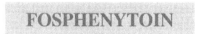

FOSPHENYTOIN

(fos′ fen i toyn)

TRADE NAME

Cerebyx®

CLASSIFICATION

Anticonvulsant (phenytoin prodrug)

APPROVED INDICATIONS FOR NEUROPSYCHOLOGICAL DISORDERS

Pharmacotherapy for the prophylactic and symptomatic management of:

- seizure disorders: partial seizures with complex symptomatology and tonic-clonic seizures

USUAL DOSAGE AND ADMINISTRATION

The manufacturer of fosphenytoin advises that the fosphenytoin dosage, concentration in solutions, and infusion rate *always* be expressed in terms of phenytoin sodium equivalents (PE). A dosage of 1.5 mg of fosphenytoin is converted after intramuscular or intravenous injection to 1 mg phenytoin (i.e., 1 PE).

Seizure Disorders: Partial Seizures With Complex Symptomatology and Tonic-Clonic Seizures

Adults: *Loading dose*, 10 to 20 mg PE/kg intramuscularly or intravenously. The intravenous dose should be infused at a rate of 100 to 150 mg PE/minute.

MAINTENANCE: 4 to 6 mg PE/kg daily intramuscularly or intravenously, usually in a single dose. Some patients may require more frequent dosing.

MAXIMAL INTRAVENOUS INFUSION RATE: 150 mg PE/minute

Women who are, or who may become, pregnant: FDA Pregnancy Category D. Safety and efficacy of fosphenytoin pharmacotherapy for women who are pregnant have not been established. However, clinical reports and studies have reported an incidence of congenital malformations (i.e., birth defects) as high as 25% among neonates exposed in utero to fosphenytoin.

For details and discussion regarding related basic principles of clinical pharmacology, readers are referred to the first text in this series, *The Pharmacologic Basis of Psychotherapeutics: An Introduction for Psychologists.*

These teratogenic effects have been characterized as the fetal hydantoin syndrome and include cardiac malformations, cleft lip and palate, CNS malformations, and developmental delay. Avoid prescribing fosphenytoin pharmacotherapy to women who are pregnant. If fosphenytoin pharmacotherapy is required, advise patients of potential benefits and possible risks to themselves and the embryo, fetus, or neonate. Collaboration with the patient's obstetrician is indicated. (See also the phenytoin monograph.)

Women who are breast-feeding: Safety and efficacy of fosphenytoin pharmacotherapy for women who are breast-feeding and their neonates and infants have not been established. Although small amounts of fosphenytoin may be excreted in breast milk, idiosyncratic reactions (e.g., cyanosis, methemoglobinemia) have been reported among breast-fed neonates and infants. Avoid prescribing fosphenytoin pharmacotherapy to women who are breast-feeding. If fosphenytoin pharmacotherapy is required, breast-feeding probably should be discontinued. Collaboration with the patient's pediatrician may be indicated.

Elderly, frail, or debilitated patients and those who have kidney or liver dysfunction: Generally prescribe lower dosages of fosphenytoin for elderly, frail, or debilitated patients. These patients may be more sensitive to the pharmacologic actions of fosphenytoin than are younger or healthier adult patients.

The rate of conversion of fosphenytoin to phenytoin may be increased among patients who have significant kidney or liver dysfunction and those who have hypoalbuminemia. The incidence and severity of ADRs may increase among these patients unless the dosage is decreased appropriately.

Children and adolescents younger than 18 years of age: Safety and efficacy of fosphenytoin pharmacotherapy for children and adolescents who are younger than 18 years of age have not been established. Fosphenytoin pharmacotherapy is *not* recommended for this indication for this age group.

Notes, Seizure Disorders: Partial Seizures With Complex Symptomatology and Tonic-Clonic Seizures

Fosphenytoin dosage is expressed in phenytoin equivalents (PE) to avoid the need for dosing conversions.

Fosphenytoin is indicated for the short-term (1 week or less) replacement of injectable or oral phenytoin pharmacotherapy when it is unavailable or is considered to be inappropriate or of less therapeutic benefit for the patient (e.g., the phenytoin injectable contains both alcohol and propylene glycol, which are associated with increased ADRs).

Intravenous fosphenytoin pharmacotherapy: Intravenous infusion of fosphenytoin, particularly at the maximal rate of infusion, has been associated with a burning, itching, or tingling sensation, predominantly in the groin area. The mechanism of this ADR has yet to be fully determined. However, it appears to be directly related to the phosphate component of fosphenytoin. No permanent related sequelae have been reported. Both the frequency of occurrence and severity of the discomfort can be minimized by slowing the rate of the infusion or by temporarily stopping the infusion. Overall, the intravenous infusion of fosphenytoin has been associated with significantly fewer incidents of this local reaction, which required the disruption of the intravenous infusion, than has intravenous pharmacotherapy with equivalent doses of phenytoin as noted in the table "Local Intolerance Associated With Intravenous Fosphenytoin and Phenytoin Pharmacotherapy."

Local intolerance associated with intravenous fosphenytoin and phenytoin pharmacotherapy.

Infusion intolerance measures	Fosphenytoin ($n = 90$)	Phenytoin ($n = 22$)
Local intolerance	9% of patients	90% of patients
Disruption of infusion	21% of patients	67% of patients
Infusion time (average)	13 minutes	44 minutes

AVAILABLE DOSAGE FORMS, STORAGE, AND COMPATIBILITY

Injectable, intramuscular and intravenous: 75 mg/ml fosphenytoin (50 mg PE)

Notes

Fosphenytoin injectable: Fosphenytoin injectable is compatible with 5% dextrose solution and 0.9% sodium chloride solution (i.e., normal saline) for injection. The fosphenytoin injectable must be diluted to a concentration ranging from 1.5 to 25 mg PE/ml *prior* to administration.

General instructions for patients: Instruct patients who are receiving fosphenytoin pharmacotherapy, or those who are assisting them with their care, to

- safely store the fosphenytoin injectable under refrigeration (2° to 8°C; 36° to 46°F). Fosphenytoin injectable formulations that are stored at room temperature for 48 hours or longer are subject to degradation and should be discarded appropriately.
- obtain an available patient information sheet regarding fosphenytoin pharmacotherapy from their pharmacist at the time that their prescription is dispensed. Encourage patients, or their caregivers, to clarify any questions that they may have regarding fosphenytoin pharmacotherapy with their pharmacist or, if needed, to consult their prescribing psychologist.

PROPOSED MECHANISM OF ACTION

Fosphenytoin is an inactive prodrug that is converted in vivo to phenytoin. Each 1.5 mg of fosphenytoin is converted to 1 mg of phenytoin (i.e., 1 mg PE).

The exact mechanism of action of fosphenytoin for the symptomatic management of seizure disorders has not yet been fully determined. However, a major component of this action appears to be related to the reduction of post-tetanic potentiation of synaptic transmission and associated limitation of seizure discharge and spread from its focus. This mechanism is believed to be mediated by the prevention of the accumulation of intracellular sodium during tetanic stimulation.

PHARMACOKINETICS/PHARMACODYNAMICS

Fosphenytoin is completely absorbed and converted to phenytoin following intramuscular injection. Peak blood concentrations are obtained within 30 minutes following intramuscular injection. Fosphenytoin is bound to plasma proteins extensively (i.e., 95% to 99%). Protein binding is saturable and concentration-dependent. The volume of distribution of fosphenytoin increases with dosage and ranges from 4.3 to 10.8 liters. Each mmol of fosphenytoin is converted to 1 mmol of phenytoin, phosphate, and formate. The half-life of conversion from fosphenytoin to phenytoin is ~15 minutes. See also the phenytoin monograph.

Therapeutic Drug Monitoring

Therapeutic blood concentrations of fosphenytoin for the suppression of tonic-clonic seizures is 10 µg/ml. Generally, the initial signs and symptoms of fosphenytoin toxicity (e.g., nystagmus) are not noted until fosphenytoin blood concentrations exceed 20 µg/ml. Severe ADRs (e.g., incoordination [ataxia]) generally are not noted until fosphenytoin blood concentrations exceed 30 µg/ml. See the phenytoin monograph.

RELATIVE CONTRAINDICATIONS

Adams–Stokes syndrome
Atrioventricular block, second and third degree
Hypersensitivity to fosphenytoin, phenytoin, or other hydantoins
Sinoatrial block
Sinus bradycardia

See also the phenytoin monograph.

CAUTIONS AND COMMENTS

Prescribe fosphenytoin pharmacotherapy cautiously to patients who

- have severe renal impairment or who require phosphate restriction. The phosphate load associated with fosphenytoin pharmacotherapy should be considered when prescribing fosphenytoin for patients who have renal impairment or who require phosphate restriction. Each 1.5 mg of fosphenytoin produces 0.0037 mmol of phosphate.

Caution patients who are receiving fosphenytoin pharmacotherapy against

- performing activities that require alertness, judgment, or physical coordination (e.g., driving an automobile, operating dangerous equipment, supervising children) until their response to fosphenytoin pharmacotherapy is known. Fosphenytoin may affect these mental and physical functions adversely.

In addition to this general precaution, caution patients who are receiving fosphenytoin pharmacotherapy to

- inform their prescribing psychologist if they begin or discontinue any other pharmacotherapy while receiving fosphenytoin pharmacotherapy.

CLINICALLY SIGNIFICANT DRUG INTERACTIONS

Concurrent fosphenytoin pharmacotherapy and the following may result in clinically significant drug interactions:

Alcohol Use

Concurrent alcohol use may increase the CNS depressant action of fosphenytoin. Advise patients to avoid, or limit, their use of alcohol while receiving fosphenytoin pharmacotherapy.

Pharmacotherapy With CNS Depressants and Other Drugs That Produce CNS Depression

Concurrent fosphenytoin pharmacotherapy and pharmacotherapy with opiate analgesics, sedative-hypnotics, or other drugs that produce CNS depression (e.g., antihistamines, phenothiazines, TCAs) may result in additive CNS depression.

ADVERSE DRUG REACTIONS

Fosphenytoin pharmacotherapy has been associated with the following ADRs, listed according to body system:

Cardiovascular: rarely, decreased systolic blood pressure
CNS: depression, dizziness, drowsiness, fatigue, headache, insomnia, irritability, mental confusion, nervousness, slurred speech, unsteadiness, and reduced performance on neuropsychological tests
Cutaneous: transient skin rashes
Genitourinary: genitourinary complaints
Hematologic: rarely, decreased hematocrit
Hepatic: abnormal liver function tests
Musculoskeletal: incoordination (ataxia) and tremor
Ophthalmic: blurred vision and double vision (diplopia)
Renal: rarely, abnormal kidney function tests
Miscellaneous: idiosyncratic reactions associated with fosphenytoin intravenous pharmacotherapy. See "Notes, Seizure Disorders: Partial Seizures With Complex Symptomatology and Tonic-Clonic Seizures" and "Intravenous Fosphenytoin Pharmacotherapy."

OVERDOSAGE

See the phenytoin monograph.

GABAPENTIN
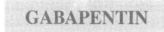

(ga′ ba pen tin)

TRADE NAME

Neurontin®

CLASSIFICATION

Anticonvulsant (GABA structural analogue)

APPROVED INDICATIONS FOR NEUROPSYCHOLOGICAL DISORDERS

Pharmacotherapy for the prophylactic and symptomatic management of:

- seizure disorders: partial seizures with or without secondary generalizations

USUAL DOSAGE AND ADMINISTRATION

Seizure Disorders: Partial Seizures With or Without Secondary Generalizations

Adults: Initially, gabapentin pharmacotherapy is prescribed according to the following schedule:

Day 1: 300 mg orally as a single dose 30 minutes before retiring for bed in the evening in order to minimize the ADRs (i.e., dizziness, fatigue, incoordination [ataxia], and somnolence) associated with the initiation of gabapentin pharmacotherapy
Day 2: 600 mg orally in two divided doses
Day 3, and thereafter: 900 mg orally in three divided doses. Gradually increase the dosage, if needed, according to individual patient response.

MAINTENANCE: The usual maintenance dosage is 1.8 to 2.4 grams daily orally in three divided doses.

MAXIMUM: 3.6 grams daily orally (generally short-term)

Women who are, or who may become, pregnant: FDA Pregnancy Category C. Safety and efficacy of gabapentin pharmacotherapy for women who are pregnant have not been established. Avoid prescribing gabapentin pharmacotherapy to women who are pregnant. If gabapentin pharmacotherapy is required, advise patients of potential benefits and possible risks to themselves and the embryo, fetus, or neonate. Collaboration with the patient's obstetrician is indicated.

For details and discussion regarding related basic principles of clinical pharmacology, readers are referred to the first text in this series, *The Pharmacologic Basis of Psychotherapeutics: An Introduction for Psychologists.*

Women who are breast-feeding: Safety and efficacy of gabapentin pharmacotherapy for women who are breast-feeding and their neonates and infants have not been established. Avoid prescribing gabapentin pharmacotherapy to women who are breast-feeding. If gabapentin pharmacotherapy is required, breast-feeding probably should be discontinued. Collaboration with the patient's pediatrician may be indicated.

Elderly, frail, or debilitated patients and those who have kidney dysfunction: Generally prescribe lower dosages for elderly, frail, or debilitated patients. Gradually increase the dosage, if needed, according to individual patient response. These patients may be more sensitive to the pharmacologic actions of gabapentin than are younger or healthier adult patients.

Gabapentin is eliminated in the urine in unchanged form. Its renal clearance is directly related to creatinine clearance. Thus, the usual recommended dosage of gabapentin must be adjusted for patients who have kidney dysfunction in order to prevent the accumulation of gabapentin and possible toxicity. See the table "Gabapentin Dosage Adjustments for Patients Who Have Renal Dysfunction."

Gabapentin dosage adjustments for patients who have renal dysfunction.

Creatinine clearance (ml/minute)	Recommended dosage (mg)
0	Initial loading dose of 300 mg. Repeat dose following each 4-hour hemodialysis session.
Less than 15	Up to 300 mg every *other* day
>15 to 30	Up to 300 mg daily
>30 to 60	Up to 600 mg daily
>60 to 90	Up to 1.2 grams daily

Children younger than 12 years of age: Safety and efficacy of gabapentin pharmacotherapy for children who are younger than 12 years of age have not been established. Gabapentin pharmacotherapy is *not* recommended for this age group.

Notes, Seizure Disorders: Partial Seizures With or Without Secondary Generalizations

Initiating and maintaining gabapentin pharmacotherapy: Gabapentin pharmacotherapy is generally indicated for short-term pharmacotherapy. Opening and mixing the contents of gabapentin capsules with food does not significantly impair absorption and may facilitate ingestion. See "Usual Dosage and Administration."

Discontinuing gabapentin pharmacotherapy: Discontinue gabapentin pharmacotherapy gradually, over a period of at least 1 week, to avoid or minimize the possible occurrence of associated withdrawal seizures, including status epilepticus.

AVAILABLE DOSAGE FORMS, STORAGE, AND COMPATIBILITY

Capsules, oral: 100, 300, 400 mg

Notes

General instructions for patients: Instruct patients who are receiving gabapentin pharmacotherapy to

- safely store gabapentin oral capsules out of the reach of children in child-resistant containers at controlled room temperature (15° to 30°C; 59° to 86°F).
- obtain an available patient information sheet regarding gabapentin pharmacotherapy from their pharmacist at the time that their prescription is dispensed. Encourage patients to clarify any questions that they may have regarding gabapentin pharmacotherapy with their pharmacist or, if needed, to consult their prescribing psychologist.

PROPOSED MECHANISM OF ACTION

The mechanism of the anticonvulsant action of gabapentin has not yet been fully determined. It appears to involve both the direct potentiation of GABA and the inhibition of voltage-dependent sodium ion channels.

PHARMACOKINETICS/PHARMACODYNAMICS

Gabapentin is moderately well absorbed following oral ingestion ($F \sim 0.6$). The ingestion of food has no effect on gabapentin absorption. However, as the dosage increases, absorption (F) decreases, presumably due to saturation of the neutral amino acid carrier (system L) that facilitates gabapentin transport across the membrane of the small intestine. Gabapentin is not bound to plasma proteins and has an apparent volume of distribution of ~ 0.8 liters/kg. Peak blood concentrations are obtained within 2 to 3 hours after administration. Gabapentin is not metabolized significantly. Thus, it is excreted primarily in unchanged form in the urine. The total body clearance is ~ 100 ml/minute (equivalent, essentially, to creatinine clearance) and the half-life of elimination is ~ 6 hours (range: 5 to 9 hours).

Therapeutic Drug Monitoring

The reported therapeutic blood concentration for gabapentin is in excess of 2 µg/ml.

RELATIVE CONTRAINDICATIONS

Hypersensitivity to gabapentin

CAUTIONS AND COMMENTS

Caution patients who are receiving gabapentin pharmacotherapy against

- performing activities that require alertness, judgment, or physical coordination (e.g., driving an automobile, operating dangerous equipment, supervising children) until their response to gabapentin pharmacotherapy is known. Gabapentin may affect these mental and physical functions adversely.

CLINICALLY SIGNIFICANT DRUG INTERACTIONS

Concurrent gabapentin pharmacotherapy and the following may result in clinically significant drug interactions:

Alcohol Use

Concurrent alcohol use may increase the CNS depressant action of gabapentin. Advise patients to avoid, or limit, their use of alcohol while receiving gabapentin pharmacotherapy.

Antacid Use

Use of an antacid (i.e., aluminum hydroxide and magnesium hydroxide) concomitantly or within 2 hours before or after the oral ingestion of gabapentin may reduce the absorption of gabapentin by 10% to 25%.

Pharmacotherapy With CNS Depressants and Other Drugs That Produce CNS Depression

Concurrent gabapentin pharmacotherapy and pharmacotherapy with opiate analgesics, sedative-hypnotics, or other drugs that produce CNS depression (e.g., antihistamines, phenothiazines, TCAs) may result in additive CNS depression.

ADVERSE DRUG REACTIONS

Gabapentin pharmacotherapy generally is well tolerated. However, gabapentin pharmacotherapy has been commonly associated with involuntary cyclical movement of the eyeball (nystagmus), dizziness, fatigue, incoordination (ataxia), and somnolence. It also has been associated with the following ADRs, listed according to body system:

Cardiovascular: peripheral edema
CNS: amnesia, behavioral disturbances, depression, nervousness, and tremor
Cutaneous: facial edema, rash, and severe itching (pruritis)
Genitourinary: glucose in the urine (glycosuria) and impotence
GI: constipation, dry mouth, dyspepsia, nausea, and vomiting
Hematologic: leukopenia and purpura
Hepatic: enlarged liver (hepatomegaly)

Metabolic/Endocrine: decreased body weight
Musculoskeletal: joint pain (arthralgia), backache, and muscle pain (myalgia)
Ophthalmic: double vision (diplopia) and reduction or dimness of vision (amblyopia)
Otic: hearing loss
Respiratory: coughing, inflammation of the pharynx (pharyngitis), pneumonia, and runny nose (rhinitis)

OVERDOSAGE

The signs and symptoms of gabapentin overdosage include diarrhea, double vision (diplopia), drowsiness, lethargy, and slurred speech. There have been no reported cases of fatal overdosages involving gabapentin. Nevertheless, gabapentin overdosage should be treated with emergency symptomatic medical support of body systems with attention to increasing gabapentin elimination. There is no known antidote.

HEROIN*
[Diacetylmorphine; Diamorphine]

(her′ o in)

TRADE NAMES

Generally available under the generic name

CLASSIFICATION

Opiate analgesic (agonist) (C-I)

See also "Opiate Analgesics, General Monograph."

APPROVED INDICATIONS FOR NEUROPSYCHOLOGICAL DISORDERS

Adjunctive pharmacotherapy for the symptomatic management of:

- pain disorders: severe pain. Heroin pharmacotherapy is indicated for the symptomatic management of severe pain, particularly that associated with cancer.

USUAL DOSAGE AND ADMINISTRATION

Pain Disorders: Severe Pain Including Cancer Pain

Adults: 0.05 to 0.1 mg/kg intramuscularly, intravenously, or subcutaneously every 4 hours, according to individual patient response

Women who are, or who may become, pregnant: FDA Pregnancy Category "not established." Safety and efficacy of heroin pharmacotherapy for women who are pregnant have not been established. Heroin crosses the placenta. However, it does not appear to be associated with the development of congenital malformations (i.e., birth defects). Neonates born to women who have received heroin pharmacotherapy, or have regularly used heroin, during their pregnancies, especially near term, will display the opiate withdrawal syndrome. Avoid prescribing heroin pharmacotherapy to women who are pregnant. If heroin pharmacotherapy is required, advise patients of potential benefits and possible risks to themselves and the embryo, fetus, or neonate. Collaboration with the patient's obstetrician, oncologist, or pediatrician is indicated.

For details and discussion regarding related basic principles of clinical pharmacology, readers are referred to the first text in this series, *The Pharmacologic Basis of Psychotherapeutics: An Introduction for Psychologists.*

Women who are breast-feeding: Safety and efficacy of heroin pharmacotherapy for women who are breast-feeding and their neonates and infants have not been established. Heroin is excreted in breast milk. Neonates and infants may display expected pharmacological actions (e.g., drowsiness, lethargy). They also may become addicted. In addition, neonatal addiction developed in utero may be prolonged among breast-fed neonates. Do not prescribe heroin pharmacotherapy to women who are breast-feeding. If heroin pharmacotherapy is required, breast-feeding should be discontinued. Collaboration with the patient's pediatrician is indicated.

Elderly, frail, or debilitated patients: Generally prescribe lower dosages for elderly, frail, or debilitated patients. Gradually increase the dosage, if needed, according to individual patient response. These patients may be more sensitive to the pharmacologic actions of heroin than are younger or healthier adult patients.

Children and adolescents: Safety and efficacy of heroin pharmacotherapy for children and adolescents have not been established. Heroin pharmacotherapy is *not* recommended for this age group.

Notes, Severe Pain Including Cancer Pain

Dosage must be individualized according to patient response. Although use has been limited in Canada and the United Kingdom, published studies regarding the use of heroin for the symptomatic management of cancer pain in other countries have not shown it to be superior to other opiates for this indication. Heroin is officially referred to as diamorphine in Canada.

AVAILABLE DOSAGE FORMS, STORAGE, AND COMPATIBILITY

Injectables, intramuscular, intravenous, or subcutaneous: 30, 100 mg/ampule. Reconstitute injectables with 1 ml of sterile water for injection. Injectable is incompatible with normal saline.

PROPOSED MECHANISM OF ACTION

Heroin elicits its analgesic and CNS and respiratory depressant actions primarily by binding to the endorphin (opiate) receptors in the CNS. The exact mechanism of these actions has not yet been fully determined. See also "Opiate Analgesics, General Monograph."

PHARMACOKINETICS/PHARMACODYNAMICS

Heroin is converted in the GI tract to morphine (see the morphine monograph) following oral ingestion. It is first converted to monoacetylmorphine and then rapidly (within minutes) converted to morphine following intramuscular, intravenous, or subcutaneous injection. The duration of action is 3 to 5 hours. The intramuscular injection of 5 mg of heroin provides approximately the same pain relief as the intramuscular injection of 10 mg of morphine (see "Opiate Analgesics, General Monograph" for other dosage equivalents). Additional data are not available.

RELATIVE CONTRAINDICATIONS

Chronic obstructive lung disease
Hypersensitivity to heroin or other opiate analgesics
Intracranial hypertension
MAOI pharmacotherapy, concurrent or within 14 days
Respiratory depression, acute

CAUTIONS AND COMMENTS

Prescribe heroin pharmacotherapy cautiously to patients who

- have histories of problematic patterns of opiate or other abusable psychotropic use. Heroin is addicting and habituating.

Caution patients who are receiving heroin pharmacotherapy to

- inform their prescribing psychologist if they begin or discontinue any other pharmacotherapy while receiving heroin pharmacotherapy.

See also "Opiate Analgesics, General Monograph."

CLINICALLY SIGNIFICANT DRUG INTERACTIONS

Concurrent heroin pharmacotherapy and the following may result in clinically significant drug interactions:

Pharmacotherapy With CNS Depressants and Other Drugs That Produce CNS Depression

Concurrent heroin pharmacotherapy and pharmacotherapy with other opiate analgesics, sedative-hypnotics, or other drugs that produce CNS depression (e.g., antihistamines, phenothiazines, TCAs) may result in additive CNS depression.

See also "Opiate Analgesics, General Monograph."

ADVERSE DRUG REACTIONS

Heroin pharmacotherapy commonly has been associated with constipation and other GI complaints, including nausea and vomiting. It also has been commonly associated with respiratory depression, sedation, and sweating (excessive).

See also "Opiate Analgesics, General Monograph."

OVERDOSAGE

Signs and symptoms of heroin overdosage include an exacerbation of its associated CNS and respiratory depressant actions (see "Opiate Analgesics, General Monograph"). Heroin overdosage requires emergency symptomatic medical support of body systems with attention to increasing heroin elimination. The opiate antagonist, naloxone (Narcan®), generally is effective in reversing associated respiratory depression.

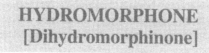

HYDROMORPHONE
[Dihydromorphinone]

(hye droe mor' fone)

TRADE NAMES

Dilaudid®
Dilaudid-HP®
Hydromorph Contin®
HydroStat®

CLASSIFICATION

Opiate analgesic (agonist) (C-II)

See also "Opiate Analgesics, General Monograph."

APPROVED INDICATIONS FOR NEUROPSYCHOLOGICAL DISORDERS

Adjunctive pharmacotherapy for the symptomatic management of:

• pain disorders: acute pain, moderate to severe, and cancer pain, moderate to severe

USUAL DOSAGE AND ADMINISTRATION

Notes, Pain Disorders: Acute Pain, Moderate to Severe, and Cancer Pain, Moderate to Severe

Adults: Initially, 2 mg orally every four to six hours; *or* 1 mg intramuscularly, intravenously, or subcutaneously every four to six hours; *or* 3 mg rectally every six to eight hours. Adjust dosage according to individual patient response. Patients who have severe pain may require 4 mg orally every four to six hours; 2 mg intramuscularly, intravenously, or subcutaneously every four to six hours; or 6 mg rectally every six to eight hours. Patients who have terminal cancer may be tolerant to opiate analgesics. Therefore, these patients may require higher dosages for adequate pain relief. A gradual increase in dosage may be required if analgesia is inadequate or if pain severity increases. For severe pain, or when prompt response is required, initially prescribe injectable formulations in adequate dosages to control pain.

For details and discussion regarding related basic principles of clinical pharmacology, readers are referred to the first text in this series, *The Pharmacologic Basis of Psychotherapeutics: An Introduction for Psychologists.*

Women who are, or who may become, pregnant: FDA Pregnancy Category C. Safety and efficacy of hydromorphone pharmacotherapy for women who are pregnant have not been established. Avoid prescribing hydromorphone pharmacotherapy to women who are pregnant. If hydromorphone pharmacotherapy is required, advise patients of potential benefits and possible risks to themselves and the embryo, fetus, or neonate. Collaboration with the patient's obstetrician or a specialist (e.g., oncologist) is indicated.

Women who are breast-feeding: Safety and efficacy of hydromorphone pharmacotherapy for women who are breast-feeding and their neonates and infants have not been established. It is unknown whether hydromorphone is excreted in breast milk. Avoid prescribing hydromorphone pharmacotherapy to women who are breast-feeding. If hydromorphone pharmacotherapy is required, breast-feeding probably should be discontinued. If desired, lactation may be maintained and breast-feeding resumed following the discontinuation of short-term hydromorphone pharmacotherapy for the management of acute pain. Collaboration with the patient's pediatrician is indicated.

Elderly, frail, or debilitated patients: Generally prescribe lower dosages for elderly, frail, or debilitated patients. Gradually increase the dosage, if needed, according to individual patient response. Dosage should be guided by the goal of optimal pain management with minimal ADRs. These patients may be more sensitive to the pharmacologic actions of hydromorphone than are younger or healthier adult patients.

Children: Safety and efficacy of hydromorphone pharmacotherapy for the management of pain disorders for children have not been established. Hydromorphone pharmacotherapy for this indication is *not* recommended for this age group.

Notes, Pain Disorders: Acute Pain, Moderate to Severe, and Cancer Pain, Moderate to Severe

Hydromorphone is an adequate drug for the symptomatic management of acute severe pain of short duration. The advantage of this drug over other opiate analgesics, such as morphine or meperidine (Demerol®), is its better oral absorption. In addition, hydromorphone rectal suppositories may provide longer duration of pain relief for some patients and obviate the need for dosing during sleeping hours.

Subcutaneous and intravenous injections are generally well tolerated. For intravenous pharmacotherapy, slowly inject over 2 to 3 minutes, depending on the dose. Rapid intravenous injection may increase associated ADRs, including hypotension and respiratory depression. Circulatory depression, peripheral circulatory collapse, and cardiac arrest also have been associated with rapid intravenous injection. Patients should lie down for injectable hydromorphone pharmacotherapy and should remain lying down for at least 30 to 60 minutes following their injections. Postural (orthostatic) hypotension and fainting may occur if patients stand up suddenly after receiving an injection of hydromorphone.

AVAILABLE DOSAGE FORMS, STORAGE, AND COMPATIBILITY

Injectables, *concentrated* intramuscular, intravenous, and subcutaneous: 10, 20, 50 mg/ml (ampules, 10 mg/ml; multidose vials, 10, 20, 50 mg/ml)

Injectables, intramuscular, intravenous, or subcutaneous: 1, 2, 4 mg/ml (ampules, 1, 2, 4 mg/ml)
Suppository, rectal: 3 mg (cocoa butter base)
Syrup, oral: 1 mg/ml (unflavored)
Tablets, oral: 1, 2, 3, 4, 8 mg

Notes

Hydromorphone injectables: The hydromorphone concentrated injectable formulations (i.e., 10, 20, and 50 mg/ml) are *only* intended for hydromorphone pharmacotherapy for patients who are tolerant to opiate analgesics and, thus, require higher dosages. *Do not confuse these concentrated injectable formulations with the less concentrated injectable formulations (i.e., 1, 2, and 4 mg/ml) because of the risk for fatal hydromorphone overdosage.*

Visually inspect hydromorphone injectables for particulate matter and discoloration prior to use. A slight yellowish discoloration may develop in hydromorphone ampules and multiple dose vials. This discoloration does *not* indicate chemical degradation nor a resultant loss of potency. However, do not use darkly discolored injectable solutions and do not use products beyond the expiration date indicated on the label.

Safely store hydromorphone injectables protected from light at controlled room temperature (15 ° to 30 °C; 59 °to 86 °F).

General instructions for patients: Instruct patients who are receiving hydromorphone pharmacotherapy, or those who are assisting them with their pharmacotherapy, to

- safely store hydromorphone oral dosage forms out of the reach of children in child- and light-resistant containers at controlled room temperature (15 ° to 30 °C; 59 °to 86 °F).
- safely store hydromorphone rectal suppositories out of the reach of children in a refrigerator at a temperature between 2 ° and 8 °C (36 ° and 46 °F).
- obtain an available patient information sheet regarding hydromorphone pharmacotherapy from their pharmacist at the time that their prescription is dispensed. Encourage patients to clarify any questions that they may have regarding hydromorphone pharmacotherapy with their pharmacist or, if needed, to consult their prescribing psychologist.

PROPOSED MECHANISM OF ACTION

Although the exact mechanism of action has not been clearly established, hydromorphone appears to elicit its analgesic, CNS depressant (e.g., drowsiness, changes in mood, and mental clouding), and respiratory depressant actions primarily by binding to the endorphin (opiate) receptors in the CNS. See also "Opiate Analgesics, General Monograph."

PHARMACOKINETICS/PHARMACODYNAMICS

Hydromorphone's analgesic action is apparent within 15 minutes after injection and may last 5 or more hours. Hydromorphone is rapidly absorbed after oral ingestion and produces analgesia within 30 minutes. Oral bioavailability is approximately 30%. Hydromorphone is metabolized extensively in the liver. The mean half-life of elimination is approximately 3 hours. Additional data are *not* available.

Although there is no intrinsic limit to hydromorphone's analgesic actions, and adequate doses will relieve even the most severe pain, hydromorphone analgesic pharmacotherapy is limited by its associated ADRs, primarily respiratory depression, nausea, and vomiting.

RELATIVE CONTRAINDICATIONS

Hypersensitivity to hydromorphone
Increased intracranial pressure
Respiratory dysfunction (including that associated with chronic obstructive lung disease, cor pulmonale, emphysema, kyphoscoliosis, pulmonary edema, status asthmaticus)

CAUTIONS AND COMMENTS

Hydromorphone is addicting and habituating and has significant abuse potential. Short-term hydromorphone pharmacotherapy for the symptomatic management of acute pain rarely results in addiction and habituation. However, several weeks of continuous pharmacotherapy may result in addiction and habituation among selected patients. Tolerance is initially noted by a shortened duration of analgesia and, subsequently, by decreases in the intensity of analgesia.

Prescribe hydromorphone pharmacotherapy cautiously to patients who

- are elderly.
- are post-operative. Hydromorphone, which also is medically prescribed as an antitussive, suppresses the cough reflex and may, thus, impede the removal of bronchial secretions and increase the risk for respiratory complications (e.g., post-operative pneumonia).
- have head injuries. Hydromorphone, like other opiate analgesics, can increase intracranial pressure. It also can obscure the clinical monitoring of these patients because of its CNS and respiratory depressant actions.
- have histories of problematic patterns of opiate or other abusable psychotropic use.
- have hypothyroidism, Addison's disease, prostatic hypertrophy, or urethral stricture.
- have kidney or liver dysfunction.
- have respiratory dysfunction or medical disorders that may make them prone to respiratory dysfunction. As with other opiate analgesics, hydromorphone can suppress the cough reflex and depress the rate and depth of respirations. Hydromorphone also produces a dose-related respiratory depression by acting directly on the respiratory center in the brainstem and centers affecting the control of respiratory rhythm. Thus, hydromorphone may produce irregular and periodic breathing (i.e., apnea).

Caution patients who are receiving hydromorphone pharmacotherapy against

- performing activities that require alertness, judgment, or physical coordination (e.g., driving an automobile, operating dangerous equipment, supervising children) until their response to hydromorphone pharmacotherapy is known. Hydromorphone may affect these mental and physical functions adversely.

In addition to this general precaution, caution patients who are receiving hydromorphone pharmacotherapy to

- inform their prescribing psychologist if they begin or discontinue any other pharmacotherapy while receiving hydromorphone pharmacotherapy.

CLINICALLY SIGNIFICANT DRUG INTERACTIONS

Concurrent hydromorphone pharmacotherapy and the following may result in clinically significant drug interactions:

Alcohol Use

Concurrent alcohol use may increase the CNS depressant action of hydromorphone. Advise patients to avoid, or limit, their use of alcohol while receiving hydromorphone pharmacotherapy.

Pharmacotherapy With CNS Depressants and Other Drugs That Produce CNS Depression

Concurrent hydromorphone pharmacotherapy and pharmacotherapy with other opiate analgesics, sedative-hypnotics, or other drugs that produce CNS depression (e.g., antihistamines, phenothiazines, TCAs) may result in additive CNS depression.

See also "Opiate Analgesics, General Monograph."

ADVERSE DRUG REACTIONS

Hydromorphone pharmacotherapy commonly has been associated with nausea, respiratory depression, and vomiting. It also has been associated with the following ADRs, listed according to body system:

Cardiovascular: postural (orthostatic) hypotension, peripheral circulatory collapse, and cardiac arrest (following rapid intravenous injection)
CNS: dizziness, drowsiness, lethargy, loss of appetite (anorexia), and sedation
Genitourinary: ureteral spasm and urinary retention
GI: constipation, nausea, and vomiting
Respiratory: respiratory depression

See also "Opiate Analgesics, General Monograph."

OVERDOSAGE

Signs and symptoms of hydromorphone overdosage include the following: respiratory depression (decreased rate and tidal volume, Cheyne–Stokes respiration, cyanosis), extreme somnolence progressing to stupor or coma, skeletal muscle flaccidity, cold and clammy skin, and, sometimes, bradycardia and hypotension. Severe overdosage, particularly that associated with the intravenous injection of hydromorphone, may result in apnea, circulatory collapse, cardiac arrest, and death.

Hydromorphone overdosage requires emergency symptomatic medical support of body systems with attention to increasing hydromorphone elimination, particularly when the overdosage has involved oral dosage forms. The opiate antagonist, naloxone (Narcan®), is the specific antidote against respiratory depression. Repeated doses of naloxone may be required during the course of the emergency medical management of hydromorphone overdosage. The duration of action of hydromorphone may exceed that of naloxone.

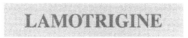
LAMOTRIGINE

(la moe' tri jeen)

TRADE NAME

Lamictal®

CLASSIFICATION

Anticonvulsant (phenyltriazine)

APPROVED INDICATIONS FOR NEUROPSYCHOLOGICAL DISORDERS

Adjunctive pharmacotherapy for the prophylactic and symptomatic management of:

- seizure disorders: partial seizures with or without complex symptomatology (i.e., psychomotor seizures) and for partial and generalized seizures associated with Lennox–Gastaut syndrome. Lamotrigine pharmacotherapy is indicated for adult patients who are refractory to less toxic anticonvulsant pharmacotherapy.

USUAL DOSAGE AND ADMINISTRATION

Seizure Disorders: Partial Seizures With or Without Complex Symptomatology Among Refractory Patients

Adults: Lamotrigine is prescribed as adjunctive pharmacotherapy with other anticonvulsants according to the table "Adjunctive Lamotrigine Pharmacotherapy: Dosage Selection."

Women who are, or who may become, pregnant: FDA Pregnancy Category C. Safety and efficacy of lamotrigine pharmacotherapy for women who are pregnant have not been established. Avoid prescribing lamotrigine pharmacotherapy to women who are pregnant. If lamotrigine pharmacotherapy is required, advise patients of potential benefits and possible risks to themselves and the embryo, fetus, or neonate. Collaboration with the patient's obstetrician is indicated.

Women who are breast-feeding: Safety and efficacy of lamotrigine pharmacotherapy for women who are breast-feeding and their neonates and infants have not been established. Lamotrigine is excreted in breast milk. Avoid prescribing lamotrigine pharmacotherapy to women who are breast-feeding. If lamotrigine pharmacotherapy is required, breast-feeding probably should be discontinued. Collaboration with the patient's pediatrician is indicated.

For details and discussion regarding related basic principles of clinical pharmacology, readers are referred to the first text in this series, *The Pharmacologic Basis of Psychotherapeutics: An Introduction for Psychologists.*

Adjunctive lamotrigine pharmacotherapy: dosage selection.

Initiation and Maintenance of Lamotrigine Pharmacotherapy	Carbamazepine, phenobarbital, phenytoin, *or* primidone *with* valproic acid	Carbamazepine, phenobarbital, phenytoin, *or* primidone *without* valproic acid
First and second weeks	25 mg lamotrigine orally every other day	50 mg lamotrigine daily orally in a single dose
Third and fourth weeks	25 mg lamotrigine daily orally in a single oral dose	100 mg lamotrigine daily orally in two divided doses
Maintenance	100 to 150 mg lamotrigine daily orally in two divided doses. Achieve the desired maintenance dosage by increasing the dosage by 25 to 50 mg every one to two weeks.	300 to 500 mg lamotrigine daily orally in two divided doses. Achieve the desired maintenance dosage by increasing the dosage by 100 mg every one to two weeks.

Elderly, frail, or debilitated patients: Generally prescribe lower dosages for elderly, frail, or debilitated patients. Lamotrigine elimination is reduced by ∼25% among elderly patients because of decreased glucuronidation, which is believed to be due to an age-related reduction in liver blood flow. Gradually increase the dosage if needed, according to individual patient response. These patients also may be more sensitive to the pharmacologic actions of lamotrigine than are younger or healthier adult patients.

Children and adolescents younger than 16 years of age: Lamotrigine pharmacotherapy is *not* recommended for children and adolescents who are younger than 16 years of age. A high incidence (∼1 in 50) of severe skin rash that may presage potentially fatal skin reactions (i.e., Stevens–Johnson syndrome and toxic epidermal necrolysis) has been reported among children and adolescents who have received lamotrigine pharmacotherapy.

Notes, Seizure Disorders: Partial Seizures With or Without Complex Symptomatology Among Refractory Patients

Lamotrigine generally is prescribed as adjunctive pharmacotherapy to other anticonvulsant pharmacotherapy (e.g., carbamazepine, phenobarbital, and phenytoin pharmacotherapy) to reduce the frequency of partial seizures. (See table "Adjunctive Lamotrigine Pharmacotherapy: Dosage Selection.") Adjunctive lamotrigine pharmacotherapy has been associated with a mean reduction in partial seizure frequency of ∼25% to 33%.

Initiating and maintaining lamotrigine pharmacotherapy: See table "Adjunctive Lamotrigine Pharmacotherapy: Dosage Selection."

Discontinuing lamotrigine pharmacotherapy: In order to decrease the risk of lamotrigine withdrawal-related seizures, gradually discontinue lamotrigine pharmacotherapy over a minimal period of 2 weeks. Reduce the dosage by ~50% each week, unless safety concerns (i.e., toxicity) require a more rapid discontinuation of lamotrigine pharmacotherapy.

AVAILABLE DOSAGE FORMS, STORAGE, AND COMPATIBILITY

Tablets, oral: 25, 100, 150, 200 mg

Notes

General instructions for patients: Instruct patients who are receiving lamotrigine pharmacotherapy to

- safely store lamotrigine oral tablets out of the reach of children in tightly closed, light- and child-resistant containers at controlled room temperature (15° to 30°C; 59° to 86°F).
- notify their prescribing psychologist immediately if any skin rash is noted (see "Cautions and Comments").
- obtain an available patient information sheet regarding lamotrigine pharmacotherapy from their pharmacist at the time that their prescription is dispensed. Encourage patients to clarify any questions that they may have regarding lamotrigine pharmacotherapy with their pharmacist or, if needed, to consult their prescribing psychologist.

PROPOSED MECHANISM OF ACTION

The exact mechanism of anticonvulsant action of lamotrigine has not yet been fully determined. It appears to involve inhibition of presynaptic voltage-dependent sodium ion channels to stabilize neuronal membranes and inhibit the release of excitatory amino acid neurotransmitters such as aspartate and glutamate.

PHARMACOKINETICS/PHARMACODYNAMICS

Lamotrigine is absorbed rapidly and completely ($F = 0.98$) from the GI tract following oral ingestion. Peak blood concentrations are achieved within 1 to 5 hours. Salivary concentrations are ~50% of the total plasma concentration. The ingestion of food slightly reduces the rate of lamotrigine absorption, but does not affect the extent of absorption. Lamotrigine is moderately bound to plasma proteins (~55%) and its mean apparent volume of distribution is ~1 liter/kg. It is metabolized primarily in the liver by glucuronic acid conjugation. Less than 20% is excreted in unchanged form in the urine. Mean total body clearance is 0.58 ml/minute/kg (range: 0.24 to 1.15 ml/minute/kg). Total body clearance (per kg) in children younger than 5 years of age is approximately twice that observed among adults. The mean half-life of elimination is ~27 hours (range: 15 to 65 hours). Additional data are not available.

Therapeutic Drug Monitoring

Among patients receiving adjunctive pharmacotherapy with one or more other anticonvulsant drugs, efficacious dosages of lamotrigine generally resulted in steady state trough blood concentrations of 1 to 4 µg/ml.

RELATIVE CONTRAINDICATIONS

Hypersensitivity to lamotrigine

CAUTIONS AND COMMENTS

Benign rashes may occur in up to 10% of patients receiving lamotrigine pharmacotherapy. However, it is *not* possible to reliably predict which rashes will be benign and which will progress to potentially life-threatening reactions (i.e., Stevens–Johnson syndrome). Therefore, lamotrigine pharmacotherapy should be discontinued immediately at the first sign of a rash and the patient referred for appropriate medical evaluation and treatment.

Prescribe lamotrigine pharmacotherapy cautiously to patients who

- have renal dysfunction. The half-life of elimination of lamotrigine may be increased (up to 100%) among patients who have renal dysfunction. Although guidelines for specific dosage adjustments have not been developed for these patients, careful prescription and monitoring of lamotrigine pharmacotherapy are required, with attention to the need for possible dosage reduction.

Caution patients who are receiving lamotrigine pharmacotherapy against

- performing activities that require alertness, judgment, or physical coordination (e.g., driving an automobile, operating dangerous equipment, supervising children) until their response to lamotrigine pharmacotherapy is known. Lamotrigine may affect these mental and physical functions adversely.

CLINICALLY SIGNIFICANT DRUG INTERACTIONS

Concurrent lamotrigine pharmacotherapy and the following may result in clinically significant drug interactions:

Acetaminophen Use

Chronic use (i.e., multiple repeated doses) of acetaminophen (Tylenol®) may result in decreased bioavailability and a decreased half-life of elimination of lamotrigine (i.e., a reduction in the half-life of 10% to 20%). The mechanism and clinical significance of this interaction are yet to be fully determined. However, occasional use of antipyretic/analgesic dosages of acetaminophen is unlikely to result in a clinically significant drug interaction.

Alcohol Use

Concurrent alcohol use may increase the CNS depressant action of lamotrigine. Advise patients to avoid, or limit, their use of alcohol while receiving lamotrigine pharmacotherapy.

Carbamazepine Pharmacotherapy

Concurrent lamotrigine and carbamazepine (Tegretol®) pharmacotherapy may result in an increase in lamotrigine total body clearance by up to 100% and a corresponding decrease in the mean half-life of elimination to ~15 hours. Increased incidence or severity of neurotoxicity (e.g., blurred vision, dizziness) also may result from concurrent pharmacotherapy. This increased incidence of toxicity may be the result of increased carbamazepine-epoxide concentrations, but currently available data are contradictory and inconclusive. See table "Adjunctive Lamotrigine Pharmacotherapy: Dosage Selection" for recommended dosage adjustments.

Pharmacotherapy With CNS Depressants and Other Drugs That Produce CNS Depression

Concurrent lamotrigine pharmacotherapy and pharmacotherapy with opiate analgesics, sedative-hypnotics, or other drugs that produce CNS depression (e.g., antihistamines, phenothiazines, TCAs) may result in additive CNS depression.

Phenobarbital Pharmacotherapy

Concurrent lamotrigine and phenobarbital (Luminal®) pharmacotherapy may result in an increase in lamotrigine total body clearance by up to 100% and a corresponding decrease in the mean half-life of elimination to ~15 hours. See table "Adjunctive Lamotrigine Pharmacotherapy: Dosage Selection" for recommended dosage adjustments.

Phenytoin Pharmacotherapy

Concurrent lamotrigine and phenytoin (Dilantin®) pharmacotherapy may result in an increase in lamotrigine total body clearance by up to 100% and a corresponding decrease in the mean half-life of elimination to ~15 hours. See table "Adjunctive Lamotrigine Pharmacotherapy: Dosage Selection" for suggested dosage adjustments.

Primidone Pharmacotherapy

See the phenobarbital monograph (phenobarbital is the active metabolite of primidone [Mysoline®]).

Valproic Acid Pharmacotherapy

Concurrent valproic acid (Depakene®) pharmacotherapy reduces the total body clearance of lamotrigine by ~50%, by means of competition for glucuronidation, and more than doubles the half-life of elimination (i.e., to a mean half-life of ~60 hours). Risk for the development of ADRs increases significantly. See table "Adjunctive Lamotrigine Pharmacotherapy: Dosage Selection" for recommended dosage adjustments.

ADVERSE DRUG REACTIONS

Lamotrigine pharmacotherapy has been associated commonly with: asthenia, blurred or double vision (diplopia), dizziness, fatigue, headache, nausea, rash, and somnolence. Lamotrigine pharmacotherapy also has been associated with the following ADRs, listed according to body system:

CNS: amnesia, anxiety, confusion, depression, drowsiness, exacerbation of the seizure disorder, insomnia, irritability, memory impairment, speech disorders, and tremor

Cutaneous: severe skin rash (~1 in 1,000 cases among adults and ~1 in 50 cases among children), which may presage Stevens–Johnson syndrome and toxic epidermal necrolysis (rare). Both of these reactions are *potentially fatal.*

Genitourinary: painful menstruation (dysmenorrhea) and inflammation of the vagina (vaginitis)

GI: diarrhea, dyspepsia, and vomiting

Musculoskeletal: joint pain (arthralgia) and incoordination (ataxia)

Respiratory: inflammation of the pharynx (pharyngitis) and runny nose (rhinitis)

Miscellaneous: accidental injury

OVERDOSAGE

The signs and symptoms of lamotrigine overdosage include coma. Lamotrigine overdosage requires emergency symptomatic medical support of body systems with attention to increasing lamotrigine elimination. There is no known antidote.

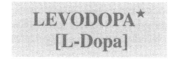

(lee voe doe' pa)

TRADE NAMES

Dopar®
Larodopa®

CLASSIFICATION

Antiparkinsonian (metabolic precursor of dopamine)

APPROVED INDICATIONS FOR NEUROPSYCHOLOGICAL DISORDERS

Pharmacotherapy for the symptomatic management of:

- Parkinson's disease: idiopathic and post-encephalitic. Levodopa pharmacotherapy also is indicated for the symptomatic management of Parkinson's disease associated with carbon monoxide and manganese poisoning.

USUAL DOSAGE AND ADMINISTRATION

Parkinson's Disease: Idiopathic, Postencephalitic, and That Associated With Carbon Monoxide and Manganese Poisoning

Adults: Initially, 500 to 1000 mg daily orally in two or more divided doses with food. Increase the initial dosage by 750 mg every three to seven days until optimal therapeutic benefit is achieved. Monitor individual patient response carefully during dosage adjustment.

MAXIMUM: 8000 mg daily orally

Women who are, or who may become, pregnant: FDA Pregnancy Category "not established." Safety and efficacy of levodopa pharmacotherapy for women who are pregnant have not been established. Avoid prescribing levodopa pharmacotherapy to women who are pregnant. If levodopa pharmacotherapy is required, advise patients of potential benefits and possible risks to themselves and the embryo, fetus, or neonate. Collaboration with the patient's obstetrician is indicated.

Women who are breast-feeding: Safety and efficacy of levodopa pharmacotherapy for women who are breast-feeding and their neonates and infants have not been established. Avoid prescribing levodopa pharmacotherapy to women who are breast-feeding. If levodopa pharmacotherapy is required, breast-feeding probably should be discontinued.

For details and discussion regarding related basic principles of clinical pharmacology, readers are referred to the first text in this series, *The Pharmacologic Basis of Psychotherapeutics: An Introduction for Psychologists.*

Elderly adults: See previous information on adult dosages. Although no special dosage adjustments generally are recommended for elderly adults, these patients may be more sensitive to the pharmacologic actions of levodopa than are younger or healthier adult patients.

Children and adolescents younger than 18 years of age: Safety and efficacy of levodopa pharmacotherapy for children and adolescents who are younger than 18 years of age have not been established. Levodopa pharmacotherapy is *not* recommended for this age group.

Notes, Parkinson's Disease: Idiopathic and Post-Encephalitic

Periodic evaluations of cardiovascular, hematologic, hepatic, and renal function are recommended for all patients who are receiving long-term levodopa pharmacotherapy. Collaboration with the patient's advanced practice nurse or family physician is required.

Levodopa pharmacotherapy in combination with peripheral decarboxylase inhibitor (e.g., benserazide, carbidopa) pharmacotherapy allows the dosage of levodopa to be decreased significantly. Associated ADRs also are decreased concomitantly in terms of both incidence and severity. Thus, it is generally recommended that levodopa pharmacotherapy be prescribed in combination with peripheral decarboxylase inhibitor (i.e., benserazide or carbidopa) pharmacotherapy whenever clinically feasible. See the levodopa and benserazide monograph and the levodopa and carbidopa monograph.

AVAILABLE DOSAGE FORMS, STORAGE, AND COMPATIBILITY

Capsules, oral: 100, 250, 500 mg
Tablets, oral: 100, 250, 500 mg

Notes

Oral levodopa pharmacotherapy: The Dopar® oral capsules contain tartrazine (FD & C Yellow No. 5). Tartrazine has been associated with hypersensitivity reactions (e.g., bronchial asthma) among susceptible patients, particularly those who have a hypersensitivity to aspirin.

General instructions for patients: Instruct patients who are receiving levodopa pharmacotherapy to

- safely store levodopa oral capsules and tablets out of the reach of children in tightly closed, light- and child-resistant containers at controlled room temperature (15° to 30°C; 59° to 86°F).
- obtain an available patient information sheet regarding levodopa pharmacotherapy from their pharmacist at the time that their prescription is dispensed. Encourage patients to clarify any questions that they may have regarding levodopa pharmacotherapy with their pharmacist or, if needed, to consult their prescribing psychologist.

PROPOSED MECHANISM OF ACTION

The signs and symptoms of Parkinson's disease appear to be related to the depletion of striatal dopamine. Dopamine does not cross the blood–brain barrier. However, levodopa, the levorotatory isomer of dopa and the metabolic precursor of dopamine, does cross the blood–brain barrier. Levodopa is converted to dopamine in the basal ganglia.

PHARMACOKINETICS/PHARMACODYNAMICS

Levodopa generally is absorbed only moderately following oral ingestion ($F = 0.4$). Extensive amounts of an oral dose of levodopa are metabolized in the lumen of the stomach and the small intestines. Concomitant carbidopa pharmacotherapy significantly increases the oral absorption of levodopa ($F = 0.9$). Thus, levodopa may be prescribed in combination with carbidopa. The apparent volume of distribution of levodopa is 1.7 liters/kg. Less than 1% of levodopa is excreted in unchanged form in the urine. The total body clearance is ∼1500 ml/minute and the mean half-life of elimination is 1.4 hours. Levodopa is metabolized in the body to dopamine and homovanillic acid (HVA). Additional data are not available.

RELATIVE CONTRAINDICATIONS

Melanoma or suspicious undiagnosed skin lesions, history of. Levodopa may activate malignant melanoma.
Hypersensitivity to levodopa
MAOI pharmacotherapy, concurrent or within the previous 14 days
Narrow-angle glaucoma

CAUTIONS AND COMMENTS

Prescribe levodopa pharmacotherapy cautiously to patients who

- have a history of active peptic ulcer disease. Levodopa pharmacotherapy has been associated with GI hemorrhage among these patients.
- have a history of myocardial infarction with residual cardiac dysrhythmias. Levodopa pharmacotherapy has been associated with serious ADRs involving the cardiovascular system. Thus, levodopa pharmacotherapy should only be initiated for these patients in situations where appropriate cardiovascular monitoring and support are readily available (e.g., a hospital cardiac or intensive care unit). Collaboration with the patient's cardiologist is required.
- have wide-angle glaucoma. Only prescribe levodopa pharmacotherapy for patients who are receiving appropriate pharmacotherapy for the treatment of wide-angle glaucoma and whose intraocular pressure is well controlled. These patients also require regular monitoring of their intraocular pressure. Collaboration with the patient's ophthalmologist is required.

CLINICALLY SIGNIFICANT DRUG INTERACTIONS

Concurrent levodopa pharmacotherapy and the following may result in clinically significant drug interactions:

Antipsychotic Pharmacotherapy

The antipsychotics, particularly the butyrophenones (e.g., haloperidol [Haldol®]) and phenothiazines (e.g., chlorpromazine [Thorazine®]), can antagonize and, thus, reduce the therapeutic action of levodopa. Patients who are receiving concurrent levodopa and antipsychotic pharmacotherapy must be carefully monitored for possible loss of antiparkinsonian effect.

MAOI Pharmacotherapy

Concurrent levodopa and MAOI pharmacotherapy may result in the hypertensive crisis. Thus, this combination of pharmacotherapy, concurrent or within 14 days, is contraindicated. See "Relative Contraindications."

Pharmacotherapy With Antihypertensive Drugs

Levodopa pharmacotherapy has been associated with postural (orthostatic) hypotension. Therefore, concurrent pharmacotherapy with antihypertensives will require careful blood pressure monitoring and a possible reduction of the dosage of the antihypertensive. Collaboration with the prescriber of the antihypertensive is indicated.

Pyridoxine Pharmacotherapy

Pyridoxine (vitamin B_6), in oral doses of 10 to 25 mg, rapidly reverses both the therapeutic and toxic effects of levodopa. Caution patients in regard to the selection and use of multiple vitamin products containing pyridoxine.

ADVERSE DRUG REACTIONS

Levodopa pharmacotherapy has been commonly associated with the following ADRs: choreiform, dystonic, and other involuntary movements; oscillations in performance, including akinesia paradoxica (hypotonic freezing), end-of-dose akinesia, and the "on–off" phenomenon; and such mental disorders as dementia, depression, paranoid ideation, and psychosis. Levodopa pharmacotherapy also has been associated with the following ADRs, listed according to body system:

Cardiovascular: angina pectoris and postural (orthostatic) hypotension
CNS: anxiety, confusion, convulsions (rare), delusions, euphoria, hallucinations, headache, incoordination (ataxia), insomnia, increased libido with serious antisocial behavior, mania, nightmares, panic attacks, and tremor
Cutaneous: dark-colored sweat, edema, hair loss (alopecia), and rash
Genitourinary: dark-colored urine, hematuria, and nocturia
GI: abdominal pain, belching or producing gas from the stomach (eructation), producing gas from the intestines (flatulence), GI bleeding, hiccups, loss of appetite (anorexia), nausea, and vomiting
Hematologic: agranulocytosis (rare), hemolytic anemia (rare), and leukopenia
Musculoskeletal: low back pain and muscle spasms and twitching. (See also CNS.)
Ophthalmic: blurred vision, dilated pupils (mydriasis), double vision (diplopia), and activation of latent Horner's syndrome
Respiratory: abnormal breathing pattern and cough
Miscellaneous: fatigue, fever, grinding of the teeth (bruxism), and malaise

OVERDOSAGE

The signs and symptoms of levodopa overdosage include abnormal involuntary movements, including choreiform and dystonic movements. Muscle twitching and blepharospasm (spasm of the orbicularis oculi muscle) may be early signs of overdosage. In general, the signs and symptoms of levodopa overdosage are qualitatively similar to the ADRs associated with levodopa pharmacotherapy. However, they are of greater magnitude. Levodopa overdosage requires emergency symptomatic medical support of body systems with attention to increasing levodopa elimination. Although theoretically feasible, the efficacy of pyridoxine (vitamin B_6) for the medical treatment of levodopa overdosage has not yet been established (see "Clinically Significant Drug Interactions").

LEVODOPA and BENSERAZIDE✻

(lee voe doe′ pa; ben ser′ a zide)

TRADE NAME

Prolopa®

CLASSIFICATION

Antiparkinsonian fixed-ratio combination (metabolic precursor of dopamine and a peripheral decarboxylase inhibitor)

APPROVED INDICATIONS FOR NEUROPSYCHOLOGICAL DISORDERS

Fixed-ratio combination pharmacotherapy for the symptomatic management of:

- Parkinson's disease: idiopathic. Note that fixed-ratio combination levodopa and benserazide pharmacotherapy is *not* indicated for the symptomatic management of drug-induced Parkinson's disease, Huntington's chorea, or intention tremor.

USUAL DOSAGE AND ADMINISTRATION

Parkinson's Disease: Idiopathic

Adults: Initially, 100:25 to 200:50 mg (levodopa:benserazide) daily orally in two divided doses. Increase the dosage according to individual patient response by 100:25 mg every three to four days until optimal therapeutic benefit is achieved without dyskinesia. As the dosage is increased, the dosing interval also should be increased to at least four times daily. Each dose should be ingested with food or immediately following a meal.

MAINTENANCE: The mean maintenance dosage is 600:150 mg (levodopa:benserazide) daily orally

MAXIMUM: 1200:300 mg (levodopa:benserazide) daily orally during the first year of pharmacotherapy

Women who are, or who may become, pregnant: FDA Pregnancy Category "not established." Safety and efficacy of fixed-ratio combination levodopa and benserazide pharmacotherapy for women who are pregnant have not been established. Avoid prescribing fixed-ratio

For details and discussion regarding related basic principles of clinical pharmacology, readers are referred to the first text in this series, *The Pharmacologic Basis of Psychotherapeutics: An Introduction for Psychologists.*

combination levodopa and benserazide pharmacotherapy to women who are pregnant. If fixed-ratio levodopa and benserazide pharmacotherapy is required, advise patients of potential benefits and possible risks to themselves and the embryo, fetus, neonate. Collaboration with the patient's obstetrician is indicated.

Women who are breast-feeding: Safety and efficacy of fixed-ratio combination levodopa and benserazide pharmacotherapy for women who are breast-feeding and their neonates and infants have not been established. Avoid prescribing fixed-ratio combination levodopa and benserazide pharmacotherapy to women who are breast-feeding. If fixed-ratio combination levodopa and benserazide pharmacotherapy is required, breast-feeding probably should be discontinued.

Elderly patients: See "Adults." Note that, although no special dosage adjustments are recommended for the elderly, these patients may be more sensitive to the pharmacologic actions of fixed-ratio combination levodopa and benserazide pharmacotherapy than are younger or healthier adult patients.

Children and adolescents younger than 18 years of age: Safety and efficacy of fixed-ratio combination levodopa and benserazide pharmacotherapy for children and adolescents who are younger than 18 years of age have not been established. Fixed-ratio combination levodopa and benserazide pharmacotherapy is *not* recommended for this age group.

Notes, Parkinson's Disease: Idiopathic

For patients whose Parkinson's disease has been managed with levodopa pharmacotherapy alone, discontinue their levodopa pharmacotherapy for at least 12 hours before initiating fixed-ratio combination levodopa and benserazide pharmacotherapy. Initiate fixed-ratio combination levodopa and benserazide pharmacotherapy at a levodopa dosage ~15% of the previous levodopa dosage (i.e., the levodopa dosage when used alone *without* benserazide).

AVAILABLE DOSAGE FORMS, STORAGE, AND COMPATIBILITY

Capsules, oral (levodopa:benserazide): 50:12.5, 100:25, 200:50 mg

Notes

The fixed-ratio combination levodopa and benserazide oral capsules are formulated in a 4 mg:1 mg ratio of levodopa to benserazide (i.e., levodopa:benserazide).

General instructions for patients: Instruct patients who are receiving fixed-ratio combination levodopa and benserazide pharmacotherapy to

- swallow fixed-ratio combination levodopa and benserazide oral capsules whole with adequate liquid chaser (i.e., 60 to 120 ml). Also instruct them *not* to chew, cut, dissolve in liquid, or open the capsules.
- safely store fixed-ratio combination levodopa and benserazide oral capsules out of the reach of children in tightly closed, light- and child-resistant containers at controlled room temperature (15° to 30°C; 59° to 86°F).

- obtain an available patient information sheet regarding fixed-ratio combination levodopa and benserazide pharmacotherapy from their pharmacist at the time that their prescription is dispensed. Encourage patients to clarify any questions that they may have regarding fixed-ratio combination levodopa and benserazide pharmacotherapy with their pharmacist or, if needed, to consult their prescribing psychologist.

PROPOSED MECHANISM OF ACTION

Levodopa, a dopamine precursor, crosses the blood–brain barrier. Thus, it is able to help to correct the akinesia associated with Parkinson's disease by forming dopamine at nigro-striatal dopaminergic sites. Unfortunately, the peripheral decarboxylation of levodopa necessitates the use of levodopa dosages that are much higher than is otherwise necessary. These higher dosages result in excessive extracerebral concentrations of dopamine which, in turn, account for several of the ADRs that have been associated with levodopa pharmacotherapy (e.g., cardiac dysrhythmias, nausea, vomiting).

Combining benserazide, a peripheral decarboxylase inhibitor, with levodopa in a fixed-ratio combination formulation allows for a significant reduction in the required dosage of levodopa and, consequently, a significant reduction in both the incidence and severity of levodopa-associated ADRs. Unfortunately, the centrally mediated ADRs associated with levodopa pharmacotherapy are *not* ameliorated (see the levodopa monograph).

PHARMACOKINETICS/PHARMACODYNAMICS

Fixed-ratio combination levodopa and benserazide pharmacotherapy results in an increase in the levodopa blood concentration to approximately 6- to 10-fold over that associated with levodopa pharmacotherapy alone.

See the levodopa monograph.

RELATIVE CONTRAINDICATIONS

Cardiovascular, endocrine, hepatic, pulmonary, or renal disease, uncompensated
Hypersensitivity to benserazide or levodopa
Melanoma or suspicious undiagnosed skin lesions, histories of. Levodopa pharmacotherapy has been associated with the activation of malignant melanoma.
MAOI pharmacotherapy, concurrent or within the previous 14 days
Narrow-angle glaucoma

See also the levodopa monograph.

CAUTIONS AND COMMENTS

Prescribe fixed-ratio combination levodopa and benserazide pharmacotherapy cautiously to patients who

- have histories of mental disorders. Fixed-ratio combination levodopa and benserazide pharmacotherapy has been associated with the occurrence of mental disorders in ~20%

of patients. Monitor patients for both exacerbation of existing mental disorders and signs and symptoms of new mental disorders.

See also the levodopa monograph.

CLINICALLY SIGNIFICANT DRUG INTERACTIONS

Concurrent fixed-ratio combination levodopa and benserazide pharmacotherapy and the following may result in clinically significant drug interactions:

Antipsychotic Pharmacotherapy

The antipsychotics, particularly the butyrophenones (e.g., haloperidol [Haldol®]) and phenothiazines (e.g., chlorpromazine [Thorazine®]), can antagonize and reduce the therapeutic action of levodopa. Thus, patients who are receiving concurrent pharmacotherapy must be monitored for possible loss of antiparkinsonian effect.

Pharmacotherapy With Antihypertensives

Fixed-ratio combination levodopa and benserazide pharmacotherapy has been associated with postural (orthostatic) hypotension. Therefore, concurrent pharmacotherapy will require blood pressure monitoring. A reduction of the dosage of the antihypertensive may be required. Collaboration with the prescriber of the antihypertensive is indicated.

ADVERSE DRUG REACTIONS

Fixed-ratio combination levodopa and benserazide pharmacotherapy commonly has been associated with choreiform, dystonic, and other involuntary movements; oscillations in performance, including akinesia paradoxica (hypotonic freezing), end-of-dose akinesia, and the "on–off" phenomenon; and various mental disorders (i.e., dementia, depression, paranoid ideation, psychotic episodes). Fixed-ratio combination levodopa and benserazide pharmacotherapy also has been associated with the following ADRs, listed according to body system:

Cardiovascular: angina pectoris and postural (orthostatic) hypotension
CNS: convulsions, euphoria, grinding of the teeth (bruxism), hallucinations, incoordination (ataxia), insomnia, increased libido with serious antisocial behavior, nightmares, and tremor
Cutaneous: dark-colored sweat, edema, hair loss (alopecia), and rash
Genitourinary: dark-colored urine, blood in the urine (hematuria), and excessive night time urination (nocturia)
GI: abdominal pain, eructation, flatulence, GI bleeding, hiccups, nausea, and vomiting
Hematologic: agranulocytosis, hemolytic anemia (rare), and leukopenia
Musculoskeletal: low back pain and muscle spasm and twitching
Ophthalmic: blurred vision, dilated pupils, double vision (diplopia), and activation of latent Horner's syndrome
Respiratory: abnormal breathing pattern and cough
Miscellaneous: fever

See also the levodopa monograph.

OVERDOSAGE

The signs and symptoms of fixed-ratio combination levodopa and benserazide overdosage include abnormal involuntary movements (e.g., choreiform and dystonic movements). Muscle twitching and blepharospasm (spastic contraction of the orbicularis oculi muscle) may be early signs of overdosage. Generally, the signs and symptoms of fixed-ratio combination levodopa and benserazide overdosage are qualitatively similar to their associated ADRs, but are more severe. Fixed-ratio combination levodopa and benserazide overdosage requires emergency symptomatic medical support of body systems with attention to increasing the elimination of levodopa and benserazide. There is no known antidote. Pyridoxine (vitamin B_6) is *ineffective* in reversing the effects of fixed-ratio combination levodopa and benserazide overdosage.

LEVODOPA and CARBIDOPA

(lee voe doe′ pa; kar bi doe′ pa)

TRADE NAMES

Apo-Levocarb®
Nu-Levocarb®
Sinemet®
Sinemet CR®

CLASSIFICATION

Antiparkinsonian fixed-ratio combination (metabolic precursor of dopamine and a peripheral decarboxylase inhibitor)

APPROVED INDICATIONS FOR NEUROPSYCHOLOGICAL DISORDERS

Fixed-ratio combination pharmacotherapy for the symptomatic management of:

- Parkinson's disease: idiopathic and post-encephalitic. Fixed-ratio combination levodopa and carbidopa pharmacotherapy also is indicated for the symptomatic management of the Parkinson's disease associated with carbon monoxide or manganese poisoning. Note that fixed-ratio combination levodopa and carbidopa pharmacotherapy is *not* indicated for the symptomatic management of drug-induced Parkinson's disease.

USUAL DOSAGE AND ADMINISTRATION

Parkinson's Disease: Idiopathic, Post-Encephalitic, and That Associated With Carbon Monoxide and Manganese Poisoning

Adults: Initially, 300:75 mg (levopa:carbidopa) daily orally in three divided doses. Gradually increase the dosage according to individual patient response by 100:25 mg every other day until optimal therapeutic benefit is achieved without dyskinesia.

MAXIMUM: 800:200 mg (levodopa:carbidopa) daily orally. The fixed-ratio combination levodopa and carbidopa extended-release formulation (i.e., Sinemet CR®) is designed to deliver fixed-ratio combination pharmacotherapy over a four- to six-hour period. Fixed-ratio combination levodopa and carbidopa extended-release tablet pharmacotherapy provides less variability in levodopa blood concentrations than is observed with the regular levodopa and carbidopa formulation (i.e., Sinemet®). However, in order to adjust for the decreased bioavailability associated with the extended-release formulation, the dosage (in terms of amount of levodopa) may need to be *increased* by 10% to 30% depending on individual patient response.

For details and discussion regarding related basic principles of clinical pharmacology, readers are referred to the first text in this series, *The Pharmacologic Basis of Psychotherapeutics: An Introduction for Psychologists.*

Women who are, or who may become, pregnant: FDA Pregnancy Category C. Safety and efficacy of fixed-ratio combination levodopa and carbidopa pharmacotherapy for women who are pregnant have not been established. Reportedly, levodopa crosses the placental barrier and is metabolized by the fetus. Avoid prescribing fixed-ratio combination levodopa and carbidopa pharmacotherapy to women who are pregnant. If fixed-ratio combination levodopa and carbidopa pharmacotherapy is required, advise patients of potential benefits and possible risks to themselves and the embryo, fetus, or neonate. Collaboration with the patient's obstetrician is indicated.

Women who are breast-feeding: Safety and efficacy of fixed-ratio combination levodopa and carbidopa pharmacotherapy for women who are breast-feeding and their neonates and infants have not been established. Avoid prescribing combination levodopa and carbidopa pharmacotherapy to women who are breast-feeding. If fixed-ratio combination levodopa and carbidopa pharmacotherapy is required, breast-feeding probably should be discontinued.

Elderly adults: See "Adults." Note that, although no special dosage adjustments are recommended for the elderly, these patients may be more sensitive to the pharmacologic actions of fixed-ratio combination levodopa and carbidopa than are younger or healthier adult patients.

Children and adolescents younger than 18 years of age: Safety and efficacy of fixed-ratio combination levodopa and carbidopa pharmacotherapy for children and adolescents who are younger than 18 years of age have not been established. Fixed-ratio combination levodopa and carbidopa pharmacotherapy is *not* recommended for this age group.

Notes, Parkinson's Disease

Initiating fixed-ratio combination levodopa and carbidopa pharmacotherapy: For patients whose Parkinson's disease has been managed with levodopa pharmacotherapy alone, discontinue their levodopa pharmacotherapy for at least 12 hours before initiating fixed-ratio combination levodopa and carbidopa pharmacotherapy. Initiate fixed-ratio combination levodopa and carbidopa pharmacotherapy at a levodopa dosage of ∼25% of the previous levodopa dosage (i.e., the levodopa dosage when used alone *without* carbidopa).

AVAILABLE DOSAGE FORMS, STORAGE, AND COMPATIBILITY

Tablets, oral (levodopa:carbidopa [Sinemet®]): 100:25, 100:10, 250:25 mg
Tablets, oral extended-release (levodopa:carbidopa [Sinemet CR®]): 100:25, 200:50 mg

Notes

Fixed-ratio combination levodopa and carbidopa oral tablets and oral extended-release tablets are formulated in ratios of 4 mg levodopa:1 mg carbidopa and 10 mg levodopa:1 mg carbidopa.

General instructions for patients: Instruct patients who are receiving fixed-ratio combination levodopa and carbidopa pharmacotherapy to

- swallow the fixed-ratio combination levodopa and carbidopa extended-release 100:25-mg tablets whole without breaking, chewing, or crushing with adequate liquid chaser (i.e., 60 to 120 ml of water). The fixed-ratio combination levodopa and carbidopa extended-release 250:25-mg tablets are scored and can be broken into two equal pieces to facilitate ingestion or to adjust the dosage more conveniently when required. However, they should *not* be otherwise broken, chewed, or crushed.
- safely store fixed-ratio combination levodopa and carbidopa oral tablets and oral extended-release tablets out of the reach of children in tightly closed, light- and child-resistant containers at controlled room temperature (15° to 30°C; 59° to 86°F).
- obtain an available patient information sheet regarding fixed-ratio combination levodopa and carbidopa pharmacotherapy from their pharmacist at the time that their prescription is dispensed. Encourage patients to clarify any questions that they may have regarding fixed-ratio combination levodopa and carbidopa pharmacotherapy with their pharmacist or, if needed, to consult their prescribing psychologist.

PROPOSED MECHANISM OF ACTION

Levodopa, a dopamine precursor, crosses the blood–brain barrier. Thus, it is able to help to correct the akinesia associated with Parkinson's disease by forming dopamine at nigro-striatal dopaminergic sites. Unfortunately, the peripheral decarboxylation of levodopa necessitates the use of levodopa dosages that are much higher than is otherwise necessary. These higher dosages result in excessive extracerebral concentrations of dopamine which, in turn, account for several of the ADRs that have been associated with levodopa pharmacotherapy (e.g., cardiac dysrhythmias, nausea, vomiting).

Combining carbidopa, a peripheral decarboxylase inhibitor, and levodopa in a fixed-ratio formulation allows for a significant reduction in the required dosage of levodopa and, consequently, a significant reduction in both the incidence and severity of levodopa-associated ADRs. Unfortunately, the centrally mediated ADRs associated with levodopa pharmacotherapy are *not* ameliorated (see the levodopa monograph).

PHARMACOKINETICS/PHARMACODYNAMICS

See the levodopa monograph.

RELATIVE CONTRAINDICATIONS

Cardiovascular, endocrine, hepatic, pulmonary, or renal disease, uncompensated
Hypersensitivity to carbidopa or levodopa
Melanoma or suspicious undiagnosed skin lesions, histories of. Levodopa pharmacotherapy has been associated with the activation of malignant melanoma.
MAOI pharmacotherapy, concurrent or within the previous 14 days
Narrow-angle glaucoma

See also the levodopa monograph.

CAUTIONS AND COMMENTS

Prescribe fixed-ratio combination levodopa and carbidopa pharmacotherapy cautiously to patients who

- have histories of mental disorders. Fixed-ratio combination levodopa and carbidopa pharmacotherapy has been associated with the occurrence of mental disorders in ~20% of patients. Monitor patients carefully for both exacerbation of existing mental disorders and signs and symptoms of new mental disorders.

See also the levodopa monograph.

CLINICALLY SIGNIFICANT DRUG INTERACTIONS

Concurrent fixed-ratio combination levodopa and carbidopa pharmacotherapy and the following may result in clinically significant drug interactions:

Antipsychotic Pharmacotherapy

The antipsychotics, particularly the butyrophenones (e.g., haloperidol [Haldol®]) and phenothiazines (e.g., chlorpromazine [Thorazine®]), can antagonize and reduce the therapeutic action of levodopa. Thus, patients who are receiving concurrent fixed-ratio combination levodopa and carbidopa pharmacotherapy and antipsychotic pharmacotherapy must be monitored carefully for possible loss of antiparkinsonian effect.

Pharmacotherapy With Antihypertensive Drugs

Fixed-ratio combination levodopa and carbidopa pharmacotherapy has been associated with postural (orthostatic) hypotension. Therefore, concurrent pharmacotherapy with antihypertensives may require blood pressure monitoring and a possible reduction of the dosage of the antihypertensive. Collaboration with the prescriber of the antihypertensive is indicated.

ADVERSE DRUG REACTIONS

Fixed-ratio combination levodopa and carbidopa pharmacotherapy commonly has been associated with choreiform, dystonic, and other involuntary movements; oscillations in performance, including akinesia paradoxica (hypotonic freezing), end-of-dose akinesia, and the "on–off" phenomenon; and various mental disorders (i.e., dementia, depression, paranoid ideation, and psychotic episodes). Fixed-ratio combination levodopa and carbidopa pharmacotherapy also has been associated with the following ADRs, listed according to body system:

Cardiovascular: angina pectoris and postural (orthostatic) hypotension
CNS: convulsions, euphoria, grinding of the teeth (bruxism), hallucinations, incoordination (ataxia), insomnia, increased libido with serious antisocial behavior, nightmares, and tremor
Cutaneous: dark-colored sweat, edema, hair loss (alopecia), and rash
Genitourinary: dark-colored urine, hematuria, and nocturia

GI: abdominal pain, eructation, flatulence, GI bleeding, hiccups, nausea, and vomiting
Hematologic: agranulocytosis, hemolytic anemia (rare), and leukopenia
Musculoskeletal: low back pain and muscle spasm and twitching
Ophthalmic: blurred vision, dilated pupils, double vision (diplopia), and activation of latent Horner's syndrome (contractions of the pupil, ptosis, and enophthalmos associated with paralysis of the cervical sympathetic nerve trunk)
Respiratory: abnormal breathing pattern and cough
Miscellaneous: fever

See also the levodopa monograph.

OVERDOSAGE

The signs and symptoms of fixed-ratio combination levodopa and carbidopa overdosage include abnormal involuntary movements such as choreiform and dystonic movements. Muscle twitching and blepharospasm may be early signs of overdosage. Generally, the signs and symptoms of fixed-ratio combination levodopa and carbidopa overdosage are similar to their associated ADRs. However, they are more severe. Fixed-ratio combination levodopa and carbidopa overdosage requires emergency symptomatic medical support of body systems with attention to increasing the elimination of levodopa and carbidopa. There is no known antidote. Pyridoxine (vitamin B_6) is *ineffective* in reversing the effects of fixed-ratio combination levodopa and carbidopa overdosage.

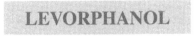

LEVORPHANOL

(lee vor' fa nole)

TRADE NAME

Levo-Dromoran®

CLASSIFICATION

Opiate analgesic (C-II)

See also "Opiate Analgesics, General Monograph."

APPROVED INDICATIONS FOR NEUROPSYCHOLOGICAL DISORDERS

Adjunctive pharmacotherapy for the symptomatic management of:

- pain disorders: acute pain, moderate to severe, and cancer pain, moderate to severe

USUAL DOSAGE AND ADMINISTRATION

Pain Disorders: Acute Pain, Moderate to Severe, and Cancer Pain, Moderate to Severe

Adults: 6 to 12 mg daily intramuscularly, orally, or subcutaneously in three or four divided doses

Women who are, or who may become, pregnant: FDA Pregnancy Category C. Safety and efficacy of levorphanol pharmacotherapy for women who are pregnant have not been established. Avoid prescribing levorphanol pharmacotherapy to women who are pregnant. If levorphanol pharmacotherapy is required, advise patients of potential benefits and possible risks to themselves and the embryo, fetus, or neonate (see "Opiate Analgesics, General Monograph"). Collaboration with the patient's obstetrician is indicated.

Women who are breast-feeding: Safety and efficacy of levorphanol pharmacotherapy for women who are breast-feeding and their neonates and infants have not been established. Avoid prescribing levorphanol pharmacotherapy to women who are breast-feeding. If levorphanol pharmacotherapy is required, breast-feeding probably should be discontinued. If desired, lactation may be maintained and breast-feeding resumed following the discontinuation of short-term levorphanol pharmacotherapy.

For details and discussion regarding related basic principles of clinical pharmacology, readers are referred to the first text in this series, *The Pharmacologic Basis of Psychotherapeutics: An Introduction for Psychologists.*

Elderly, frail, or debilitated patients and those who have respiratory dysfunction: 3 to 6 mg daily orally or subcutaneously in three or four divided doses. Note: Dosage is 50% of the recommended adult dosage. Generally prescribe lower dosages for elderly, frail, or debilitated patients and those who have respiratory dysfunction. Gradually increase the dosage, if needed, according to individual patient response. These patients may be more sensitive to the pharmacologic actions of levorphanol than are younger or healthier adult patients.

Children and adolescents younger than 18 years of age: Safety and efficacy of levorphanol pharmacotherapy for children and adolescents have not been established. Levorphanol pharmacotherapy is *not* recommended for this age group.

Notes, Pain Disorders: Acute Pain and Cancer Pain, Moderate to Severe

Adjust the levorphanol dosage according to the severity of the patient's pain and his or her age and weight; concurrent pharmacotherapy; and clinical condition, including kidney and liver function. Higher dosages of levorphanol may be required for patients who are tolerant to opiate analgesics.

Injectable levorphanol pharmacotherapy: Levorphanol is injected intramuscularly or subcutaneously for the symptomatic management of pain disorders. Although the injectable formulation may be injected intravenously, intravenous pharmacotherapy generally is reserved for use as a supplement to general anesthesia.

AVAILABLE DOSAGE FORMS, STORAGE, AND COMPATIBILITY

Injectable, intramuscular, intravenous, or subcutaneous: 2 mg/ml
Tablets, oral: 2 mg

Notes

Safely store the levorphanol injectable formulation at room temperature below 40 °C (104 °F). The levorphanol injectable formulation is chemically or physically incompatible with aminophylline, ammonium chloride, amobarbital (Amytal®), chlorothiazide (Diuril®), heparin, methicillin (Staphcillin®), nitrofurantoin (Macrodantin®), pentobarbital (Nembutal®), phenobarbital (Luminal®), phenytoin (Dilantin®), secobarbital (Seconal®), sodium bicarbonate, sodium iodide, and thiopental (Pentothal®).

General instructions for patients: Instruct patients who are receiving levorphanol pharmacotherapy to

• safely store levorphanol oral tablets out of the reach of children in tightly closed child- and light-resistant containers at controlled room temperature (15 ° to 30 °C; 59 ° to 86 °F).
• obtain an available patient information sheet regarding levorphanol pharmacotherapy from their pharmacist at the time that their prescription is dispensed. Encourage patients to clarify any questions that they may have regarding levorphanol pharmacotherapy with their pharmacist or, if needed, to consult their prescribing psychologist.

PROPOSED MECHANISM OF ACTION

Levorphanol primarily elicits its analgesic, CNS depressant, and respiratory depressant actions by binding to the endorphin receptors in the CNS. However, the exact mechanisms of its actions have not yet been fully determined. See also "Opiate Analgesics, General Monograph."

PHARMACOKINETICS/PHARMACODYNAMICS

Levorphanol appears to be well absorbed following intramuscular injection or oral ingestion. Peak blood concentrations are achieved within ~1 hour after oral ingestion. Levorphanol is ~40% plasma protein bound. The mean half-life of elimination is 12 hours (range: 11 to 16 hours) and the mean total body clearance is 1 liter/minute (range: 0.8 to 1.3 liters/minute). Additional data are not available.

RELATIVE CONTRAINDICATIONS

Alcoholism, acute
Anoxia
Bronchial asthma
Hypersensitivity to levorphanol
Intracranial pressure, increased
Respiratory depression

CAUTIONS AND COMMENTS

Levorphanol is addicting and habituating. Long-term levorphanol pharmacotherapy, or regular personal use, may result in addiction and habituation. Abrupt discontinuation after long-term pharmacotherapy, or regular personal use, may result in a reportedly mild form of the opiate analgesic withdrawal syndrome.

Prescribe levorphanol pharmacotherapy cautiously to patients who

- have acute cholecystitis or pancreatitis or will be undergoing surgery of the biliary tract. Opiate analgesics generally increase biliary tract pressure. Levorphanol may cause a moderate to marked elevation of biliary pressure. Caution is advised.
- have head injuries, intracranial lesions, or other medical disorders associated with increased intracranial pressure. The respiratory depressant action associated with levorphanol and its potential for elevating cerebrospinal fluid pressure may markedly increase intracranial pressure among these patients. Levorphanol's analgesic and sedative actions also may obscure the clinical course of these patients.
- have histories of problematic patterns of abusable psychotropic use, including levorphanol or other opiate analgesic use. Prescribe the least quantity of drug to help avoid problematic patterns of use, including unadvised patient increases in dosage or frequency of use.
- have liver dysfunction. Serious liver dysfunction appears to predispose patients to a higher incidence of ADRs (e.g., anxiety, dizziness, drowsiness, marked apprehension) even when usual recommended dosages are prescribed. These ADRs may be the result of decreased levorphanol metabolism by the liver and resultant accumulation.
- have respiratory depression, limited respiratory function (e.g., severely limited respiratory reserve, severe bronchial asthma, other obstructive respiratory conditions), or cyanosis.

The respiratory depressant action of levorphanol may further compromise the respiratory function of these patients.

Caution patients who are receiving levorphanol pharmacotherapy against

- performing activities that require alertness, judgment, and physical coordination (e.g., driving an automobile, operating dangerous equipment, supervising children) until their response to levorphanol pharmacotherapy is known. The CNS depressant action of levorphanol may affect these mental and physical functions adversely.

In addition to this general precaution, caution patients who are receiving levorphanol pharmacotherapy to

- inform their prescribing psychologist if they begin or discontinue any other pharmacotherapy while receiving levorphanol pharmacotherapy.

CLINICALLY SIGNIFICANT DRUG INTERACTIONS

Concurrent levorphanol pharmacotherapy and the following may result in clinically significant drug interactions:

Alcohol Use

Concurrent alcohol use may increase the CNS depressant action of levorphanol. Advise patients to avoid, or limit, their use of alcohol while receiving levorphanol pharmacotherapy.

Pharmacotherapy With CNS Depressants and Other Drugs That Produce CNS Depression

Concurrent levorphanol pharmacotherapy and pharmacotherapy with other opiate analgesics, sedative-hypnotics, or other drugs that produce CNS depression (e.g., antihistamines, phenothiazines, TCAs) may result in additive CNS depression.

See also "Opiate Analgesics, General Monograph."

ADVERSE DRUG REACTIONS

Levorphanol pharmacotherapy commonly has been associated with dizziness, nausea, and vomiting. It also has been associated with the following ADRs, listed according to body system:

Cardiovascular: dysrhythmias (e.g., bradycardia, cardiac arrest, tachycardia)
CNS: abnormal dreams, amnesia, confusion, depression, and lethargy
Cutaneous: flushing, hives, itching, local irritation at the injection site, rash, and sweating (excessive)
Genitourinary: difficult or painful urination (dysuria) and urinary retention
GI: constipation, dry mouth, and dyspepsia

Ocular: double vision (diplopia) and reduction or dimness of vision (amblyopia)
Respiratory: apnea and hypoventilation

See also "Opiate Analgesics, General Monograph."

OVERDOSAGE

Signs and symptoms of levorphanol overdosage are similar to the signs and symptoms associated with other opiate analgesic overdosage (see "Opiate Analgesics, General Monograph"). Levorphanol overdosage requires emergency symptomatic medical support of body systems with attention to increasing levorphanol elimination. Naloxone (Narcan®) is a specific and effective antidote.

(lor a′ ze pam)

TRADE NAMES

Ativan®
Novo-Lorazem®
Nu-Loraz®

CLASSIFICATION

Anticonvulsant (sedative-hypnotic) (benzodiazepine) (C-IV)

See also "Benzodiazepines, General Monograph."

APPROVED INDICATIONS FOR NEUROPSYCHOLOGICAL DISORDERS

Pharmacotherapy for the symptomatic management of:

• seizure disorders: status epilepticus

USUAL DOSAGE AND ADMINISTRATION

Seizure Disorders: Status Epilepticus

Adults: Initially, 0.05 mg/kg by slow intravenous injection. If seizures continue or recur, two additional doses may be administered at 10- to 15-minute intervals.

MAXIMUM: 4 mg intravenously per dose; 8 mg intravenously per 12-hour period.

Women who are, or who may become, pregnant: FDA Pregnancy Category D. Safety and efficacy of lorazepam pharmacotherapy for women who are pregnant have not been established (see "Benzodiazepines, General Monograph"). Maternal use of lorazepam near term has resulted in lethargy and respiratory depression among neonates. Avoid prescribing lorazepam pharmacotherapy to women who are pregnant. If lorazepam pharmacotherapy is required, advise patients of potential benefits and possible risks to themselves and the embryo, fetus, or neonate. Collaboration with the patient's obstetrician is indicated.

For details and discussion regarding related basic principles of clinical pharmacology, readers are referred to the first text in this series, *The Pharmacologic Basis of Psychotherapeutics: An Introduction for Psychologists.*

Women who are breast-feeding: Safety and efficacy of lorazepam pharmacotherapy for women who are breast-feeding and their neonates and infants have not been established (see "Benzodiazepines, General Monograph"). Avoid prescribing lorazepam pharmacotherapy for women who are breast-feeding. If lorazepam pharmacotherapy is required, breast-feeding probably should be discontinued. If desired, lactation may be maintained and breast-feeding resumed following the discontinuation of short-term lorazepam pharmacotherapy.

Elderly, frail, or debilitated patients and those who have organic brain syndrome: Generally prescribe lower dosages for elderly, frail, or debilitated patients and those who have organic brain syndrome. Reportedly, these patients are more sensitive to lorazepam's CNS depressant action than are younger or healthier adult patients, even when lower dosages are prescribed.

Children and adolescents younger than 18 years of age: Safety and efficacy of lorazepam pharmacotherapy for children and adolescents have not been established. Lorazepam pharmacotherapy is *not* recommended for this age group.

Notes, Seizure Disorders: Status Epilepticus

Lorazepam intravenous pharmacotherapy usually is indicated for the initial control of seizures among patients who have status epilepticus. The intravenous injection of lorazepam should *not* exceed a rate of 2 mg/minute. Availability of appropriate emergency equipment and properly trained personnel *must* be assured prior to the intravenous administration of lorazepam because of the possibility of heavy sedation and associated partial airway obstruction.

AVAILABLE DOSAGE FORMS, STORAGE, AND COMPATIBILITY

Injectables, intramuscular or intravenous: 1, 2, 4 mg/ml

Notes

In addition to the injectable formulation, lorazepam is available in various other dosage forms including a concentrated oral solution, oral tablets, and sublingual tablets. However, these dosage forms are *not* indicated for patients who require lorazepam pharmacotherapy for the symptomatic management of status epilepticus.

The lorazepam injectable should be diluted with an equal volume of a sterile compatible solution for intravenous injection immediately prior to intravenous administration. The lorazepam injectable is compatible with bacteriostatic water for injection, 5% dextrose injection, sodium chloride injection, and sterile water for injection.

The lorazepam injectable should be refrigerated at a temperature between 2° and 8°C (36° and 46°F) and protected from light.

Discard, in a safe and appropriate manner, injectable dosage forms that are discolored or that contain a precipitate.

PROPOSED MECHANISM OF ACTION

Lorazepam has anticonvulsant, anxiolytic, and sedative actions. The exact mechanisms of these actions have not yet been fully determined. However, they appear to be mediated by or work in concert with the inhibitory neurotransmitter, GABA. Thus, lorazepam's actions appear to be accomplished by binding to benzodiazepine receptors within the GABA complex. See also "Benzodiazepines, General Monograph."

PHARMACOKINETICS/PHARMACODYNAMICS

Lorazepam is well absorbed following oral ingestion with a mean bioavailability of 93%. Peak blood concentrations of lorazepam are achieved within 2 hours after oral ingestion and 60 minutes after sublingual placement. Lorazepam is 85% bound to plasma proteins. Its mean apparent volume of distribution is 1.3 liters/kg. It is rapidly conjugated to an inactive glucuronide. Less than 1% of lorazepam is excreted in unchanged form in the urine. The mean half-life of elimination is ~16 hours and the mean total body clearance is ~80 ml/minute.

RELATIVE CONTRAINDICATIONS

Glaucoma, acute narrow-angle (See "Benzodiazepines, General Monograph.")
Hypersensitivity to lorazepam or other benzodiazepines
Myasthenia gravis

CAUTIONS AND COMMENTS

See "Benzodiazepines, General Monograph."

CLINICALLY SIGNIFICANT DRUG INTERACTIONS

Concurrent lorazepam pharmacotherapy and the following may result in clinically significant drug interactions:

Alcohol Use

Concurrent alcohol use may significantly increase the CNS depressant action of lorazepam.

Pharmacotherapy With CNS Depressants and Other Drugs That Produce CNS Depression

Concurrent lorazepam pharmacotherapy and pharmacotherapy with opiate analgesics, other sedative-hypnotics, or other drugs that produce CNS depression (e.g., antihistamines, phenothiazines, TCAs) may result in significant additive CNS depression.

See also "Benzodiazepines, General Monograph."

ADVERSE DRUG REACTIONS

Lorazepam pharmacotherapy commonly has been associated with dizziness, drowsiness, sedation, unsteadiness, and weakness. The incidence of sedation and unsteadiness increase with age. A dose-related anterograde amnesia (decreased or lack of ability to recall events during the period of drug action) also has been associated with lorazepam pharmacotherapy. Other ADRs, listed according to body system, include:

CNS: agitation, confusion, depression, disorientation, fatigue, lethargy, and sleep disturbances

Cutaneous: skin rash

Hematologic: rarely, a reduction in the number of circulating white blood cells (leukopenia)

See also "Benzodiazepines, General Monograph."

OVERDOSAGE

Signs and symptoms of lorazepam overdosage include somnolence, confusion, and coma. Lorazepam overdosage requires emergency symptomatic medical support of body systems with attention to increasing lorazepam elimination. The benzodiazepine antagonist, flumazenil (Anexate®, Romazicon®), may be required. Note that patients whose seizure disorders have been managed with benzodiazepine pharmacotherapy may be at increased risk for the occurrence of seizures when their benzodiazepine overdosage is treated with flumazenil pharmacotherapy.

MAGNESIUM SULFATE

(mag nee′ zee um sul fate)

TRADE NAMES

Generally available under the generic name, magnesium sulfate

CLASSIFICATION

Anticonvulsant (inorganic salt)

APPROVED INDICATIONS FOR NEUROPSYCHOLOGICAL DISORDERS

Pharmacotherapy for the symptomatic management of:

- seizure disorders. Magnesium pharmacotherapy is indicated for the symptomatic medical management of seizure disorders associated with glomerulonephritis among children, particularly when associated with low blood concentrations of magnesium (i.e., hypomagnesemia). It also is indicated for the control of seizures associated with severe toxemia of pregnancy (i.e., eclampsia).

USUAL DOSAGE AND ADMINISTRATION

Seizure Disorders

Adults: Initially, 4 grams intravenously. Subsequently, 4 grams intramuscularly every four hours according to individual patient response. Injections should be made into large healthy muscle sites (e.g., dorsogluteal site). When more than one injection is required, rotate intramuscular injection sites to minimize tissue damage.

MAXIMUM: 32 grams daily intramuscularly or intravenously

Women who are, or who may become, pregnant: FDA Pregnancy Category B. Safety and efficacy of magnesium pharmacotherapy for women who are pregnant have not been established. Magnesium freely crosses the placental barrier and may cause fetal bradycardia and neonatal CNS depression when administered for the management of pre-eclampsia or eclampsia. However, the extent of both maternal and neonatal CNS depression may generally be less than that associated with other anticonvulsant pharmacotherapy. Avoid prescribing magnesium pharmacotherapy to women who are pregnant. If magnesium pharmacotherapy is required, advise patients of potential benefits and possible risks to themselves and the embryo, fetus, or neonate. Collaboration with the patient's obstetrician is indicated.

For details and discussion regarding related basic principles of clinical pharmacology, readers are referred to the first text in this series, *The Pharmacologic Basis of Psychotherapeutics: An Introduction for Psychologists.*

Women who are breast-feeding: Although magnesium is excreted in breast milk, the amount ingested by breast-fed neonates and infants generally is only ~2 mg more magnesium per day than would be ingested if their mothers were not receiving magnesium pharmacotherapy. The amount excreted in breast milk generally is considered to be clinically insignificant. Breast milk concentrations of magnesium return to normal within 24 hours after the discontinuation of maternal magnesium pharmacotherapy.

Elderly, frail, or debilitated patients: Initially prescribe lower dosages for elderly, frail, or debilitated patients. Gradually increase the dosage, if needed, according to individual patient response. These patients may be more sensitive to the pharmacologic actions of magnesium sulfate than are younger or healthier adult patients.

Children and adolescents younger than 18 years of age: Initially, 25 to 50 mg/kg/dose intramuscularly or intravenously every four to six hours, as needed for seizure control

MAXIMUM: Initially, 2 grams/dose intramuscularly or intravenously

MAINTENANCE: 30 to 60 mg/kg daily intravenously

MAXIMUM: Maintenance, 1 gram daily intravenously

Notes, Seizure Disorders

Injectable magnesium sulfate pharmacotherapy: Monitor magnesium blood concentrations. *Ensure adequate dosage reduction to account for any existing kidney dysfunction.*

INTRAMUSCULAR MAGNESIUM SULFATE PHARMACOTHERAPY: For intramuscular magnesium pharmacotherapy, the concentration of magnesium sulfate should not exceed 500 mg/ml (50%) for *adults*. It should *not* exceed 200 mg/ml (20%) for *children*.

INTRAVENOUS MAGNESIUM SULFATE PHARMACOTHERAPY: For intravenous magnesium pharmacotherapy, the concentration of magnesium sulfate should not exceed 200 mg/ml (20%) nor should the rate of infusion exceed 150 mg/minute (i.e., 1.5 ml of a 10% concentration, or equivalent, per minute).

Generally, it is recommended that intravenous magnesium sulfate pharmacotherapy be restricted to hospitalized patients who can be monitored appropriately (including blood pressure, electrocardiogram, and respiratory function) and for whom magnesium blood concentrations can be obtained easily and rapidly. An intravenous formulation of calcium gluconate should be readily available to reverse the ADRs or toxicity associated with magnesium sulfate pharmacotherapy (e.g., heart block or respiratory depression). Appropriate symptomatic medical support of body systems also is required.

AVAILABLE DOSAGE FORMS, STORAGE, AND COMPATIBILITY

Injectable, intramuscular or intravenous: 10%, 12.5%, 50%
Injectable, intravenous *only*: 1%, 2%, 4%, 8%. The 1% and 2% intravenous formulations are prepared in 5% dextrose solutions.

Notes

Magnesium sulfate is incompatible with alkali carbonates, alkali hydroxides, and salicylates. Safely store injectables at controlled room temperature (15° to 30 °C; 59° to 86 °F).

PROPOSED MECHANISM OF ACTION

The exact mechanism of anticonvulsant action of magnesium sulfate has not yet been fully determined. However, magnesium blood concentrations greater than 2.5 mEq/liter (i.e., hypermagnesemia) block peripheral neuromuscular transmission and depress the CNS, resulting in anticonvulsant action. At a molecular level, hypermagnesemia appears to decrease the amount of acetylcholine released at the motor nerve end plate in response to motor nerve impulses.

PHARMACOKINETICS/PHARMACODYNAMICS

The onset of action of magnesium sulfate following intravenous injection is immediate, with effects lasting ~30 minutes. Following intramuscular injection, the onset of action is ~1 hour, with effects lasting 3 to 4 hours. Magnesium sulfate is not metabolized. It is excreted 100% in unchanged form in the urine in direct proportion to the glomerular filtration rate. Additional data are not available.

Therapeutic Drug Monitoring

Magnesium blood concentrations of 2.5 to 7.5 mEq/liter are generally adequate for the symptomatic management of seizures associated with hypomagnesemia and toxemia of pregnancy. Blood concentrations of 10 mEq/liter have been associated with the suppression of deep-tendon reflexes, heart block, and respiratory paralysis. Blood concentrations exceeding 12 mEq/liter may be fatal.

RELATIVE CONTRAINDICATIONS

Deep-tendon reflexes, absence of
Heart block
Myocardial damage, severe
Respiratory rate less than 16 respirations per minute
Toxemia of pregnancy, *during* the 2 hours immediately preceding delivery

CAUTIONS AND COMMENTS

Caution patients who are receiving magnesium sulfate pharmacotherapy against

- performing activities that require alertness, judgment, or physical coordination (e.g., driving an automobile, operating dangerous equipment, supervising children) until their response to magnesium sulfate pharmacotherapy is known. Magnesium sulfate may affect these mental and physical functions adversely.

Prescribe magnesium sulfate pharmacotherapy cautiously to patients who

- have kidney dysfunction. Magnesium sulfate is 100% excreted in unchanged form in the urine. Therefore, it may accumulate, leading to severe magnesium toxicity among patients who have kidney dysfunction if appropriate dosage reductions are not implemented.

CLINICALLY SIGNIFICANT DRUG INTERACTIONS

Concurrent magnesium sulfate pharmacotherapy and the following may result in clinically significant drug interactions:

Cardiac Glycoside

If calcium pharmacotherapy is required to treat magnesium intoxication among digitalized patients, heart block may result. Collaboration with the prescriber of the cardiac glycoside (e.g., digoxin [Lanoxin®]) is indicated. See "Overdosage."

Pharmacotherapy With CNS Depressants and Other Drugs That Produce CNS Depression

Concurrent magnesium sulfate pharmacotherapy and pharmacotherapy with opiate analgesics, sedative-hypnotics, or other drugs that produce CNS depression (e.g., antihistamines, phenothiazines, TCAs) may result in additive CNS depression.

Pharmacotherapy With Drugs That Produce Neuromuscular Blockade

Concurrent magnesium sulfate pharmacotherapy and pharmacotherapy with succinylcholine (Anectine®), tubocurarine, or other neuromuscular blockers may result in additive neuromuscular blockade and resultant apnea. Collaboration with the prescriber of the neuromuscular blocker (generally the patient's surgeon) is indicated.

ADVERSE DRUG REACTIONS

Magnesium sulfate pharmacotherapy generally is well tolerated. Adverse drug reactions generally do not occur at blood concentrations below 4 mEq/liter. However, ADRs commonly are associated with hypermagnesemia. These ADRs include the following: depressed cardiac function, circulatory collapse, CNS depression, depressed reflexes, flaccid paralysis, flushing, hypotension, hypothermia, and sweating.

OVERDOSAGE

Signs and symptoms of magnesium sulfate overdosage include the disappearance of the patellar reflex, heart block, hypotension, and respiratory paralysis. Magnesium sulfate overdosage requires emergency symptomatic medical support of body systems with attention to increasing magnesium sulfate elimination. Calcium salts (generally intravenously administered calcium gluconate) are antidotes for magnesium sulfate overdosage and usually will reverse associated heart block and respiratory depression.

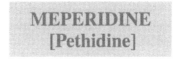

**MEPERIDINE
[Pethidine]**

(me per′ i deen)

TRADE NAME

Demerol®

CLASSIFICATION

Opiate analgesic (C-II)

See also "Opiate Analgesics, General Monograph."

APPROVED INDICATIONS FOR NEUROPSYCHOLOGICAL DISORDERS

Adjunctive pharmacotherapy for the short-term symptomatic management of:

• pain disorders: acute pain, moderate to severe, and cancer pain, moderate to severe

USUAL DOSAGE AND ADMINISTRATION

Pain Disorders: Acute Pain, Moderate to Severe, and Cancer Pain, Moderate to Severe

Adults: 1 to 3 mg/kg orally every three or four hours, as needed; *or* 0.5 to 1.5 mg/kg intramuscularly, intravenously, or subcutaneously every three or four hours, as needed

MAXIMUM: 3 mg/kg/dose intramuscularly, intravenously, or subcutaneously to a maximum of 150 mg/dose

Women who are, or who may become, pregnant: FDA Pregnancy Category B. Safety and efficacy of meperidine pharmacotherapy for women who are pregnant have not been established. Neonatal addiction and withdrawal are associated with maternal meperidine pharmacotherapy, or regular personal use, near term. Avoid prescribing meperidine pharmacotherapy to women who are pregnant. If meperidine pharmacotherapy is required, advise patients of potential benefits and possible risks to themselves and the embryo, fetus, or neonate. Collaboration with the patient's obstetrician is indicated.

For details and discussion regarding related basic principles of clinical pharmacology, readers are referred to the first text in this series, *The Pharmacologic Basis of Psychotherapeutics: An Introduction for Psychologists.*

Women who are breast-feeding: Safety and efficacy of meperidine pharmacotherapy for women who are breast-feeding and their neonates and infants have not been established. Meperidine is excreted into breast milk. Repeated doses can result in significant concentrations in breast milk of both meperidine and its active metabolite, normeperidine. These concentrations may place breast-fed neonates and infants at risk for expected pharmacologic actions (e.g., drowsiness, lethargy, poor sucking) and addiction. Avoid prescribing meperidine pharmacotherapy to women who are breast-feeding. If meperidine pharmacotherapy is required, breast-feeding probably should be discontinued. If desired, lactation may be maintained and breast-feeding resumed following the discontinuation of short-term meperidine pharmacotherapy. Collaboration with the patient's pediatrician is indicated.

Elderly, frail, or debilitated patients: Generally prescribe lower dosages for elderly, frail, or debilitated patients. Gradually increase the dosage, if needed, according to individual patient response. These patients may be more sensitive to the pharmacologic actions of meperidine than are younger or healthier adult patients.

Children: 1 to 3 mg/kg orally every three or four hours, as needed; *or* 0.5 to 1.5 mg/kg intramuscularly, intravenously, or subcutaneously every three or four hours, as needed

MAXIMUM: 2 mg/kg/dose intramuscularly, intravenously, or subcutaneously to a maximum of 100 mg/dose

Adolescents: 1 to 1.5 mg/kg intramuscularly, intravenously, or subcutaneously every three or four hours, as needed

MAXIMUM: 4 mg/kg/dose intramuscularly, intravenously, or subcutaneously to a maximum of 150 mg/dose

Notes, Pain Disorders

Adjust the dosage according to the severity of pain and individual patient response. Note the difference between recommended oral and injectable dosages. Meperidine is less effective when ingested orally than when injected intramuscularly, intravenously, or subcutaneously. Poor drug absorption following oral ingestion generally requires higher oral dosages. Following intravenous injection, meperidine is excreted into the stomach and reabsorbed and, thus, may have a late increased action. As tolerance to meperidine's analgesic action develops, do *not* exceed recommended dosages. Higher dosages have been associated with seizures, even among patients who have no previous history of seizure disorders.

Note: Meperidine pharmacotherapy is recommended *only* for short-term symptomatic pain management. Repeated doses result in the accumulation of a toxic metabolite, normeperidine. Normeperidine has a relatively long half-life of elimination (mean ~16 hours) and can cause several problematic ADRs including dysphoria, irritability, myoclonus, and seizures. The incidence and severity of these ADRs associated with normeperidine increase significantly with: 1) the administration of repeated doses of the parent drug, meperidine; and 2) the presence of reduced kidney function. In these and related clinical situations, morphine pharmacotherapy should be considered as a possible therapeutic substitute for meperidine pharmacotherapy (see morphine monograph).

Injectable meperidine pharmacotherapy

INTRAMUSCULAR MEPERIDINE PHARMACOTHERAPY: Absorption from intra-muscular injection sites may be variable. Inject meperidine into healthy muscle sites. The dorsogluteal and ventrogluteal sites are recommended. Carefully identify recommended sites before injection. Inadvertent injection at a nerve trunk may result in sensory-motor paralysis (usually transitory). Intramuscular injections of meperidine also have been associated with pain at the injection site. Carefully rotate injection sites when repeated injections are required.

INTRAVENOUS MEPERIDINE PHARMACOTHERAPY: Dilute the meperidine injectable prior to intravenous injection. Slowly inject over 3 to 5 minutes with the patient lying down. Rapid intravenous injection increases the incidence of associated ADRs, including apnea, hypotension, peripheral circulatory collapse, severe respiratory depression, and cardiac arrest. Do *not* inject meperidine intravenously unless an opiate antagonist (i.e., naloxone [Narcan®]) and the facilities and equipment needed for emergency symptomatic medical support of body systems, including equipment for assisted respiration, are immediately available.

SUBCUTANEOUS PHARMACOTHERAPY: Avoid subcutaneous injections because they are generally painful and have been associated with local tissue irritation and induration, particularly when repeated injections are required. Subcutaneous injection may be used occasionally. However, intramuscular injection is preferred when repeated doses are required.

AVAILABLE DOSAGE FORMS, STORAGE, AND COMPATIBILITY

Injectables, intramuscular, intravenous, or subcutaneous: 10, 25, 50, 75, 100 mg/ml
Syrup, oral: 50 mg/5 ml (banana flavored)
Tablets, oral: 50, 100 mg

Notes and General Instructions for Patients

Meperidine injectable formulations: Do *not* combine the meperidine injectable solution with the barbiturate injectable solution because they are physically incompatible. Safely store injectables at room temperature (15° to 25 °C; 50° to 77 °F).

Meperidine oral formulations: Instruct patients who are receiving meperidine oral pharmacotherapy to

- ingest each dose of the meperidine oral syrup with sufficient water (30 to 60 ml [1 or 2 ounces]) to minimize the associated topical anesthestic effect on the oral passages.
- safely store meperidine oral syrup and oral tablets out of the reach of children in tightly closed, child- and light-resistant containers at controlled room temperature (15° to 30 °C; 59° to 86 °F).
- obtain an available patient information sheet regarding meperidine pharmacotherapy from their pharmacist at the time that their prescription is dispensed. Encourage patients to clarify any questions that they may have regarding meperidine pharmacotherapy with their pharmacist or, if needed, to consult their prescribing psychologist.

PROPOSED MECHANISM OF ACTION

Meperidine appears to elicit its analgesic and CNS and respiratory depressant actions primarily by binding to the endorphin receptors in the CNS. However, the exact mechanism of action has not yet been fully determined. See also "Opiate Analgesics, General Monograph."

PHARMACOKINETICS/PHARMACODYNAMICS

Meperidine has several therapeutic actions qualitatively similar to those of morphine, one of which is analgesia. When injected in doses of 80 to 100 mg, meperidine is approximately equivalent in analgesic action to 10 mg of morphine. The onset of action is slightly more rapid than that for morphine, although the duration of action is slightly shorter. Meperidine is significantly less effective following oral ingestion than when injected. However, the exact ratio of oral to injectable analgesia has not been determined.

Meperidine is moderately absorbed (~52%) following oral ingestion. Peak analgesia generally occurs within 1 hour after oral ingestion or intramuscular, intravenous, or subcutaneous injection. Analgesia may last for up to 2 to 4 hours. Meperidine is moderately (~60%) bound to plasma proteins and has a mean apparent volume of distribution of ~4.5 liters/kg. Meperidine is extensively metabolized, primarily in the liver, with ~5% eliminated in unchanged form in the urine. Total body clearance is ~850 ml/minute. The mean half-life of elimination is ~3 hours. Normeperidine, an active metabolite of meperidine, is associated with CNS excitation and may accumulate in patients who have kidney dysfunction. Meperidine is a weak acid. Therefore, alkalinization of the urine will decrease its excretion, and acidification of the urine will increase its excretion. These changes in urinary pH may significantly affect the total body clearance and the half-life of elimination of meperidine and its metabolite. Additional data are not available.

RELATIVE CONTRAINDICATIONS

Coma

Hypersensitivity to meperidine

MAOI pharmacotherapy, concurrent or within 14 days. Concurrent pharmacotherapy may result in the occurrence of serious ADRs. Some reactions resemble acute opiate analgesic overdosage and are characterized by coma, cyanosis, hypotension, and respiratory depression. Other reactions have been predominantly associated with convulsions, hyperexcitability, hyperpyrexia (body temperature of 41 °C [106 °F]), hypertension, and tachycardia. The mechanism of these reactions is unknown. However, they may be related to a pre-existing hyperphenylalaninemia. If opiate analgesic pharmacotherapy is required for patients who are receiving MAOI pharmacotherapy, or have received such pharmacotherapy within 14 days, a morphine sensitivity test should be performed prior to initiating meperidine or other opiate analgesic pharmacotherapy. Small, repeated incremental doses of morphine are injected over the course of several hours with direct medical monitoring of body systems. Collaboration with the patient's family physician or a specialist in morphine sensitivity testing is required.

Porphyria. Meperidine pharmacotherapy can precipitate an acute attack of porphyria among patients who have histories of porphyria.

Ritonavir pharmacotherapy (see "Clinically Significant Drug Interactions").

CAUTIONS AND COMMENTS

Meperidine also is referred to in Canada and the United Kingdom as "pethidine." Meperidine can produce addiction and habituation similar to that associated with morphine and other opiate analgesics. Thus, it has high abuse potential (see the opiate analgesic general monograph).

Prescribe meperidine pharmacotherapy cautiously, and in reduced dosages, to patients who

- have acute abdominal disorders (e.g., appendicitis). Meperidine may obscure the medical diagnosis or clinical course of these disorders.
- have atrial flutter and other supraventricular tachycardias. Meperidine pharmacotherapy may cause a vagolytic action that may produce a significant increase in the ventricular response rate among these patients.
- have head injuries, other medical disorders associated with increased intracranial pressure, or preexisting increased intracranial pressure. The respiratory depressant action of meperidine and its ability to increase cerebrospinal fluid pressure may be markedly exaggerated among these patients. Opiate analgesics also produce ADRs that may obscure the clinical course of these patients. Meperidine must be prescribed with extreme caution for these patients.
- have histories of problematic patterns of meperidine or other abusable psychotropic use. Meperidine has high abuse potential. Prescribe meperidine pharmacotherapy cautiously to these patients and monitor closely for problematic patterns of use.
- have seizure disorders. Meperidine pharmacotherapy may aggravate seizure disorders among these patients.
- regularly drink alcoholic beverages or are receiving concurrent pharmacotherapy with other opiate analgesics, sedative-hypnotics, or other drugs that depress the CNS (e.g., phenothiazines, TCAs). Hypotension, profound sedation, respiratory depression, and coma may occur among these patients.
- have severe kidney or liver dysfunction because of the potential accumulation of meperidine's metabolite normeperidine. Observe for associated signs and symptoms of CNS stimulation (e.g., agitation, irritability, nervousness, seizures).
- have status asthmaticus (acute asthmatic attack), chronic obstructive lung disease, cor pulmonale, substantially decreased respiratory reserve, or pre-existing respiratory depression, hypoxia, or hypercapnia. Even usual recommended dosages of meperidine for these patients may decrease their respiratory drive while simultaneously increasing airway resistance to the point of apnea.

Caution patients who are receiving meperidine pharmacotherapy against

- performing activities that require alertness, judgment, and physical coordination (e.g., driving an automobile, operating dangerous equipment, supervising children) until their response to meperidine is known. Meperidine may affect these mental and physical functions adversely.

In addition to this general precaution, caution patients who are receiving meperidine pharmacotherapy to

- inform their prescribing psychologist if they begin or discontinue any other pharmacotherapy while receiving meperidine pharmacotherapy.

CLINICALLY SIGNIFICANT DRUG INTERACTIONS

Concurrent meperidine pharmacotherapy and the following may result in clinically significant drug interactions:

Alcohol Use

Concurrent alcohol use may increase the CNS depressant action of meperidine. Advise patients to avoid, or limit, their use of alcohol while receiving meperidine pharmacotherapy.

MAOI Pharmacotherapy

See "Relative Contraindications."

Pharmacotherapy With CNS Depressants and Other Drugs That Produce CNS Depression

Concurrent meperidine pharmacotherapy and pharmacotherapy with other opiate analgesics, sedative-hypnotics, or other drugs that produce CNS depression (e.g., antihistamines, phenothiazines, TCAs) may result in additive CNS depression.

Ritonavir Pharmacotherapy

Ritonavir (Norvir®), an antiretroviral drug indicated for the pharmacologic management of HIV infection, can significantly inhibit the hepatic microsomal enzyme metabolism of meperidine (Demerol®). This interaction may result in severe toxicity, including cardiac dysrhythmias and seizures. Concurrent meperidine and ritonavir pharmacotherapy is *contraindicated.*

See also "Opiate Analgesics, General Monograph."

ADVERSE DRUG REACTIONS

The most serious ADRs associated with meperidine pharmacotherapy include respiratory depression, circulatory depression, respiratory arrest, shock, and cardiac arrest. Other ADRs are listed according to body system. Reportedly, some of these ADRs are more common among nonhospitalized or ambulatory patients and those who are not experiencing severe pain. Prescribing lower dosages or advising these patients to lie down following the administration of meperidine may be of benefit.

Cardiovascular: bradycardia, cardiovascular depression, fainting (syncope), hypotension, palpitations, phlebitis (following intravenous injection), and tachycardia
CNS: agitation, CNS depression, disorientation, dizziness, dysphoria, euphoria, hallucinations (transient), headache, lightheadedness, sedation, and seizures (severe)
Cutaneous: hives (urticaria), severe itching (pruritus), and other skin rashes; sweating (excessive); and wheal and flare at intravenous injection sites
Genitourinary: diminished amount of urine formation (oliguria) and urinary retention

GI: biliary tract spasm, constipation, dry mouth, nausea, and vomiting
Musculoskeletal: incoordinated muscle movements (ataxia), tremor, and weakness
Ocular: visual disturbances
Respiratory: respiratory depression

See also "Opiate Analgesics, General Monograph."

OVERDOSAGE

Signs and symptoms of meperidine overdosage include: respiratory depression with a decrease in rate and tidal volume, Cheyne–Stokes respiration, cyanosis, extreme somnolence progressing to stupor or coma, skeletal muscle flaccidity, cold and clammy skin, and, sometimes, bradycardia and hypotension. In severe overdosage, particularly that involving intravenous injection, apnea, circulatory collapse, cardiac arrest, and death may occur. Meperidine overdosage requires emergency symptomatic medical support of respiratory and other body systems with attention to increasing meperidine elimination. The opiate antagonist, naloxone (Narcan®), is a specific antidote for treating the respiratory depression associated with meperidine and other opiate analgesic overdosage. If patients are addicted to opiates, the use of the opiate antagonist will precipitate an acute opiate analgesic withdrawal syndrome. The severity of the opiate analgesic withdrawal syndrome depends on the patient's degree of opiate analgesic addiction, the amount of opiate analgesic involved in the overdosage, the time elapsed before seeking emergency treatment, and the dose of the antagonist injected. Generally, lower dosages of the opiate analgesic antagonist (10% to 20% of the usual recommended initial dosage) are recommended for these patients.

MEPHENYTOIN*
[Methoin; Methylphenylethylhydantoin; Phenantoin]

(me fen' i toyn)

TRADE NAME

Mesantoin®

CLASSIFICATION

Anticonvulsant (hydantoin derivative)

APPROVED INDICATIONS FOR NEUROPSYCHOLOGICAL DISORDERS

Pharmacotherapy for the prophylactic and symptomatic management of:

- seizure disorders. Mephenytoin pharmacotherapy is indicated for partial seizures (e.g., Jacksonian seizures, psychomotor seizures) and tonic-clonic (grand mal) seizures among patients who are refractory to, or otherwise cannot be prescribed, less toxic anticonvulsants.

USUAL DOSAGE AND ADMINISTRATION

Seizure Disorders: Partial and Tonic-Clonic Seizures Among Patients Who Are Refractory to Other Pharmacotherapy

Adults: Initially, 50 to 100 mg daily orally in a single dose for one week. Increase the dosage weekly by 50- to 100-mg increments, if necessary, according to individual patient response.

MAINTENANCE: 200 to 600 mg daily orally in three divided doses

Women who are, or who may become, pregnant: FDA Pregnancy Category C. Teratogenic effects associated with mephenytoin are similar to those associated with phenytoin and include developmental delay, hydrocephalus, inguinal hernia, large fontanelles, and various heart defects. If mephenytoin pharmacotherapy is required, advise patients of potential benefits and possible risks to themselves and the embryo, fetus, or neonate. Collaboration with the patient's obstetrician is indicated.

For details and discussion regarding related basic principles of clinical pharmacology, readers are referred to the first text in this series, *The Pharmacologic Basis of Psychotherapeutics: An Introduction for Psychologists.*

Women who are breast-feeding: Safety and efficacy of mephenytoin pharmacotherapy for women who are breast-feeding and their neonates and infants have not been established. Avoid prescribing mephenytoin pharmacotherapy to women who are breast-feeding. If mephenytoin pharmacotherapy is required, breast-feeding probably should be discontinued. Collaboration with the patient's pediatrician may be indicated.

Elderly, frail, or debilitated patients: Initially prescribe lower dosages of mephenytoin for elderly, frail, or debilitated patients. Gradually increase the dosage if needed, according to individual patient response. These patients may be more sensitive to the pharmacologic actions of mephenytoin than are younger or healthier adult patients.

Children and adolescents younger than 18 years of age: Initially, 50 mg daily orally in a single dose for one week. Increase the dosage weekly by 50- to 100-mg increments, if needed, according to individual patient response.

MAINTENANCE: 100 to 400 mg daily orally in three divided doses; *or* 3 to 15 mg/kg daily orally in three divided doses

Notes, Seizure Disorders: Partial and Tonic-Clonic Seizures Among Patients Who Are Refractory to Other Pharmacotherapy

Mephenytoin pharmacotherapy usually is prescribed in combination with other anticonvulsant pharmacotherapy, particularly phenytoin pharmacotherapy.

AVAILABLE DOSAGE FORMS, STORAGE, AND COMPATIBILITY

Tablets, oral: 100 mg

Notes

General instructions for patients: Instruct patients who are receiving mephenytoin pharmacotherapy to

- safely store mephenytoin oral tablets out of the reach of children in tightly closed, child-resistant containers at controlled room temperature (15° to 30°C; 59° to 86°F).
- obtain an available patient information sheet regarding mephenytoin pharmacotherapy from their pharmacist at the time that their prescription is dispensed. Encourage patients to clarify any questions that they may have regarding mephenytoin pharmacotherapy with their pharmacist or, if needed, to consult their prescribing psychologist.

PROPOSED MECHANISM OF ACTION

The exact mechanism of the anticonvulsant action of mephenytoin has not yet been clearly established. Its other pharmacological actions, including behavioral and electroencephalographic effects, are similar to those associated with phenytoin and the barbiturates.

PHARMACOKINETICS/PHARMACODYNAMICS

Mephenytoin has an onset of action of 30 minutes and a duration of action of 24 to 48 hours following oral ingestion. Mephenytoin is metabolized in the liver to its principal active and toxic metabolite, 5,5-ethylphenylhydantoin. Additional data are not available.

Therapeutic Drug Monitoring

Precise therapeutic blood concentrations for mephenytoin have not yet been determined. However, total blood concentrations of mephenytoin and its major metabolite, 5,5-ethyl-phenylhydantoin, of 25 to 40 µg/ml are reportedly associated with adequate seizure control without signs and symptoms of clinical intoxication.

RELATIVE CONTRAINDICATIONS

Blood disorders, history of
Hypersensitivity to mephenytoin or other hydantoins (e.g., phenytoin)

CAUTIONS AND COMMENTS

Prescribe mephenytoin pharmacotherapy cautiously to *all* patients. Mephenytoin pharmacotherapy has been associated with serious and potentially fatal blood disorders (i.e., agranulocytosis, leukopenia, neutropenia, pancytopenia, and thrombocytopenia). Prescribing psychologists should

- obtain complete blood and platelet counts prior to initiating mephenytoin pharmacotherapy, after the initial 2 weeks of pharmacotherapy, after 2 weeks of the established maintenance dosage, every month thereafter for 1 year, and at 3-month intervals for the remaining duration of pharmacotherapy. Collaboration with the patient's family physician or a specialist (e.g., hematologist) is indicated.

Caution patients who are receiving mephenytoin pharmacotherapy against

- performing activities that require alertness, judgment, or physical coordination (e.g., driving an automobile, operating dangerous equipment, supervising children) until their response to mephenytoin pharmacotherapy is known. Mephenytoin may affect these mental and physical functions adversely.

In addition to this general precaution, caution patients who are receiving mephenytoin pharmacotherapy to

- report any new or unusual signs and symptoms (e.g., easy bruising, enlarged lymph nodes, fever, mucous membrane bleeding, skin rash, sore throat) that may indicate blood disorders. If noted, patients should be immediately referred to their family physician or specialist (e.g., hematologist) for hematologic evaluation and any related necessary medical management.

CLINICALLY SIGNIFICANT DRUG INTERACTIONS

Concurrent mephenytoin pharmacotherapy and the following may result in clinically significant drug interactions:

Alcohol Use

Concurrent alcohol use may increase the CNS depressant action of mephenytoin. Advise patients to avoid, or limit, their use of alcohol while receiving mephenytoin pharmacotherapy.

Pharmacotherapy With CNS Depressants and Other Drugs That Produce CNS Depression

Concurrent mephenytoin pharmacotherapy and pharmacotherapy with opiate analgesics, sedative-hypnotics, or other drugs that produce CNS depression (e.g., antihistamines, phenothiazines, TCAs) may result in additive CNS depression.

ADVERSE DRUG REACTIONS

Mephenytoin pharmacotherapy commonly has been associated with drowsiness, which is generally dose related. It also has been associated with the following ADRs, listed according to body system:

CNS: confusion, depression, dizziness, fatigue, incoordination (ataxia), insomnia, irritability, nervousness, and psychosis

Cutaneous: edema, erythema multiforme (Stevens–Johnson syndrome), exfoliative dermatitis, hair loss (alopecia), skin pigmentation, skin rashes, and toxic epidermal necrolysis (potentially fatal)

Hematologic: see "Cautions and Comments."

Musculoskeletal: choreiform movements, difficult and defective speech due to impairment of the tongue or other muscles essential to speech (dysarthria), and tremor

Ophthalmic: conjunctivitis; constant involuntary, rapid cyclical movement of the eyeball in any direction (nystagmus); double vision (diplopia); and sensitivity to light (photophobia)

Miscellaneous: weight gain

OVERDOSAGE

Signs and symptoms of mephenytoin overdosage are similar to the signs and symptoms associated with phenytoin overdosage (see the phenytoin monograph). Mephenytoin overdosage requires emergency symptomatic medical support of body systems with attention to increasing mephenytoin elimination. There is no known antidote.

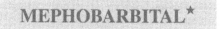

MEPHOBARBITAL*

(me foe bar′ bi tal)

TRADE NAME

Mebaral®

CLASSIFICATION

Sedative-hypnotic (barbiturate) (C-IV)

See also "Barbiturates, General Monograph."

APPROVED INDICATIONS FOR NEUROPSYCHOLOGICAL DISORDERS

Pharmacotherapy for the prophylactic and symptomatic management of:

- seizure disorders: absence (petit mal) and tonic-clonic (grand mal) seizures

USUAL DOSAGE AND ADMINISTRATION

Seizure Disorders: Absence and Tonic-Clonic Seizures

Adults: Initially, 96 to 400 mg daily orally in three or four divided doses. Gradually increase the dosage each day over a 5- to 7-day period, according to individual patient response, until optimal dosage is obtained.

MAINTENANCE: Usual adult maintenance dosage is 400 to 600 mg daily orally in divided doses. If preferred, the maintenance dosage may be prescribed as a single daily dose 30 minutes before retiring for bed in the evening.

Women who are, or who may become, pregnant: FDA Pregnancy Category D. Safety and efficacy of mephobarbital pharmacotherapy for women who are pregnant have not been established. Mephobarbital readily crosses the placenta after injection resulting in fetal blood concentrations that approach maternal blood concentrations. Its use during pregnancy has been associated with a wide variety of congenital malformations (i.e., birth defects). These malformations include the following: atrial septal defect, cleft lip and palate, congenital hip dislocation, inguinal hernia, talipes equinus, and ventricular septal defect. Do *not* prescribe mephobarbital pharmacotherapy to women who are pregnant.

For details and discussion regarding related basic principles of clinical pharmacology, readers are referred to the first text in this series, *The Pharmacologic Basis of Psychotherapeutics: An Introduction for Psychologists.*

Women who are breast-feeding: Safety and efficacy of mephobarbital pharmacotherapy for women who are breast-feeding and their neonates and infants have not been established. Small amounts of barbiturates are excreted in breast milk. Avoid prescribing mephobarbital pharmacotherapy to women who are breast-feeding. If mephobarbital pharmacotherapy is required, breast-feeding probably should be discontinued. Collaboration with the patient's pediatrician is indicated.

Elderly, frail, or debilitated patients and those who have kidney or liver dysfunction: Generally prescribe lower dosages for elderly, frail, or debilitated patients and those who have kidney or liver dysfunction. Gradually increase the dosage, if needed, according to individual patient response. These patients may be more sensitive to the pharmacologic actions of mephobarbital than are younger or healthier adult patients.

Infants and children younger than 5 years of age: 48 to 128 mg daily orally in three or four divided doses

Children 5 years of age and older and adolescents: 96 to 256 mg daily orally in three or four divided doses

AVAILABLE DOSAGE FORMS, STORAGE, AND COMPATIBILITY

Tablets, oral: 32, 50, 100 mg

Notes

General instructions for patients: Instruct patients who are receiving mephobarbital pharmacotherapy to

- safely store mephobarbital oral tablets out of the reach of children in tightly closed, child- and light-resistant containers.
- obtain an available patient information sheet regarding mephobarbital pharmacotherapy from their pharmacist at the time that their prescription is dispensed. Encourage patients to clarify any questions that they may have regarding mephobarbital pharmacotherapy with their pharmacist or, if needed, to consult their prescribing psychologist.

PROPOSED MECHANISM OF ACTION

The exact mechanism of mephobarbital's anticonvulsant action has not yet been fully determined. However, mephobarbital appears to act primarily at the level of the thalamus, where it interferes with impulse transmission to the cortex by increasing the threshold for electrical stimulation. See also "Barbiturates, General Monograph."

PHARMACOKINETICS/PHARMACODYNAMICS

Mephobarbital has strong sedative action, but relatively weak hypnotic action. Thus, mephobarbital pharmacotherapy usually is associated with little or no drowsiness or lassitude. After oral ingestion, approximately half of the mephobarbital dose is absorbed from the GI tract. It has an onset of action of 30 to 60 minutes after oral ingestion and its duration of action is 10 to 16 hours.

The lipid solubility of barbiturates, such as mephobarbital, results in their rapid and widespread distribution throughout the body. Particularly high concentrations are achieved in the brain, kidneys, and liver. Therapeutic blood concentrations have not been established nor has the half-life of elimination. Mephobarbital is primarily metabolized to phenobarbital (i.e., ~75% of a single dose in 24 hours) by the microsomal enzymes of the liver. The phenobarbital is excreted in the urine in unchanged form or as glucuronide or sulfate conjugates. Thus, long-term mephobarbital pharmacotherapy, such as that required for the symptomatic management of seizure disorders, may result in the accumulation of phenobarbital in the blood. It is unclear whether mephobarbital or phenobarbital is the active drug during long-term mephobarbital pharmacotherapy. (See also the phenobarbital monograph.)

Therapeutic Drug Monitoring

Mephobarbital blood concentrations for the symptomatic management of seizure disorders are not established. See also "Barbiturates, General Monograph."

RELATIVE CONTRAINDICATIONS

Hypersensitivity to mephobarbital or other barbiturates
Liver dysfunction, severe
Porphyria, active or latent
Pregnancy

CAUTIONS AND COMMENTS

Addiction and habituation have been associated with long-term mephobarbital pharmacotherapy and regular personal use. Abrupt discontinuation of long-term mephobarbital pharmacotherapy, or regular personal use, may result in the signs and symptoms of the barbiturate withdrawal syndrome. These signs and symptoms include status epilepticus. Prescribe the smallest quantity of mephobarbital feasible for dispensing at one time to minimize the possible development of problematic patterns of use or overdosage.

Prescribe mephobarbital pharmacotherapy cautiously for patients who

- are receiving oral anticoagulant pharmacotherapy because of the associated difficulty in stabilizing prothrombin times. Avoid prescribing mephobarbital pharmacotherapy to patients who are receiving oral anticoagulant pharmacotherapy. If mephobarbital pharmacotherapy is required, collaboration with the prescriber of the anticoagulant is indicated.
- have CNS depression. Mephobarbital pharmacotherapy may increase CNS depression among these patients.
- have kidney dysfunction. Adjust the dosage for these patients carefully.
- have liver dysfunction. Adjust the dosage for these patients carefully.
- have respiratory dysfunction, including respiratory depression.

Caution patients who are receiving mephobarbital pharmacotherapy against

- drinking alcohol or using other drugs that produce CNS depression. Concurrent use of alcohol or other drugs that produce CNS depression may result in excessive CNS depression.

- performing activities that require alertness, judgment, and physical coordination (e.g., driving an automobile, operating dangerous equipment, supervising children) until their response to mephobarbital pharmacotherapy is known. Mephobarbital may affect these mental and physical functions adversely.

In addition to these general precautions, caution patients who are receiving mephobarbital pharmacotherapy to

- inform their prescribing psychologist if they begin or discontinue any other pharmacotherapy while receiving mephobarbital pharmacotherapy.

CLINICALLY SIGNIFICANT DRUG INTERACTIONS

Concurrent mephobarbital pharmacotherapy and the following may result in clinically significant drug interactions:

Alcohol Use

Concurrent alcohol use may increase the CNS depressant action of mephobarbital. Advise patients to avoid, or limit, their use of alcohol while receiving mephobarbital pharmacotherapy.

Pharmacotherapy With Drugs That Are Primarily Metabolized in the Liver

Mephobarbital may stimulate the production of the hepatic microsomal enzymes that are responsible for the metabolism of many different drugs. Whenever mephobarbital is added to or removed from a patient's pharmacotherapy, attention must be given to the effect on concurrent pharmacotherapy (e.g., corticosteroid, oral anticoagulant, oral contraceptive, or quinidine [Biquin®] pharmacotherapy). Dosage adjustments (i.e., an increase or decrease in dosage) may be required. Collaboration with the patient's family physician or other prescribers (e.g., advanced practice nurse, dentist) is indicated.

Pharmacotherapy With CNS Depressants and Other Drugs That Produce CNS Depression

Concurrent mephobarbital pharmacotherapy and pharmacotherapy with opiate analgesics, sedative-hypnotics, or other drugs that produce CNS depression (e.g., antihistamines, phenothiazines, TCAs) may result in additive CNS depression.

See also "Barbiturates, General Monograph."

ADVERSE DRUG REACTIONS

Mephobarbital pharmacotherapy has been associated with drowsiness, and, rarely, vertigo. It also may cause ADRs that generally are associated with other barbiturates because of its chemical and pharmacological similarity to the other barbiturates.

See also "Barbiturates, General Monograph."

OVERDOSAGE

The signs and symptoms of mephobarbital overdosage include CNS and respiratory depression and other signs and symptoms that are similar to those associated with other barbiturate overdosage (see "Barbiturates, General Monograph"). Mephobarbital overdosage requires emergency symptomatic medical support of body systems with attention to increasing mephobarbital elimination. There is no known antidote.

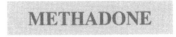

METHADONE

(meth′ a done)

TRADE NAMES

Dolophine®
Methadose®

CLASSIFICATION

Opiate analgesic (C-II)

See also "Opiate Analgesics, General Monograph."

APPROVED INDICATIONS FOR NEUROPSYCHOLOGICAL DISORDERS

Adjunctive pharmacotherapy for the symptomatic management of:

- pain disorders: acute pain, moderate to severe

USUAL DOSAGE AND ADMINISTRATION

Acute Pain, Moderate to Severe

Adults: 0.1 mg/kg (generally 2.5 to 10 mg) intramuscularly, orally, or subcutaneously every three or four hours, as needed

MAXIMUM: 10 mg/dose

Women who are, or who may become, pregnant: FDA Pregnancy Category C. Safety and efficacy of methadone pharmacotherapy for women who are pregnant have not been established. Methadone crosses the placenta. Although physical malformations generally have not been associated with methadone use during pregnancy, long-term pharmacotherapy, or regular personal use, during pregnancy will likely result in the neonatal opiate analgesic withdrawal syndrome. Avoid prescribing methadone pharmacotherapy to women who are pregnant. If methadone pharmacotherapy is required, advise patients of potential benefits and possible risks to themselves and the embryo, fetus, or neonate. Collaboration with the patient's obstetrician is indicated.

For details and discussion regarding related basic principles of clinical pharmacology, readers are referred to the first text in this series, *The Pharmacologic Basis of Psychotherapeutics: An Introduction for Psychologists.*

Women who are breast-feeding: Safety and efficacy of methadone pharmacotherapy for women who are breast-feeding and their neonates and infants have not been established. Methadone is excreted in breast milk in concentrations up to 85% of those in the maternal blood. Expected pharmacologic actions may be observed among breast-fed neonates and infants (e.g., drowsiness, lethargy, respiratory depression), who also may become addicted. Avoid prescribing methadone pharmacotherapy to women who are breast-feeding. If methadone pharmacotherapy is required, breast-feeding probably should be discontinued. If desired, lactation may be maintained and breast-feeding resumed following the discontinuation of short-term methadone pharmacotherapy. Collaboration with the patient's pediatrician is indicated.

Elderly, frail, or debilitated patients and those who have kidney dysfunction: Generally prescribe lower dosages for elderly, frail, or debilitated patients. Gradually increase the dosage, if needed, according to individual patient response. These patients may be more sensitive to the pharmacologic actions of methadone than are younger or healthier adult patients. Patients who have kidney dysfunction also may require lower dosages.

Children: Safety and efficacy of methadone pharmacotherapy for the symptomatic management of acute pain for children have not been established. Methadone pharmacotherapy for this indication is *not* recommended for this age group.

Notes, Acute Pain, Moderate to Severe

Adjust dosage according to the severity of the patient's pain and individual response to methadone pharmacotherapy. Patients who have severe pain, or those who have developed a tolerance to the analgesic action of methadone or other opiate analgesics, may require dosages that exceed the usual recommended dosages. When adjusting dosages, or replacing injectable pharmacotherapy with oral pharmacotherapy, note the differences in the bioavailability and the differences in duration of action for injectable and oral dosage forms (see "Pharmacokinetics/Pharmacodynamics").

Injectable methadone pharmacotherapy: An injectable dose of 10 mg of methadone is approximately equivalent in analgesic action to 10 mg of morphine. Intramuscular injection is preferred when repeated doses are required for patients who are unable to swallow, are vomiting, or for any other reason are unable to ingest the oral dosage form. Subcutaneous injection is suitable for occasional use.

Oral methadone pharmacotherapy: Too-frequent oral dosing over a few days may result in signs and symptoms of drug accumulation and toxicity (e.g., somnolence, respiratory depression).

AVAILABLE DOSAGE FORMS, STORAGE, AND COMPATIBILITY

Injectable, intramuscular or subcutaneous: 10 mg/ml
Solution, oral: 1, 2 mg/ml (contains 8% alcohol) (citrus flavored)
Solution, oral concentrate (Methadone Intensol®, Methadose Concentrate®): 10 mg/ml (for opiate addiction maintenance program use *only*)
Syrup, oral: 5 mg/15 ml

Tablets, oral: 5, 10 mg
Tablets, oral dispersible (Methadone Diskets®): 40 mg

Notes

General instructions for patients: Instruct patients who are receiving methadone pharmacotherapy, as appropriate, to

- safely store methadone oral syrup and tablets out of the reach of children in tightly closed, child- and light-resistant containers. Safely store oral and injectable formulations at controlled room temperature (15° to 30 °C; 59° to 86 °F). All methadone dosage forms should be stored and used in accordance with federal regulations for controlled substances.
- obtain an available patient information sheet regarding methadone pharmacotherapy from their pharmacist at the time that their prescription is dispensed. Encourage patients to clarify any questions that they may have regarding methadone pharmacotherapy with their pharmacist or, if needed, to consult their prescribing psychologist.

PROPOSED MECHANISM OF ACTION

Methadone is a synthetic opiate analgesic with multiple actions quantitatively similar to those of morphine. Its most prominent actions involve the CNS and body organs composed of smooth muscle (e.g., intestines, lungs). However, one of the major actions of concern to psychologists is its analgesic action and use as adjunctive pharmacotherapy for the symptomatic management of acute pain disorders. Methadone elicits its analgesic action primarily by binding to the endorphin receptors in the CNS. However, the exact mechanism of action has not yet been fully determined. See "Opiate Analgesics, General Monograph."

PHARMACOKINETICS/PHARMACODYNAMICS

Methadone is well absorbed (~90%) following oral ingestion. However, when ingested orally, methadone is approximately one-half as potent as when injected, presumably because of its significant first-pass hepatic metabolism. Oral ingestion is associated with a delay in onset of action, a lowering of the peak blood concentration, and an increase in the duration of analgesic action. Methadone's duration of action is 3 to 5 hours intramuscularly or subcutaneously. Following oral ingestion, it is 6 to 8 hours. A prolonged duration of action makes methadone an effective drug for the symptomatic management of cancer pain and for the maintenance of opiate addiction. Methadone is ~90% bound to plasma proteins and has a mean apparent volume of distribution of ~4 liters/kg. Approximately 25% of methadone is excreted in unchanged form in the urine. This percentage can change by 50% in inverse correlation with changes in urinary pH. The total body clearance is ~90 ml/minute and the mean half-life of elimination is ~36 hours.

RELATIVE CONTRAINDICATIONS

Hypersensitivity to methadone

See also "Opiate Analgesics, General Monograph."

CAUTIONS AND COMMENTS

Methadone is addicting and habituating and has the potential to be highly abused. Prescribe methadone pharmacotherapy cautiously to patients who have histories of problematic patterns of opiate or other abusable psychotropic use. Also prescribe methadone pharmacotherapy cautiously to patients who

- have acute abdominal conditions (e.g., appendicitis) for which the use of methadone may obscure the monitoring of the clinical course of these disorders.
- regularly drink alcohol or are receiving concurrent pharmacotherapy with other drugs that produce CNS depression (e.g., antihistamines, phenothiazines, sedative-hypnotics). Additive actions may result in hypotension, respiratory depression, and profound sedation or coma. Avoid prescribing methadone pharmacotherapy to patients who are unable to abstain from drinking alcohol or are receiving pharmacotherapy with other opiate analgesics.
- have difficulty maintaining normal blood pressure (e.g., have a depleted blood volume or are concurrently receiving phenothiazines or other pharmacotherapy that can lower blood pressure). Methadone pharmacotherapy for these patients may result in severe hypotension.
- have head injuries or other medical disorders associated with increased intracranial pressure. Methadone's associated respiratory depressant actions and its ability to elevate cerebrospinal fluid pressure may be exaggerated among these patients. Methadone pharmacotherapy also may obscure the clinical course of these patients. In addition, methadone has been associated with postural hypotension among these patients. Prescribe methadone pharmacotherapy cautiously to patients who have head injuries or other medical disorders associated with increased intracranial pressure.
- have status asthmaticus, chronic obstructive lung disease, cor pulmonale, substantially reduced respiratory reserve, pre-existing respiratory depression, hypoxia, or hypercapnia. Even usual therapeutic dosages of methadone for these patients may decrease respiratory drive while simultaneously increasing airway resistance to the point of apnea.

Caution patients who are receiving methadone pharmacotherapy against

- performing activities that require alertness, judgment, and physical coordination (e.g., driving an automobile, operating dangerous equipment, supervising children) until their response to methadone pharmacotherapy is known. Methadone may affect these mental and physical functions adversely.

CLINICALLY SIGNIFICANT DRUG INTERACTIONS

Concurrent methadone pharmacotherapy and the following may result in clinically significant drug interactions:

Alcohol Use

Concurrent alcohol use may increase the CNS depressant action of methadone. Advise patients to avoid, or limit, their use of alcohol while receiving methadone pharmacotherapy.

Pharmacotherapy With CNS Depressants and Other Drugs That Produce CNS Depression

Concurrent methadone pharmacotherapy and pharmacotherapy with other opiate analgesics, sedative-hypnotics, and other drugs that produce CNS depression (e.g., antihistamines, phenothiazines, TCAs) may result in additive CNS depression.

Phenytoin Pharmacotherapy

Phenytoin (Dilantin®), an anticonvulsant, may increase the hepatic metabolism of methadone, resulting in decreased blood concentrations and diminished pharmacologic action.

Rifampin Pharmacotherapy

Rifampin (Rimactane®), an antibacterial, may increase the hepatic metabolism of methadone, resulting in decreased blood concentrations and diminished pharmacologic action.

See also "Opiate Analgesics, General Monograph."

ADVERSE DRUG REACTIONS

Methadone has a low incidence of ADRs when compared to morphine and produces less euphoria than heroin. Methadone pharmacotherapy commonly is associated with dizziness, drowsiness, excessive sweating, GI complaints, lightheadedness, nausea, sedation, and vomiting. Methadone also may produce the ADRs commonly associated with other opiate analgesics because of its chemical and pharmacological similarity to these opiate analgesics (see "Opiate Analgesics, General Monograph"). In addition, methadone pharmacotherapy has been associated with the following ADRs, listed according to body system:

Cardiovascular: bradycardia, fainting (syncope), flushing of the face, and palpitation
CNS: agitation, disorientation, and dysphoria
Cutaneous: edema, hives (urticaria), severe itching (pruritus), and skin rashes
Genitourinary: antidiuretic effect, decreased sex drive, and urinary retention
GI: biliary tract spasm, constipation, dry mouth, and loss of appetite (anorexia)
Ocular: blurred vision
Miscellaneous: decreased sex drive

OVERDOSAGE

Signs and symptoms of methadone overdosage are similar to those observed with morphine overdosage. These signs and symptoms, which begin within seconds after intravenous injection or within minutes of oral ingestion, include: abnormal contraction of the pupils (miosis); coma; cool, clammy skin; respiratory depression; skeletal muscle flaccidity; and somnolence. In severe overdosage, these signs and symptoms can progress to apnea, bradycardia, hypotension, and death.

Methadone overdosage requires emergency symptomatic medical support of body systems with attention to increasing methadone elimination. The opiate antagonist naloxone (Narcan®), is an essential component of the emergency medical management of methadone and other opiate analgesic overdosage. *Repeated doses* of naloxone usually are required because the duration of methadone action is prolonged (36 to 48 hours) and that of naloxone is short (1 to 3 hours).

Naloxone pharmacotherapy will precipitate the opiate analgesic withdrawal syndrome among patients who are addicted to methadone, including those who are enrolled in opiate addiction maintenance programs. The signs and symptoms of the opiate analgesic withdrawal syndrome include: abdominal cramps, diarrhea, dilated pupils, piloerection (goose flesh), restlessness, salivation, sweating, tearing, vomiting, and yawning. These signs and symptoms generally remit as the action of naloxone abates. See also "Opiate Analgesics, General Monograph" and the naloxone monograph.

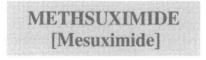

METHSUXIMIDE
[Mesuximide]

(meth sux′ i mide)

TRADE NAME

Celontin®

CLASSIFICATION

Anticonvulsant (succinimide derivative)

APPROVED INDICATIONS FOR NEUROPSYCHOLOGICAL DISORDERS

Pharmacotherapy for the prophylactic and symptomatic management of:

• seizure disorders. Methsuximide pharmacotherapy is indicated for absence (petit mal) seizures and partial seizures among patients who are refractory to other anticonvulsant pharmacotherapy.

USUAL DOSAGE AND ADMINISTRATION

Seizure Disorders: Absence Seizures or Partial Seizures Among Patients Who Are Refractory to Other Pharmacotherapy

Adults: Initially, 300 mg daily orally in a single dose for one week. Increase the daily dosage by 300 mg at weekly intervals, if necessary, according to individual patient response.

MAXIMUM: 1200 mg daily orally

Women who are, or who may become, pregnant: FDA Pregnancy Category C. Safety and efficacy of methsuximide pharmacotherapy for women who are pregnant have not been established. Methsuximide pharmacotherapy has been associated with hypoplasia of the nails and distal phalanges, delayed development, and neonatal hemorrhage. The overall incidence of these congenital malformations (i.e., birth defects) is ~5%. Avoid prescribing methsuximide pharmacotherapy to women who are pregnant. If methsuximide pharmacotherapy is required, advise patients of potential benefits and possible risks to themselves and the embryo, fetus, or neonate. Collaboration with the patient's obstetrician is indicated.

For details and discussion regarding related basic principles of clinical pharmacology, readers are referred to the first text in this series, *The Pharmacologic Basis of Psychotherapeutics: An Introduction for Psychologists.*

Women who are breast-feeding: Safety and efficacy of methsuximide pharmacotherapy for women who are breast-feeding and their neonates and infants have not been established. Avoid prescribing methsuximide pharmacotherapy to women who are breast-feeding. If methsuximide pharmacotherapy is required, breast-feeding probably should be discontinued. Collaboration with the patient's pediatrician is indicated.

Elderly, frail, or debilitated patients: Initially prescribe lower dosages for elderly, frail, or debilitated patients. Gradually increase the dosage if needed, according to individual patient response. These patients may be more sensitive to the pharmacologic actions of methsuximide than are younger or healthier adult patients.

Children and adolescents younger than 18 years of age: Same dosage as for adults; alternatively, a maintenance dosage of 10 mg/kg daily orally

Notes, Seizure Disorders: Absence Seizures and Partial Seizures Among Patients Who Are Refractory to Other Pharmacotherapy

Methsuximide may be prescribed in combination with other anticonvulsants (e.g., phenobarbital, phenytoin) for the prophylactic and symptomatic management of absence seizures or partial seizures with complex symptomatology when other anticonvulsant pharmacotherapy alone has failed to provide adequate seizure control.

See "Cautions and Comments."

AVAILABLE DOSAGE FORMS, STORAGE, AND COMPATIBILITY

Capsules, oral: 150, 300 mg

Notes

General instructions for patients: Instruct patients who are receiving methsuximide pharmacotherapy to

- ingest each dose of the methsuximide oral capsules with food to decrease associated gastric irritation.
- safely store methsuximide oral capsules out of the reach of children in tightly closed, light- and child-resistant containers at controlled room temperature (15° to 30°C; 59° to 86°F).
- obtain an available patient information sheet regarding methsuximide pharmacotherapy from their pharmacist at the time that their prescription is dispensed. Encourage patients to clarify any questions that they may have regarding methsuximide pharmacotherapy with their pharmacist or, if needed, to consult their prescribing psychologist.

PROPOSED MECHANISM OF ACTION

The exact mechanism of anticonvulsant action of methsuximide has not yet been fully determined. However, it appears to involve depression of the motor cortex and elevation of the seizure threshold. Methsuximide suppresses the paroxysmal three-cycle-per-second spike and wave activity that is associated with lapses of consciousness, which occur commonly with absence seizures.

PHARMACOKINETICS/PHARMACODYNAMICS

Methsuximide is fairly well absorbed following oral ingestion and achieves peak blood concentrations within 1 to 3 hours. It is extensively metabolized in the liver to several metabolites, including the active metabolite, N-demethylmethsuximide. Less than 1% of methsuximide is excreted in unchanged form in the urine. The half-life of elimination is ~3 hours. Additional data are not available.

RELATIVE CONTRAINDICATIONS

Hypersensitivity to methsuximide or other succinimides.

CAUTIONS AND COMMENTS

Prescribe methsuximide pharmacotherapy cautiously to *all* patients. Methsuximide has increased potential for toxicity (see "Adverse Drug Reactions"). Prior to initiating methsuximide pharmacotherapy, obtain complete blood counts, hepatic function tests, and urinalysis. Periodically monitor these tests for the remaining duration of methsuximide pharmacotherapy. Collaboration with the patient's family physician is indicated.

Caution patients who are receiving methsuximide pharmacotherapy against

* performing activities that require alertness, judgment, or physical coordination (e.g., driving an automobile, operating dangerous equipment, supervising children) until their response to methsuximide pharmacotherapy is known. Methsuximide may affect these mental and physical functions adversely.

CLINICALLY SIGNIFICANT DRUG INTERACTIONS

Concurrent methsuximide pharmacotherapy and the following may result in clinically significant drug interactions:

Alcohol Use

Concurrent alcohol use may increase the CNS depressant action of methsuximide. Advise patients to avoid, or limit, their use of alcohol while receiving methsuximide pharmacotherapy.

Antidepressant Pharmacotherapy

Antidepressant pharmacotherapy may precipitate seizures. Therefore, patients who have seizure disorders and who are receiving antidepressant pharmacotherapy, should be monitored for decreased seizure control. The dosage of methsuximide should be adjusted as indicated by individual patient response.

Pharmacotherapy With CNS Depressants and Other Drugs That Produce CNS Depression

Concurrent methsuximide pharmacotherapy and pharmacotherapy with opiate analgesics, sedative-hypnotics, or other drugs that produce CNS depression (e.g., antihistamines, phenothiazines, TCAs) may result in additive CNS depression.

ADVERSE DRUG REACTIONS

Methsuximide pharmacotherapy commonly has been associated with dizziness, drowsiness, incoordination (ataxia), loss of appetite (anorexia), nausea, and vomiting. Methsuximide pharmacotherapy also has been associated with the following ADRs, listed according to body system:

CNS: aggressiveness, depression, insomnia, irritability, mental confusion, nervousness, and, rarely, psychosis

Cutaneous: hives (urticaria), rash, severe itching (pruritus), and Stevens–Johnson syndrome

Genitourinary: microscopic hematuria and proteinuria

GI: abdominal pain, diarrhea, hiccups, and weight loss

Hematologic: eosinophilia, leukopenia, monocytosis, and pancytopenia

Ophthalmic: blurred vision and sensitivity to light (photophobia)

OVERDOSAGE

Signs and symptoms of acute methsuximide overdosage include coma, nausea, respiratory depression, and vomiting. The active N-demethylmethsuximide metabolite of methsuximide is believed to be responsible for the observed toxicity. Blood concentrations of the metabolite exceeding 40 µg/ml are associated with toxicity and those exceeding 150 µg/ml are associated with coma. Acute methsuximide overdosage requires emergency symptomatic medical support of body systems with attention to increasing methsuximide elimination. There is no known antidote.

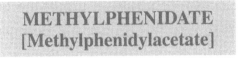

METHYLPHENIDATE
[Methylphenidylacetate]

(meth il fen' i date)

TRADE NAMES

Ritalin®
Ritalin-SR®

CLASSIFICATION

CNS stimulant (C-II)

APPROVED INDICATIONS FOR NEUROPSYCHOLOGICAL DISORDERS

Pharmacotherapy for the symptomatic management of:

- sleep disorders: narcolepsy

USUAL DOSAGE AND ADMINISTRATION

Narcolepsy

Adults: 20 to 60 mg daily orally in two or three divided doses 30 to 45 minutes before eating. Some patients may prefer to ingest their last daily dose before 6 p.m. (1800 hours) to prevent associated insomnia.

Women who are, or who may become, pregnant: FDA Pregnancy Category C. Safety and efficacy of methylphenidate pharmacotherapy for women who are pregnant have not been established. Avoid prescribing methylphenidate pharmacotherapy to women who are pregnant. If methylphenidate pharmacotherapy is required, advise patients of potential benefits and possible risks to themselves and the embryo, fetus, or neonate. Collaboration with the patient's obstetrician may be indicated.

Women who are breast-feeding: Safety and efficacy of methylphenidate pharmacotherapy for women who are breast-feeding and their neonates and infants have not been established. Avoid prescribing methylphenidate pharmacotherapy to women who are breast-feeding. If methylphenidate pharmacotherapy is required, breast-feeding probably should be discontinued. Collaboration with the patient's pediatrician may be indicated.

For details and discussion regarding related basic principles of clinical pharmacology, readers are referred to the first text in this series, *The Pharmacologic Basis of Psychotherapeutics: An Introduction for Psychologists.*

Elderly, frail, or debilitated patients: Generally prescribe lower dosages for elderly, frail, or debilitated patients. Gradually increase the dosage according to individual patient response. These patients may be more sensitive to the pharmacologic actions of methylphenidate than are younger or healthier adult patients.

Children younger than 12 years of age: Safety and efficacy of methylphenidate pharmacotherapy for the symptomatic management of narcolepsy have not been established for children younger than 12 years of age. Methylphenidate pharmacotherapy for this indication is *not* recommended for this age group.

Notes, Narcolepsy

If paradoxical signs and symptoms or other troublesome ADRs occur, reduce the dosage. If necessary, discontinue methylphenidate pharmacotherapy.

AVAILABLE DOSAGE FORMS, STORAGE, AND COMPATIBILITY

Tablets, oral: 5, 10, 20 mg
Tablets, oral extended-release (i.e., Ritalin-SR®): 20 mg

Notes

Methylphenidate oral extended-release tablets: The methylphenidate oral extended-release tablets (Ritalin-SR®) have a duration of action of approximately 8 hours. These tablets are indicated for patients whose signs and symptoms have been managed with regular methylphenidate oral tablets (Ritalin®) and who prefer 8-hour dosing.

General instructions for patients: Instruct patients who are receiving methylphenidate pharmacotherapy to

- ingest each dose of the methylphenidate oral tablets on an empty stomach 30 to 45 minutes before eating in order to obtain maximal GI absorption.
- swallow methylphenidate oral extended-release tablets whole without breaking, chewing, or crushing.
- safely store methylphenidate oral tablets out of the reach of children at a temperature below 30 °C (86 °F) in tightly closed, child- and light-resistant containers protected from moisture.
- obtain an available patient information sheet regarding methylphenidate pharmacotherapy from their pharmacist at the time that their prescription is dispensed. Encourage patients to clarify any questions that they may have regarding methylphenidate pharmacotherapy with their pharmacist or, if needed, to consult their prescribing psychologist.

PROPOSED MECHANISM OF ACTION

The exact mechanism of methylphenidate's CNS stimulant action for the symptomatic management of narcolepsy has not yet been fully determined. However, it appears to primarily involve stimulation of the CNS by activation of the brainstem arousal system and cortex.

PHARMACOKINETICS/PHARMACODYNAMICS

Methylphenidate is rapidly and well absorbed following oral ingestion. However, bioavailability is low (i.e., $F = 0.3$) and peak blood concentrations are variable because of extensive hepatic first-pass metabolism. When compared to regular methylphenidate oral tablets (i.e., Ritalin®), methylphenidate oral extended-release tablets (i.e., Ritalin-SR®) are absorbed more slowly, but to the same extent. Methylphenidate is mainly excreted into the urine as metabolites with less than 5% excreted in unchanged form. Methylphenidate has a mean half-life of elimination of ~2 hours. Additional data are not available.

RELATIVE CONTRAINDICATIONS

Agitation
Angina pectoris, severe
Anxiety
Glaucoma
Heart disease, severe
Hypersensitivity to methylphenidate
MAOI pharmacotherapy, concurrent or within 14 days
Tachycardia
Thyrotoxicosis
Tourette's disorder (Gilles de la Tourette's syndrome), or family history of

CAUTIONS AND COMMENTS

Long-term methylphenidate pharmacotherapy, or regular personal use, may result in addiction and habituation. Prescribe methylphenidate pharmacotherapy cautiously to patients who have histories of problematic patterns of abusable psychotropic use. Also prescribe methylphenidate pharmacotherapy cautiously to patients who

- have histories of seizure disorders or EEG abnormalities in the absence of seizures that are being managed with anticonvulsant pharmacotherapy. The safety and efficacy of concurrent methylphenidate and anticonvulsant pharmacotherapy have not been established. If seizures occur, methylphenidate pharmacotherapy should be discontinued.
- have hypertension. Methylphenidate pharmacotherapy may exacerbate this medical disorder. Avoid prescribing methylphenidate pharmacotherapy to patients who have hypertension. If methylphenidate pharmacotherapy is required, monitor blood pressure regularly. Collaboration with the patient's advanced practice nurse or family physician is indicated.

Caution patients who are receiving methylphenidate pharmacotherapy against

- performing activities that require alertness, judgment, and physical coordination (e.g., driving an automobile, operating dangerous equipment, supervising children) until their response to methylphenidate pharmacotherapy is known. Methylphenidate may affect these mental and physical functions adversely.

In addition to this general precaution, caution patients to

- inform their prescribing psychologist if they begin or discontinue any other pharmacotherapy while receiving methylphenidate pharmacotherapy.

CLINICALLY SIGNIFICANT DRUG INTERACTIONS

Concurrent methylphenidate pharmacotherapy and the following may result in clinically significant drug interactions:

Anticoagulant (Oral) Pharmacotherapy

Concurrent methylphenidate pharmacotherapy may inhibit the metabolism of oral anticoagulants (i.e., coumadin [Warfarin®]). Lower dosages of the anticoagulant may be required. Collaboration with the prescriber of the anticoagulant pharmacotherapy is indicated.

Anticonvulsant Pharmacotherapy

Concurrent methylphenidate pharmacotherapy may inhibit the metabolism of anticonvulsants (e.g., diphenylhydantoin [Dilantin®], phenobarbital [Luminal®], primidone [Mysoline®]). Lower dosages of the anticonvulsant may be required. Collaboration with the prescriber of the anticonvulsant pharmacotherapy is indicated.

Clonidine Pharmacotherapy

Sudden death has occurred among several children who received concurrent clonidine (Catapres®) and methylphenidate pharmacotherapy for the treatment of attention-deficit/hyperactivity disorder (note that clonidine pharmacotherapy currently is *not* approved for this indication). Although the nature of this possible drug interaction has not been conclusively determined, its seriousness warrants precaution and careful monitoring of blood pressure whenever clonidine and methylphenidate pharmacotherapy is initiated or adjusted (i.e., dosages are increased or decreased).

Guanethidine Pharmacotherapy

Methylphenidate may decrease the antihypertensive action of guanethidine (Ismelin®). Higher dosages of the antihypertensive may be required. Collaboration with the prescriber of the guanethidine pharmacotherapy is indicated.

MAOI Pharmacotherapy

Methylphenidate may interact with MAOIs (e.g., phenelzine [Nardil®]), resulting in the release of large amounts of catecholamines and the hypertensive crisis. The hypertensive crisis is characterized by severe headache and hypertension. Thus, methylphenidate pharmacotherapy, concurrent or within 14 days of MAOI pharmacotherapy, **is contraindicated**.

Phenylbutazone Pharmacotherapy

Concurrent methylphenidate pharmacotherapy may inhibit the metabolism of phenylbutazone (Novo-Butazone®). Lower dosages of phenylbutazone may be required. Collaboration with the prescriber of the phenylbutazone is indicated.

TCA Pharmacotherapy

Concurrent methylphenidate and TCA (e.g., desipramine [Norpramin®], imipramine [Tofranil®]) pharmacotherapy may result in the inhibition of the metabolism of the TCA. Lower dosages of the TCA may be required.

ADVERSE DRUG REACTIONS

Methylphenidate pharmacotherapy is commonly associated with insomnia, particularly if the last daily dose is ingested late in the day. This ADR may be managed by reducing the dosage of methylphenidate or by omitting the afternoon or evening dose. Anorexia (loss of appetite), which is usually transient, and nervousness also occur commonly. The latter may be managed with a reduction in dosage. Other ADRs associated with methylphenidate pharmacotherapy, listed according to body system, include:

Cardiovascular: angina, blood pressure changes (increase or decrease), cardiac dysrhythmias (e.g., tachycardia), and changes in pulse rate (increase or decrease)

CNS: addiction and habituation with long-term pharmacotherapy; anxiety; convulsions; depressed mood (transient); dizziness; drowsiness; dyskinesia; encephalopathy; hallucinations; headache; insomnia; psychotic episodes, including hallucinations; tics, or their exacerbation; and Tourette's disorder (i.e., Gilles de la Tourette's syndrome). Psychotic episodes and Tourette's disorder usually subside with the discontinuation of methylphenidate pharmacotherapy. See also information regarding the musculoskeletal system, following.

Cutaneous: hair loss (alopecia); itchy hives or wheals (urticaria); rash; and severe itching (pruritus). Rarely, abnormal decrease in the number of blood platelets (thrombocytopenia purpura); reddened areas of the skin, usually involving the extremities (erythema multiforme) with inflammation and necrosis of the blood or lymph vessels (necrotizing vasculitis); and redness of the skin followed by scaling and loss of skin with associated enlargement of the liver, fever, and edema (exfoliative dermatitis)

GI: initially, abdominal pain, loss of appetite (anorexia), and nausea. These ADRs may be relieved by ingesting each dose of methylphenidate with food.

Hematologic: rarely, abnormal decrease in the number of red blood cells (anemia), abnormal decrease in the number of white blood cells (leukopenia), and abnormal decrease in the number of blood platelets (thrombocytopenia)

Metabolic/Endocrine: weight loss

Musculoskeletal: defect in voluntary movement (dyskinesia), growth retardation among children (minor, usually associated with long-term pharmacotherapy), and joint pain (arthralgia). Rarely, choreoathetoid movements (e.g., extreme range of motion; jerky, involuntary movement more proximal than distal; fluctuating muscle tone from hypo- to hypertonia)

Ocular: blurring of the vision and difficulties with accommodation (adjustment of the eye for seeing various distances)

Miscellaneous: fever

OVERDOSAGE

Signs and symptoms of acute methylphenidate overdosage are associated with its CNS stimulant and sympathomimetic actions. These signs and symptoms may include: abnormal dilation of the pupil (mydriasis), agitation, cardiac dysrhythmias, confusion, convulsions, delirium, dryness of the mouth and other mucous membranes, euphoria, flushing, hallucinations, headache, increase in body temperature above 41.1 °C (106 °F) (hyperpyrexia), increased action of the reflexes (hyperreflexia), hypertension, muscle twitching, palpitations, sweating, tremors, tachycardia, and vomiting. Acute methylphenidate overdosage requires emergency symptomatic medical support of body systems with attention to increasing methylphenidate elimination, particularly when overdosage involves the oral extended-release tablets. There is no known antidote.

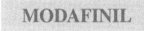
MODAFINIL

(moe daf' en il)

TRADE NAMES

Alertec®
Provigil®

CLASSIFICATION

CNS stimulant (C-IV)

APPROVED INDICATIONS FOR NEUROPSYCHOLOGICAL DISORDERS

Pharmacotherapy for the symptomatic management of:

- sleep disorders: narcolepsy

Note: Modafinil pharmacotherapy is indicated solely for the symptomatic management of excessive daytime sleepiness associated with narcolepsy. It is *not* indicated for the treatment of normal fatigue states. Modafinil does *not* reduce the incidence or severity of cataplectic seizures that commonly are associated with narcolepsy.

USUAL DOSAGE AND ADMINISTRATION

Narcolepsy:

Adults: *Canada*: Initially, 200 mg orally daily in two divided doses, morning and noon. Increase dosage in increments of 100 mg according to individual patient response. *United States*: 200 mg orally daily as a single morning dose.

Maximum: *Canada*: Single oral dose of 300 mg and total daily oral dosage of 400 mg. *United States*: 400 mg orally daily.

Women who are, or who may become, pregnant: FDA Pregnancy Category C. Safety and efficacy of modafinil pharmacotherapy for women who are pregnant have not been established. Avoid prescribing modafinil pharmacotherapy to women who are pregnant. If modafinil pharmacotherapy is required, advise patients of potential benefits and possible risks to themselves and the embryo, fetus, or neonate. Collaboration with the patient's obstetrician may be indicated.

For details and discussion regarding related basic principles of clinical pharmacology, readers are referred to the first text in this series, *The Pharmacologic Basis of Psychotherapeutics: An Introduction for Psychologists.*

Women who are breast-feeding: Safety and efficacy of modafinil pharmacotherapy for women who are breast-feeding and their neonates and infants have not been established. Avoid prescribing modafinil pharmacotherapy to women who are breast-feeding. If modafinil pharmacotherapy is required, breast-feeding probably should be discontinued. Collaboration with the patient's pediatrician may be indicated.

Elderly, frail, or debilitated patients: Generally prescribe lower dosages for elderly, frail, or debilitated patients. Gradually increase the dosage according to individual patient response. These patients may be more sensitive to the pharmacologic actions of modafinil than younger or healthier adult patients.

Adult patients who have liver dysfunction: The half-life of elimination may be doubled among patients with significant liver dysfunction. Initial dosages should be reduced by half. Carefully monitor patients and adjust subsequent dosages, as required, according to individual patient response.

Children and adolescents younger than 16 years of age: Safety and efficacy of modafinil pharmacotherapy for the symptomatic management of narcolepsy have not been established for children and adolescents younger than 16 years of age. Modafinil pharmacotherapy for this indication is *not* recommended for this age group.

Notes, Narcolepsy

Approved dosages differ slightly in Canada and the United States. *Canada*: The second daily dose generally should be ingested at noon or in the early afternoon in order to avoid associated insomnia. The occasional patient who has narcolepsy may require and tolerate dosages of 500 mg orally daily. However, for the majority of patients the incidence and severity of ADRs increase significantly when the stated maximum dosage is exceeded.

AVAILABLE DOSAGE FORMS, STORAGE, AND COMPATIBILITY

Tablets, oral: 100, 200 mg

Notes

General instructions for patients: Instruct patients who are receiving modafinil pharmacotherapy to

- safely store modafinil oral tablets out of the reach of children between 15° and 25 °C (59° and 77 °F) in tightly closed, child-resistant containers.
- obtain an available patient information sheet regarding modafinil pharmacotherapy from their pharmacist at the time that their prescription is dispensed. Encourage patients to clarify any questions that they may have regarding modafinil pharmacotherapy with their pharmacist or, if needed, to consult their prescribing psychologist.

PROPOSED MECHANISM OF ACTION

The exact mechanism of modafinil's CNS stimulant action for the symptomatic management of narcolepsy has not yet fully been determined. However, it appears primarily to involve: 1) stimulation of α-1 adrenergic receptors; 2) increase in the metabolism (turnover rate) of serotonin (5-HT); and 3) inhibition of the activity of GABA neurons. On EEG, modafinil increases high frequency α waves and decreases δ and θ waves (i.e., produces EEG changes that are consistent with measures of increased mental alertness).

PHARMACOKINETICS/PHARMACODYNAMICS

Modafinil is absorbed fairly rapidly following oral ingestion. Peak blood concentrations are achieved in ~3 hours. The ingestion of food may decrease the rate, but not the extent, of modafinil absorption. Modafinil is bound moderately to plasma proteins (~60%) and has an apparent volume of distribution of ~66 liters (i.e., ~0.9 liters/kg). It is metabolized extensively in the liver and is excreted mainly into the urine as inactive metabolites. Long-term modafinil pharmacotherapy may result in autoinduction (i.e., stimulation of its own metabolism) (see also "Significant Drug Interactions"). Less than 10% is excreted in unchanged form in the urine. Modafinil has a mean half-life of elimination of 10 to 15 hours and its total body clearance is ~5 liters/hour.

RELATIVE CONTRAINDICATIONS

Agitation
Anxiety, severe
Hypersensitivity to modafinil
Liver dysfunction, severe

CAUTIONS AND COMMENTS

Although currently available data suggest that the risk is relatively low, long-term modafinil pharmacotherapy, or regular personal use, may result in addiction and habituation. Prescribe modafinil pharmacotherapy cautiously to patients who have histories of problematic patterns of abusable psychotropic use. Also prescribe modafinil pharmacotherapy cautiously to patients who

- have histories of seizure disorders or EEG abnormalities in the absence of seizures that are being managed with anticonvulsant pharmacotherapy. The safety and efficacy of concurrent modafinil and anticonvulsant pharmacotherapy have not been established. If seizures occur, modafinil pharmacotherapy should be discontinued.
- have coronary artery disease, mitral valve prolapse, recent history of myocardial infarction, and unstable angina. Modafinil pharmacotherapy may exacerbate these cardiovascular disorders. Avoid prescribing modafinil pharmacotherapy to patients who have these disorders. If modafinil pharmacotherapy is required, ensure that patients are monitored closely. Collaboration with the patient's family physician or cardiologist is indicated.

Caution patients who are receiving modafinil pharmacotherapy against

- performing activities that require alertness, judgment, and physical coordination (e.g., driving an automobile, operating dangerous equipment, supervising children) until their response to modafinil pharmacotherapy is known. Modafinil has been associated with overstimulation and overconfidence, which may affect these mental and physical functions adversely.

In addition to this general precaution, caution patients to

- inform their prescribing psychologist if they begin or discontinue any other pharmacotherapy while receiving modafinil pharmacotherapy.

CLINICALLY SIGNIFICANT DRUG INTERACTIONS

Note: *Modafinil has been demonstrated "in vitro" to variably affect the cytochrome P-450 isoenzymes associated with drug metabolism. For most of these isoenzymes, this action appears to have no significant effect. However, it does appear to 1) induce CYP-3A4 and 2) inhibit CYP-2C19. Because of these "mixed" effects upon the cytochrome P-450 isoenzymes and the lack of sufficient clinical experience to date with modafinil, it is recommended that 1) the drug interactions listed here be interpreted with caution and 2) all patients, who are receiving modafinil pharmacotherapy, carefully be monitored for possible drug interactions.* Concurrent modafinil pharmacotherapy and the following may result in clinically significant drug interactions:

Anticoagulant (Oral) Pharmacotherapy

Concurrent modafinil pharmacotherapy may induce the metabolism of oral anticoagulants (i.e., coumadin [Warfarin®]). Higher dosages of the anticoagulant may be required. Collaboration with the prescriber of the anticoagulant pharmacotherapy is indicated.

Anticonvulsant Pharmacotherapy

Concurrent modafinil pharmacotherapy may induce the metabolism of certain anticonvulsants (e.g., phenobarbital [Luminal®], primidone [Mysoline®]) by means of induction of CYP-3A4. Similarly, concurrent modafinil pharmacotherapy may inhibit the metabolism of certain anticonvulsants (e.g., diazepam [Valium®], mephenytoin [Mesantoin®], phenytoin [Dilantin®]) by means of inhibition of CYP-2C19. Concurrent pharmacotherapy with various anticonvulsants (e.g., carbamazepine [Tegretol®], phenobarbital [Luminal®]) also may affect modafinil blood concentrations by means of their induction of hepatic microsomal enzymes, particularly CYP-3A4. Thus, careful patient monitoring and dosage adjustment of the anticonvulsants and modafinil, as indicated by patient response, is required. Collaboration with the prescriber of the anticonvulsant pharmacotherapy is indicated.

Oral Contraceptive Pharmacotherapy

Concurrent modafinil pharmacotherapy may induce the metabolism of oral contraceptives and result in contraceptive failure. Higher dosages of the oral contraceptive, and/or other alternative methods of contraception, may be required. Collaboration with the prescriber of the oral contraceptive is indicated.

TCA Pharmacotherapy

Concurrent modafinil and TCA (e.g., clomipramine [Anafranil®], desipramine [Norpramin®], imipramine [Tofranil®]) pharmacotherapy may result in the inhibition of the metabolism of the TCA by means of inhibition of CYP-2C19. This effect appears to be particularly significant among patients who are already deficient in CYP-2D6 (i.e., poor metabolizers of debrisoquine) and, thus, increasingly dependent on CYP-2C19 as a major route of hepatic metabolism for the TCAs. Carefully monitor patient response and TCA blood concentrations, as appropriate. Lower dosages of the TCA may be required.

ADVERSE DRUG REACTIONS

Generally, modafinil pharmacotherapy is well tolerated. However, it commonly has been associated with headache and insomnia. Other ADRs associated with modafinil pharmacotherapy, listed according to body system, include

> **Cardiovascular:** chest pain, hypertension, and palpitation (Note: cardiovascular ADRs are significantly more likely to occur when the recommended maximal dosages are exceeded, particularly among patients who have pre-existing cardiovascular disorders.)
> **CNS:** anxiety, dizziness, dyskinesia (particularly among elderly patients), euphoria, and nervousness
> **GI:** diarrhea, dry mouth, and dyspepsia

OVERDOSAGE

Signs and symptoms of acute modafinil overdosage are associated with its CNS stimulant and sympathomimetic actions. These signs and symptoms may include anxiety, agitation, excitation, headache, hypertension (systolic), hypertonia, insomnia, irritability, palpitations, tachycardia, and tremor. Acute modafinil overdosage requires emergency symptomatic medical support of body systems with attention to increasing modafinil elimination. There is no known antidote.

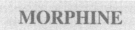

MORPHINE

(mor' feen)

TRADE NAMES

Duramorph®
Morphitec®
M.O.S.®
MS Contin®
MSIR®
Oramorph SR®

CLASSIFICATION

Opiate analgesic (C-II)

See also "Opiate Analgesics, General Monograph."

APPROVED INDICATIONS FOR NEUROPSYCHOLOGICAL DISORDERS

Adjunctive pharmacotherapy for the symptomatic management of:

- pain disorders: acute pain, moderate to severe, and chronic cancer pain, moderate to severe. Dosage generally is prescribed according to type and severity of pain, method of administration, and individual patient response.

USUAL DOSAGE AND ADMINISTRATION

Acute Pain, Moderate to Severe

Adults: Initially, 5 to 20 mg intramuscularly; *or* 2.5 to 15 mg intravenously, slowly, over four to five minutes; *or* 10 to 30 mg orally; *or* 10 to 20 mg rectally. Repeat the initial dose every four hours, as needed, according to individual patient response. (See "Notes, Pain Disorders: Acute Pain, Moderate to Severe, and Chronic Cancer Pain, Moderate to Severe.")

Women who are, or who may become, pregnant: FDA Pregnancy Category C. Safety and efficacy of morphine pharmacotherapy for women who are pregnant have not been established. Although morphine pharmacotherapy during pregnancy has not been associated with congenital malformations (i.e., birth defects), high-dosage pharmacotherapy, or regular personal use, near term may result in the neonatal opiate analgesic withdrawal syndrome (see "Opiate Analgesics, General Monograph"). Avoid prescribing morphine pharmacotherapy to women who are

---

For details and discussion regarding related basic principles of clinical pharmacology, readers are referred to the first text in this series, *The Pharmacologic Basis of Psychotherapeutics: An Introduction for Psychologists.*

pregnant. If morphine pharmacotherapy is required, advise patients of potential benefits and possible risks to themselves and the embryo, fetus, or neonate. Collaboration with the patient's advanced practice nurse, midwife, or obstetrician is indicated. Morphine pharmacotherapy is *not* recommended for pregnant women prior to labor unless potential benefits outweigh possible risks to the embryo, fetus, or neonate. Opiate pharmacotherapy during labor may result in drowsiness and other expected pharmacologic actions (e.g., respiratory depression) among neonates.

Women who are breast-feeding: Safety and efficacy of morphine pharmacotherapy for women who are breast-feeding and their neonates and infants have not been established. Morphine is excreted into breast milk. The concentration of morphine in breast milk is generally higher than the concentration in maternal blood. Expected pharmacologic actions (e.g., CNS or respiratory depression, constipation) may be observed among breast-fed neonates and infants, who also may become addicted (see "Opiate Analgesics, General Monograph"). Avoid prescribing morphine pharmacotherapy to women who are breast-feeding. If morphine pharmacotherapy is required, breast-feeding should be discontinued. If desired, lactation may be maintained and breast-feeding resumed following the discontinuation of short-term morphine pharmacotherapy. Collaboration with the patient's pediatrician is indicated.

Elderly, frail, or debilitated patients: Generally prescribe lower dosages for elderly, frail, or debilitated patients. Gradually increase the dosage, if needed, according to individual patient response. These patients may be more sensitive to the pharmacologic actions of morphine than are younger or healthier adult patients.

Children: Initially, 0.1 to 0.2 mg/kg intramuscularly or subcutaneously; *or* 0.05 to 0.1 mg/kg intravenously, slowly, over four to five minutes; *or* 0.15 to 0.3 mg/kg orally; *or* 0.15 to 0.3 mg/kg rectally. Repeat the initial dose every four hours, as needed, according to individual patient response. (See "Notes, Pain Disorders: Acute Pain, Moderate to Severe and Chronic Cancer Pain, Moderate to Severe.")

MAXIMUM: 15 mg/dose

Slow Intravenous or Subcutaneous Injection

Adults: 2.5 to 15 mg intravenously or subcutaneously. For intravenous injection, dilute in 4 to 5 ml of sterile water for injection and inject slowly over 4 to 5 minutes, with the patient lying down.

Children: 0.1 to 0.2 mg/kg subcutaneously every 4 hours, as needed

MAXIMUM: 15 mg/dose

Continuous Intravenous or Subcutaneous Infusion

Loading dose, for patients whose pain is poorly controlled: 1 to 2 mg/minute until pain is relieved. Dilute in 4 to 5 ml of sterile intravenous solution and infuse slowly over 1 minute while monitoring heart rate, respiratory rate, and blood pressure. Withhold morphine pharmacotherapy if respiratory rate slows to less than 10 respirations per minute or if the diastolic pressure decreases more than 10%. Resume morphine pharmacotherapy when respiratory rate and blood pressure have stabilized.

Loading dose, for patients whose pain is presently controlled: Using the previous day's 24-hour opiate requirement, calculate hourly dose with attention to method of administration and analgesic equivalents.

Continuous intravenous or subcutaneous infusion for relief of severe chronic pain associated with cancer: Individualize dosage according to individual patient response.

ADULTS: Initially, 0.8 to 10 mg/hour. Adjust to lowest effective dosage. An intravenous loading dose of 15 mg or more can be injected for initial relief of pain prior to initiating continuous intravenous infusion.

Maintenance   0.8 to 80 mg/hour. Dosages of 150 mg/hour have occasionally been required. Relatively high dosages (275 to 440 mg/hour) occasionally have been infused for several hours or days to provide relief of exacerbations of chronic pain among adults previously stabilized on lower dosages or whose dosage had been gradually titrated to relatively high dosages. Subsequent dosage reductions, according to patient response, were generally possible.

Multiple, Slow Intravenous Injection for Patient Controlled Analgesia (PCA)

Dosage is adjusted according to severity of pain and individual patient response. Assure that the patient understands the use of the PCA infusion device. Care must be exercised to avoid overdosage and resultant respiratory depression. Also avoid inadvertent abrupt cessation of pharmacotherapy. Abrupt cessation of pharmacotherapy may result in a loss of analgesia and the opiate withdrawal syndrome.

Chronic Cancer Pain: Moderate to Severe

Adults: Initially, 0.2 to 0.4 mg/kg orally or rectally every four to six hours, as needed. Once the patient has been stabilized, it may be of benefit to replace short-acting oral or rectal morphine pharmacotherapy with long-acting pharmacotherapy with an oral extended-release formulation. (See Notes, "Pain Disorders: Acute Pain, Moderate to Severe and Chronic Cancer Pain, Moderate to Severe.")

Women who are, or who may become, pregnant: FDA Pregnancy Category C. Safety and efficacy of morphine pharmacotherapy for women who are pregnant have not been established. Although morphine pharmacotherapy during pregnancy has not been associated with congenital malformations (i.e., birth defects), high-dosage pharmacotherapy, or regular personal use, near term may result in the neonatal opiate analgesic withdrawal syndrome (see "Opiate Analgesics, General Monograph"). Avoid prescribing morphine pharmacotherapy to women who are pregnant. If morphine pharmacotherapy is required, advise patients of potential benefits and possible risks to themselves and the embryo, fetus, or neonate. Collaboration with the patient's obstetrician is indicated.

Women who are breast-feeding: Safety and efficacy of morphine pharmacotherapy for women who are breast-feeding and their neonates and infants have not been established. Morphine is excreted into breast milk. The concentration of morphine in breast milk is generally higher than that in maternal blood. Expected pharmacological actions (e.g., CNS or respiratory depression, constipation) may be observed among breast-fed infants, who also may become addicted (see also "Opiate Analgesics, General Monograph"). Avoid prescribing morphine pharmacotherapy to women who are breast-feeding. If morphine pharmacotherapy is required, breast-feeding should be discontinued. Collaboration with the patient's pediatrician may be indicated.

Elderly, frail, or debilitated patients: Generally prescribe lower dosages for elderly, frail, or debilitated patients. Gradually increase the dosage, if needed, according to individual patient response. These patients may be more sensitive to the pharmacologic actions of morphine than are younger or healthier adult patients.

Children: 0.2 to 0.4 mg/kg orally or rectally every four to six hours, as needed. *Note*: dosage is the same as for adults.

Intravenous Analgesia

Adults: 0.05 to 0.1 mg/kg intravenously. Slowly inject intravenously over three to five minutes.

Women who are, or who may become, pregnant: FDA Pregnancy Category C. Safety and efficacy of morphine pharmacotherapy for women who are pregnant have not been established. Although morphine pharmacotherapy during pregnancy has not been associated with congenital malformations (i.e., birth defects), maternal morphine pharmacotherapy, or regular personal use, near term may result in the neonatal opiate analgesic withdrawal syndrome (see "Opiate Analgesics, General Monograph"). Collaboration with the patient's obstetrician is indicated.

Women who are breast-feeding: Safety and efficacy of morphine pharmacotherapy for women who are breast-feeding and their neonates and infants have not been established. Morphine is excreted into breast milk. The concentration of morphine in breast milk is generally higher than that in maternal blood. Expected pharmacological actions (e.g., CNS or respiratory depression, constipation) may be observed among breast-fed infants who also may become addicted (see also "Opiate Analgesics, General Monograph"). Avoid prescribing morphine pharmacotherapy to women who are breast-feeding. If morphine pharmacotherapy is required, breast-feeding should be discontinued. If desired, lactation may be maintained and breast-feeding resumed following the discontinuation of short-term intravenous morphine pharmacotherapy. Collaboration with the patient's pediatrician is indicated.

Elderly, frail, or debilitated patients: Generally prescribe lower dosages for elderly, frail, or debilitated patients. Gradually increase the dosage, if needed, according to individual patient response. These patients may be more sensitive to the pharmacologic actions of morphine than are younger or healthier adult patients.

Children: 0.05 to 0.1 mg/kg intravenously. Slowly inject intravenously over three to five minutes. *Note*: dosage is the same as for adults.

MAXIMUM: 15 mg/dose

Notes, Pain Disorders: Acute Pain, Moderate to Severe and Chronic Cancer Pain, Moderate to Severe

Prescribe morphine pharmacotherapy at regular intervals throughout the 24-hour day for the symptomatic management of moderate to severe acute pain. Do *not* prescribe morphine on an "as needed" basis. This recommendation is particularly important for patients who have chronic pain associated with malignant disease. These patients usually need to be awakened during the night to maintain pain management so that they will not awaken with morning pain. The dosage range for morphine is wide. There is no "usual" recommended dosage because of such variable factors as general health, pharmacokinetic parameters, and individual factors associated with the experience of pain, including its cause, intensity, and duration. A general rule is to prescribe the lowest effective dosage as infrequently as possible. This recommendation will help to provide optimal therapeutic benefit while minimizing the development of tolerance to morphine's analgesic action.

When adjusting the dosage, do not increase the dosage more frequently than every 24 hours. It generally takes approximately five morphine half-lives to attain a new steady-state concentration among patients who have normal kidney and liver function. Monitor patients closely following all increases in dosage for ADRs, particularly constipation, hypotension, sedation, nausea, respiratory depression, and vomiting.

During the first 2 to 3 days of effective pain management, patients may sleep for several hours. This somnolence may be incorrectly attributed to excessive CNS depression rather than effective pain management among exhausted patients who previously had ineffective pain management. Maintain the dosage for ~3 days before reducing the dose, given that respiratory function and other physiological parameters are adequate. Following the relief of severe pain, periodically attempt to reduce the morphine dosage. Lower dosages or complete discontinuation of morphine pharmacotherapy may become possible as a result of physiological change or improved psychological health among patients.

Injectable morphine pharmacotherapy: Injectable morphine pharmacotherapy may be prescribed for intramuscular or subcutaneous injection or for intravenous infusion with a portable infusion pump. It also may be prescribed by slow intravenous injection over 3 to 5 minutes or by continuous intravenous infusion.

INTRAMUSCULAR MORPHINE PHARMACOTHERAPY: Usually prescribe intramuscular morphine pharmacotherapy every 4 hours, around the clock.

INTRAVENOUS MORPHINE PHARMACOTHERAPY: Dilute each dose in intravenous solution (dextrose 5% in water or sodium chloride injection) to the desired concentration (usually 0.1 to 0.5 mg/ml) before injection. Slowly inject intravenously over 3 to 5 minutes. Rapid intravenous injection may result in an increased severity and frequency of associated ADRs, including: apnea, cardiac arrest, chest wall rigidity, hypotension, peripheral circulatory collapse, possible anaphylaxis, and severe respiratory depression. The opiate antagonist, naloxone (Narcan®), emergency supportive equipment for assisted breathing, and trained medical personnel should be immediately available whenever intravenous morphine pharmacotherapy is administered.

SUBCUTANEOUS MORPHINE INFUSION WITH PUMP: Subcutaneous morphine infusion is indicated for patients who have limited muscle mass or inadequate or inaccessible peripheral veins. When replacing intravenous morphine pharmacotherapy with subcutaneous infusion, use the same dose and monitor the same parameters. The maximum dosage has not been determined, but dosages as high as 480 mg daily may be required. Erythema, bruising, induration, or tenderness around the subcutaneous injection site may occur. Inspect the subcutaneous injection site daily for these ADRs and for leakage of drug around the site. Irritation at subcutaneous injection sites may be minimized by changing needle sites every 7 to 10 days (some prescribers prefer every 48 hours).

Morphine Oral Pharmacotherapy: Prescribe oral morphine pharmacotherapy rather than injectable morphine pharmacotherapy whenever possible, with the end goal of ultimate pain relief. As a general rule, when replacing injectable morphine pharmacotherapy with oral morphine pharmacotherapy, double the dose (e.g., 5 mg intravenously = 10 mg orally) because of the decreased oral bioavailability of morphine. Whenever possible, prescribe the oral extended-release tablets or capsules, which will allow some patients to be dosed every 8 to 12 hours (MS Contin® and Oramorph SR® extended-release tablets) or every 24 hours (Kadian® extended-release capsules).

EXTENDED-RELEASE FORMULATIONS: Morphine pharmacotherapy with the oral extended-release formulations is indicated for patients who have been stabilized on a dosage of morphine. To replace this pharmacotherapy with the oral extended-release formulations, approximate the dosage according to the entire daily dosage in either a single dose with the extended-release *capsules* or two or three equally divided doses with the extended-release tablets every 12 or 8 hours, respectively. Generally, do not adjust the dosage more frequently than every 48 hours because of the pharmacokinetic properties of the oral morphine extended-release formulations. A short-acting opiate analgesic may be required during the interim 48 hours in order to provide relief for breakthrough pain. If the oral extended-release formulation is replacing a different opiate analgesic, use the approximate analgesic equivalents to determine the initial daily dosage requirements provided in the "Opiate Analgesics, General Monograph."

Following the management of chronic, severe cancer pain, periodically attempt to reduce the dosage or discontinue morphine pharmacotherapy. Always prescribe the lowest effective dosage of the extended-release formulation according to individual patient response. Unfortunately, oral formulations may not achieve therapeutic efficacy among patients who have chronic cancer pain.

AVAILABLE DOSAGE FORMS, STORAGE, AND COMPATIBILITY

Capsules, oral: 15, 30 mg
Capsules, oral extended-release: 20, 50, 100 mg. Oral extended-release capsules generally are indicated for the symptomatic management of moderate to severe chronic cancer pain.
Concentrate, oral with calibrated dropper (M.O.S.®, M.O.S.-SR®, Roxanol® concentrated oral solution): 20, 50 mg/ml (unflavored)
Injectables, intramuscular, intravenous, or subcutaneous: 0.5, 1, 2, 3, 4, 5, 8, 10, 15, 25, 30, 50 mg/ml. Morphine injectable is incompatible with aminophylline, calcium chloride, heparin, or sodium bicarbonate.
Injectables, cartridges: 1, 5 mg/ml
Injectables, cartridges for PCA infusor: 1, 2, 3, 5 mg in 30 ml
Injectables, Rapiject® prefilled single-dose syringe: 1, 2, 50 mg in 50 ml (the 50-mg injectable is formulated without a preservative)
Solutions, oral: 5, 10, 20 mg/5 ml
Suppositories, rectal (RMS®): 5, 10, 20, 30 mg
Syrups, oral: 1, 5, 10, 20 mg/ml (orange-flavored, contains 5% alcohol; unflavored, alcohol free)

Tablets, oral: 5, 10, 15, 20, 25, 30, 35, 40, 50, 60 mg

Tablets, oral extended-release (MS Contin®, Oramorph SR®): 15, 30, 60, 100, 200 mg. The oral extended-release tablets are generally indicated for the symptomatic management of moderate to severe chronic cancer pain.

Notes

Injectable formulations: Safely store injectables between 15° and 30 °C (59° to 86 °F). Do *not* autoclave. No loss of potency or increased toxicity has been associated with a discolored injectable solution of morphine.

Some injectable formulations (e.g., those manufactured by Abbott or Faulding) contain sodium metabisulfite. Sulfites may cause hypersensitivity reactions, including anaphylactic reactions, among susceptible patients. Although relatively uncommon, these reactions appear to occur with a higher incidence among patients who have asthma.

MORPHINE INJECTABLES (1, 2 mg/ml):   When stored at room temperature, morphine injection diluted to concentrations of 0.1 to 0.5 mg/ml in polyvinyl chloride (PVC) bags containing dextrose 5% injection or sterile water for injection should be used within 24 hours after dilution in order to avoid risk of microbial contamination. Morphine injectables and dilutions in dextrose 5% injection or sodium chloride 0.9% injection may be stored in portable infusion pump cassettes, syringes, or PVC infusion bags. Protected from light, they will remain stable for 24 hours at room temperature or for 72 hours when refrigerated. Proper aseptic technique for the preparation and handling of solutions is required to prevent contamination.

As with all injectables, intravenous admixtures should be inspected visually, whenever packaging permits, for clarity, particulate matter, precipitates, and leakage prior to use. Do not use solutions that are hazy or those that contain particulate matter or precipitates, or are leaking. Discard these solutions appropriately. A yellow discoloration does not indicate a loss of potency or toxicity.

HIGHLY CONCENTRATED INJECTABLE SOLUTIONS: Highly concentrated solutions of morphine for injection (e.g., Morphine HP®) may be used with or without dilution. These injectable formulations are indicated exclusively for the relief of severe pain among patients who require intramuscular or subcutaneous opiate analgesia in doses higher than those usually required (i.e., patients who are tolerant to opiate analgesics). These formulations allow smaller injection volumes and, thus, less discomfort, usually associated with the injection of larger volumes of drug at subcutaneous or intramuscular injection sites. It is recommended strongly that the use of these highly concentrated formulations be avoided for patients who are not opiate-tolerant because of the potential for overdosage error. When a less concentrated morphine injection is being replaced with the highly concentrated solution formulation, similar dosages should be prescribed, depending on individual patient need and response. If a highly concentrated morphine solution is replacing a different opiate analgesic, an equivalency table (see "Opiate Analgesics, General Monograph") should be used as a guide to determine the appropriate initial dose.

Do not confuse concentrated solutions of morphine for injection with non-concentrated injectable formulations, which have lower dosage strengths. *Fatal overdosage may result.*

PREFILLED SYRINGES: The Rapiject® prefilled syringe is considered to be sterile as long as it is in a sealed intact system with caps in place. This formulation contains no bacteriostatics or antimicrobials and is intended for use as a single-dose unit. Any unused portion should be discarded appropriately. Store at room temperature below 25 °C (77 °F). Protect from light. Do not autoclave.

Directions for Rapiject® prefilled syringe

- Remove protective caps from vial and injector.
- Insert vial into injector.
- Rotate vial three turns in clockwise direction until some resistance occurs.
- Rotate vial another turn or two. The needle will then be in contact with the morphine solution.
- Remove the needle cap and expel the air.
- The Rapiject® is ready for use.

Morphine oral formulations: Do not confuse the regular morphine capsules, tablets, oral solutions, or oral syrups with the morphine oral extended-release capsules and tablets or the more concentrated oral solutions. *Fatal overdosage may result.*

EXTENDED-RELEASE CAPSULES AND TABLETS: The extended-release *capsules* are formulated to be dosed every 12 hours. The extended-release *tablets* are formulated to be dosed every 8 or 12 hours depending on individual patient requirements.

SYRUPS: The Morphitec® syrup contains tartrazine (FD & C No. 5). Tartrazine has been associated with hypersensitivity reactions, including bronchial asthma, among susceptible patients. These reactions appear to occur more commonly among patients who have a hypersensitivity to aspirin.

The M.O.S.® syrup contains sodium metabisulfite. Sulfites have been associated with hypersensitivity reactions, including anaphylactic reactions, among susceptible patients. Although relatively uncommon, these reactions appear to occur with a higher incidence among patients who have asthma. The M.O.S. flavored syrup also contains 5% alcohol.

General instructions for patients: Instruct patients who are receiving morphine pharmacotherapy to

- safely store morphine oral capsules, tablets, and other oral dosage forms out of the reach of children in tightly closed child- and light-resistant containers at controlled room temperature (15 ° to 30 °C; 59 ° to 86 °F).
- swallow each dose of morphine oral extended-release capsules and tablets whole without breaking, chewing, or crushing. Breaking, chewing, or crushing these formulations could result in the rapid release and absorption of large doses of morphine and associated toxicity. Also instruct patients to ingest each dose of their oral capsules and tablets with adequate liquid chaser (i.e., 60 to 120 ml of water). If patients have difficulty swallowing the oral extended-release capsules, instruct them to take the capsule apart gently and sprinkle the timed beads onto a small amount of applesauce, pudding, jam, yogurt, or other cold soft food within 30 minutes of ingestion. To assure that the entire dose is ingested, advise them to rinse their mouth with water or another beverage immediately following the ingestion of the timed beads and to swallow the rinse. Caution them not to chew or crush the timed beads.
- obtain an available patient information sheet regarding morphine pharmacotherapy from their pharmacist at the time that their prescription is dispensed. Encourage patients to clarify any questions that they may have regarding morphine pharmacotherapy with their pharmacist or, if needed, to consult their prescribing psychologist.

PROPOSED MECHANISM OF ACTION

Morphine acts as an agonist at specific opiate receptor sites in the CNS producing analgesia. It also produces alterations in endocrine and autonomic nervous system function (e.g., decreased GI motility), drowsiness, mood changes, nausea, respiratory depression, and vomiting. See also "Opiate Analgesics, General Monograph."

PHARMACOKINETICS/PHARMACODYNAMICS

Morphine is absorbed fairly well following oral ingestion. However, only about 40% reaches the systemic circulation because of significant first-pass hepatic metabolism. Thus, oral morphine pharmacotherapy is less adequate than intramuscular or subcutaneous morphine pharmacotherapy. Plasma protein binding is low (~36%). The mean apparent volume of distribution is ~3 liters/kg (range: 1 to 5 liters/kg). Among elderly patients, the volume of distribution is considerably smaller and initial concentrations of morphine are, thus, correspondingly higher. Peak analgesic action occurs within 20 minutes following intravenous injection and within 1 hour following intramuscular, oral, rectal, or subcutaneous administration. Morphine is rapidly and extensively metabolized, primarily in the liver. Less than 10% is eliminated in unchanged form in the urine. Morphine's total body clearance ranges from 900 to 1200 ml/minute. The half-life of elimination is ~2 to 4 hours. Morphine's duration of action is 4 to 5 hours when administered by the oral or injectable routes.

RELATIVE CONTRAINDICATIONS

Alcoholism, acute
Biliary tract surgery or biliary or renal colic. Morphine causes smooth muscle spasms.
Cirrhosis, severe
CNS depression, severe
Delirium tremens
Heart failure secondary to chronic obstructive lung disease
Hypersensitivity to morphine or any of the components of the morphine formulation (e.g., the Rapiject® prefilled syringe formulation contains sodium metabisulfite, which may cause hypersensitivity reactions among susceptible patients, particularly those who have a history of asthma).
Hypotension, severe. Opiate analgesics may exacerbate this medical disorder.
MAOI pharmacotherapy, concurrent or within 14 days
Respiratory depression, severe
Respiratory disorders characterized by hypoxia, such as status asthmaticus (acute asthma attack), chronic obstructive lung disease, or cor pulmonale, or, for any other reason, a substantially decreased respiratory reserve (e.g., pre-existing respiratory depression, hypoxia, or hypercapnia). Among these patients, even low therapeutic doses of morphine may decrease respiratory drive while simultaneously increasing airway resistance to the point of apnea.
Upper airway obstruction

CAUTIONS AND COMMENTS

Morphine generally is considered the prototype for all opiate analgesics and, thus, is the measure by which they are compared. Morphine has high abuse potential, and long-term morphine pharmacotherapy, or regular personal use, may result in addiction and habituation. Prescribe morphine pharmacotherapy cautiously to patients who have histories of substance-use disorders or who

- have acute abdominal conditions (e.g., acute appendicitis). Morphine pharmacotherapy may obscure the medical diagnosis or clinical course of these conditions.
- are elderly, frail, or debilitated or have severe kidney or liver dysfunction. Morphine may have prolonged duration and cumulative actions among these patients.
- are in shock. Associated impaired perfusion may prevent absorption after intramuscular or subcutaneous morphine injection. Repeated injections may result in overdosage due to an excessive amount of morphine being absorbed when the patient's circulation is restored.
- have atrial flutter and other supraventricular tachycardias. Morphine's vagolytic action may produce a significant increase in the ventricular response rate among these patients.
- have compromised ability to maintain blood pressure due to excessive blood loss (e.g., injury, surgery) or are receiving phenothiazine pharmacotherapy or other pharmacotherapy with drugs that can lower blood pressure. Morphine pharmacotherapy may produce severe hypotension among these patients.
- have head injuries, brain tumors, other intracranial lesions, or pre-existing increased intracranial pressure. The respiratory depressant action of morphine and its ability to increase cerebrospinal fluid pressure may be markedly exaggerated among these patients. Morphine pharmacotherapy also may obscure the clinical course of these medical disorders.
- have hypothyroidism, Addison's disease, prostatic hypertrophy, or urethral stricture. Morphine pharmacotherapy may exacerbate these medical disorders.
- regularly drink alcohol or are concurrently receiving pharmacotherapy with other opiate analgesics, phenothiazines, sedative-hypnotics, TCAs, or other drugs that produce CNS depression. Additive CNS depression may occur among these patients.

Caution patients who are receiving morphine pharmacotherapy against

- performing activities that require alertness, judgment, and physical coordination (e.g., driving an automobile, operating dangerous equipment, supervising children) until their response to morphine is known. The CNS depressant action of morphine may affect these mental and physical functions adversely.

In addition to this general precaution, caution patients who are receiving morphine pharmacotherapy to

- inform their prescribing psychologist if they begin or discontinue any other pharmacotherapy while receiving morphine pharmacotherapy.

CLINICALLY SIGNIFICANT DRUG INTERACTIONS

Concurrent morphine pharmacotherapy and the following may result in clinically significant drug interactions:

Alcohol Use

Concurrent alcohol use may increase the CNS depressant action of morphine. Advise patients to avoid, or limit, their use or alcohol while receiving morphine pharmacotherapy. Caution patients that their usual response to alcohol may be exaggerated.

Pharmacotherapy With CNS Depressants and Other Drugs That Produce CNS Depression

Concurrent morphine pharmacotherapy and pharmacotherapy with other opiate analgesics, sedative-hypnotics, or other drugs that produce CNS depression (e.g., antihistamines, phenothiazines, TCAs) may result in additive CNS depression. When concurrent pharmacotherapy is required, dosage of one or both drugs should be reduced.

Pharmacotherapy With Drugs That Acidify the Urine

The renal elimination of morphine is decreased by drugs that acidify the urine (e.g., ammonium chloride).

Pharmacotherapy With Drugs That Alkalinize the Urine

The renal elimination of morphine is enhanced by drugs that alkalinize the urine (e.g., sodium bicarbonate). Thus, this interaction may result in increased morphine elimination, a shortened half-life of elimination, and decreased pain relief.

Rifampin Pharmacotherapy

Rifampin (Rifadin®), an antibiotic primarily used for the therapeutic management of active tuberculosis, is a potent inducer of hepatic microsomal enzymes. Concurrent rifampin and morphine pharmacotherapy can result in a significant decrease in both the bioavailability of morphine (mean reduction ~25%) and the peak plasma concentration of morphine (mean reduction ~50%). These effects may result in a loss of the analgesic efficacy of morphine and necessitate the selection and use of an alternative analgesic (see "Opiate Analgesics, General Monograph").

See also "Opiate Analgesics, General Monograph."

ADVERSE DRUG REACTIONS

Morphine pharmacotherapy has been associated with serious ADRs. These ADRs include cardiac arrest, circulatory depression, respiratory arrest, and shock. Morphine pharmacotherapy also commonly has been associated with constipation, dizziness, lightheadedness, nausea, sedation, sweating, and vomiting.

See also "Opiate Analgesics, General Monograph."

OVERDOSAGE

Signs and symptoms of morphine overdosage include respiratory depression (i.e., decrease in respiratory rate and tidal volume, Cheyne–Stokes respiration, cyanosis), extreme somnolence progressing to stupor or coma, skeletal muscle flaccidity, and cold and clammy skin. Bradycardia and hypotension also may occur. Severe morphine overdosage may result in apnea, cardiac arrest, circulatory collapse, and death.

Morphine overdosage requires emergency symptomatic medical support of body systems with attention to increasing morphine elimination. The opiate antagonist, naloxone (Narcan®), is the specific antidote against respiratory depression. Usual dosages of naloxone will precipitate the opiate withdrawal syndrome among patients addicted to morphine. The severity of the syndrome depends on the degree of the patient's addiction and the dose administered. For these patients, 10% to 20% of the usual dosage initially should be administered and then adjusted (increased) according to individual patient response.

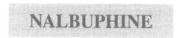

NALBUPHINE

(nal′ byoo feen)

TRADE NAME

Nubain®

CLASSIFICATION

Opiate analgesic (mixed agonist/antagonist)

See also "Opiate Analgesics, General Monograph."

APPROVED INDICATIONS FOR NEUROPSYCHOLOGICAL DISORDERS

Adjunctive pharmacotherapy for the symptomatic management of:

- pain disorders: acute or chronic pain, moderate to severe

USUAL DOSAGE AND ADMINISTRATION

Acute Pain, Moderate to Severe

Adults: 40 to 80 mg daily intramuscularly, intravenously, or subcutaneously in four to eight divided doses

MAXIMUM: 20 mg/dose; 160 mg daily

Women who are, or who may become, pregnant: FDA Pregnancy Category B. Safety and efficacy of nalbuphine pharmacotherapy for women who are pregnant have not been established. Nalbuphine rapidly crosses the placenta and may achieve fetal blood concentrations approximately equivalent to maternal blood concentrations. Associated fetal and neonatal effects have been reported, including fetal bradycardia and neonatal bradycardia and respiratory depression (see also "Opiate Analgesics, General Monograph"). Avoid prescribing nalbuphine pharmacotherapy to women who are pregnant. If nalbuphine pharmacotherapy is required, advise patients of potential benefits and possible risks to themselves and the embryo, fetus, or neonate. Collaboration with the patient's obstetrician is indicated.

For details and discussion regarding related basic principles of clinical pharmacology, readers are referred to the first text in this series, *The Pharmacologic Basis of Psychotherapeutics: An Introduction for Psychologists.*

Women who are breast-feeding: Safety and efficacy of nalbuphine pharmacotherapy for women who are breast-feeding and their neonates and infants have not been established (see "Opiate Analgesics, General Monograph"). Avoid prescribing nalbuphine pharmacotherapy to women who are breast-feeding. If nalbuphine pharmacotherapy is required, breast-feeding probably should be discontinued. If desired, lactation may be maintained and breast-feeding resumed following the discontinuation of short-term nalbuphine pharmacotherapy. Collaboration with the patient's pediatrician is indicated.

Elderly, frail, or debilitated patients: Generally prescribe lower dosages for elderly, frail, or debilitated patients. Gradually increase the dosage, if needed, according to individual patient response. These patients may be more sensitive to the pharmacologic actions of nalbuphine than are younger or healthier adult patients.

Children and adolescents younger than 18 years of age: Safety and efficacy of nalbuphine pharmacotherapy for children and adolescents have not been established. Nalbuphine pharmacotherapy is *not* recommended for this age group.

AVAILABLE DOSAGE FORMS, STORAGE, AND COMPATIBILITY

Injectables, intramuscular, intravenous, or subcutaneous: 10, 20 mg/ml

Notes

The injectable formulations of some manufacturers (e.g., Astra and Du Pont) contain sodium metabisulfite. Sulfites have been associated with hypersensitivity reactions, including anaphylactic reactions, among susceptible patients. Although relatively uncommon, these reactions appear to occur with a higher incidence among patients who have asthma.

Safely store nalbuphine injectable formulations protected from light at controlled room temperature (15° to 30 °C; 59° to 86 °F).

PROPOSED MECHANISM OF ACTION

Nalbuphine elicits its analgesic, CNS depressant, and respiratory depressant actions primarily by binding to the endorphin receptors in the CNS. However, the exact mechanism of action has not yet been fully determined. See also "Opiate Analgesics, General Monograph."

PHARMACOKINETICS/PHARMACODYNAMICS

Nalbuphine has limited oral bioavailability (~20%). Thus, injectable pharmacotherapy is required for optimal bioavailability. Onset of action occurs within 3 minutes following intravenous injection and within 15 minutes following intramuscular or subcutaneous injection. The mean apparent volume of distribution is 4 liters/kg. Nalbuphine is metabolized in the liver and less than 5% is excreted in unchanged form in the urine. The mean half-life of elimination is ~5 hours and the mean total body clearance is 1.5 liters/minute.

RELATIVE CONTRAINDICATIONS

Hypersensitivity to nalbuphine

See also "Opiate Analgesics, General Monograph."

CAUTIONS AND COMMENTS

Nalbuphine is addicting and habituating. Long-term nalbuphine pharmacotherapy, or regular personal use, may result in addiction and habituation. Abrupt discontinuation after long-term pharmacotherapy, or regular personal use, may result in a reportedly mild form of the opiate withdrawal syndrome. Nalbuphine also may cause signs and symptoms of the opiate withdrawal syndrome among patients who are receiving long-term opiate analgesic pharmacotherapy with pure opiate agonists (e.g., morphine) because it has mixed opiate agonist/antagonist actions.

Prescribe nalbuphine pharmacotherapy cautiously for patients who have histories of substance-use disorders or who

- have acute cholecystitis or pancreatitis or will be undergoing surgery of the biliary tract. Opiate analgesics generally increase biliary tract pressure. Nalbuphine may cause spasms of the circular muscle constricting the opening of the common bile duct (i.e., sphincter of Oddi).
- have head injuries, intracranial lesions, or other conditions associated with increased intracranial pressure. The respiratory depressant action associated with nalbuphine and its potential for elevating cerebrospinal fluid pressure may markedly increase intracranial pressure among these patients. Nalbuphine's analgesic and sedative actions also may obscure the clinical course of these conditions.
- have histories of problematic patterns of opiate analgesic or other abusable psychotropic use (i.e., substance-use disorders). These patients may be at risk for developing problematic patterns of use. In addition, patients who are addicted to opiates may experience signs and symptoms of the opiate withdrawal syndrome. Nalbuphine, a mixed agonist/antagonist, has weak opiate antagonist action.
- have liver dysfunction. Serious liver dysfunction appears to predispose patients to a higher incidence of ADRs (e.g., anxiety, dizziness, drowsiness, marked apprehension) even when usual recommended dosages are prescribed. These ADRs may be the result of decreased nalbuphine metabolism by the liver and resultant accumulation.
- have respiratory depression, limited respiratory function (e.g., severely limited respiratory reserve, severe bronchial asthma, other obstructive respiratory conditions), or cyanosis. The respiratory depressant action of nalbuphine may further compromise the respiratory function of these patients.

Caution patients who are receiving nalbuphine pharmacotherapy against

- performing activities that require alertness, judgment, and physical coordination (e.g., driving an automobile, operating dangerous equipment, supervising children) until their response to nalbuphine is known. The CNS depressant action of nalbuphine may affect these mental and physical functions adversely.

In addition to this general precaution, caution patients to

- inform their prescribing psychologist if they begin or discontinue any other pharmacotherapy while receiving nalbuphine pharmacotherapy.

CLINICALLY SIGNIFICANT DRUG INTERACTIONS

Concurrent nalbuphine pharmacotherapy and the following may result in clinically significant drug interactions:

Alcohol Use

Concurrent alcohol use may increase the CNS depressant action of nalbuphine. Advise patients to avoid, or limit, their use of alcohol while receiving nalbuphine pharmacotherapy.

Pharmacotherapy With CNS Depressants and Other Drugs That Produce CNS Depression

Concurrent nalbuphine pharmacotherapy and pharmacotherapy with other opiate analgesics, sedative-hypnotics, or other drugs that produce CNS depression (e.g., antihistamines, phenothiazines, TCAs) may result in additive CNS depression.

ADVERSE DRUG REACTIONS

Nalbuphine pharmacotherapy commonly has been associated with dizziness, nausea, sedation, a sweaty-clammy feeling, and vomiting. It also has been associated with the following ADRs, listed according to body system:

Cardiovascular: hypertension and tachycardia
CNS: depression and headache
Cutaneous: flushing, hives, and itching (severe)
Genitourinary: urinary urgency
GI: constipation, cramps, and dyspepsia
Ocular: blurred vision
Respiratory: labored or difficult breathing (dyspnea) and respiratory depression

See also "Opiate Analgesics, General Monograph."

OVERDOSAGE

Signs and symptoms of nalbuphine overdosage are similar to the signs and symptoms associated with other opiate analgesic overdosage, although respiratory depression reportedly is less severe. Nalbuphine overdosage requires emergency symptomatic medical support of body systems with attention to increasing nalbuphine elimination. Naloxone (Narcan®) is a specific and effective antidote.

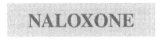

NALOXONE

(nal ox' own)

TRADE NAME

Narcan®

CLASSIFICATION

Opiate antagonist

APPROVED INDICATIONS FOR NEUROPSYCHOLOGICAL DISORDERS

Adjunctive pharmacotherapy for the symptomatic management of:

- substance-related disorders: opiate analgesic overdosage, known or suspected. *Note*: Naloxone is an opiate antagonist that produces complete or partial reversal of the signs and symptoms of opiate overdosage, particularly respiratory depression. Naloxone also is indicated for the diagnosis of suspected acute opiate overdosage. Although overdosages involving opiate analgesics and other psychotropic drugs require emergency symptomatic *medical* support of body systems, prescribing psychologists require a knowledge of the use and action of naloxone and other antagonists, such as those indicated for the emergency symptomatic medical management of benzodiazepine overdosage (e.g., flumazenil [Anexate®, Romazicon®]).

USUAL DOSAGE AND ADMINISTRATION

Opiate Analgesic Overdosage, Known or Suspected

Adults: 0.4 to 2 mg intravenously. If therapeutic response is not achieved, repeat at 2- to 3-minute intervals. If therapeutic response is not noted after 10 mg, reevaluate the diagnosis of opiate analgesic overdosage. Intramuscular or subcutaneous injection may be required if intravenous injection is not feasible.

INTRAVENOUS INFUSION: 2 mg per 500 ml of sterile 5% dextrose or normal saline intravenous solution to obtain a concentration of 4 µg/ml (0.004 mg/ml). Use admixture within 24 hours. Discard remaining admixture after 24 hours. Generally infuse at 100 ml/hour (0.4 mg/hour). Infusion is generally initiated for opiate analgesic overdosage associated with long-acting opiate analgesics (e.g., methadone, propoxyphene). Individualize the solution concentration and infusion rate to obtain desired antagonist response without fluid overload or precipitation of the acute opiate analgesic withdrawal syndrome.

For details and discussion regarding related basic principles of clinical pharmacology, readers are referred to the first text in this series, *The Pharmacologic Basis of Psychotherapeutics: An Introduction for Psychologists.*

Women who are, or who may become, pregnant: FDA Pregnancy Category B. Safety and efficacy of naloxone pharmacotherapy for women who are pregnant (other than during labor) have not been established. Naloxone has no known direct pharmacologic action other than its opiate antagonist action. When indicated for the symptomatic management of acute opiate analgesic overdosage, potential benefits significantly outweigh minor potential risks to the embryo, fetus, or neonate. Collaboration with the patient's obstetrician is indicated.

Women who are breast-feeding: Safety and efficacy of naloxone pharmacotherapy for women who are breast-feeding and their neonates and infants have not been established. It is unknown whether naloxone is excreted in breast milk. However, risk to breast-fed neonates and infants, other than reversal of opiate analgesic action, appears minimal. Collaboration with the patient's pediatrician is indicated.

Elderly, frail, or debilitated patients: Same dosage and administration as generally recommended for younger or healthier adults. See information for adults, previous.

Children: 0.01 mg/kg intravenously. If therapeutic response is not achieved, a subsequent dose of 0.1 mg/kg may be injected. This dosage may be repeated at two to three minute intervals, if needed, according to individual patient response. Intramuscular or subcutaneous injection may be required in divided doses if intravenous injection is not feasible. If necessary, may dilute naloxone with sterile water for injection.

INTRAVENOUS INFUSION: Intravenous infusion generally is initiated for opiate analgesic overdosage involving long-acting opiate analgesics (e.g., methadone [Dolophine®], propoxyphene [Darvon®]). The infusion rate for children should be adjusted according to individual patient factors (e.g., body weight; heart, kidney, and liver function) and clinical response.

Neonates: 0.01 mg/kg intravenously. If therapeutic response is not achieved, inject a subsequent dose of 0.1 mg/kg. Intramuscular or subcutaneous injection may be required in divided doses if intravenous injection is not feasible. If necessary, may dilute naloxone with sterile water for injection.

INTRAVENOUS INFUSION: Intravenous infusion generally is initiated for opiate analgesic overdosage involving long-acting opiate analgesics (e.g., methadone [Dolophine®], propoxyphene [Darvon®]). The infusion rate for neonates should be adjusted according to individual patient factors (e.g., body weight; heart, kidney, and liver function) and clinical response.

Notes, Acute Opiate Analgesic Overdosage

Generally, naloxone may be prescribed for intramuscular, intravenous, or subcutaneous pharmacotherapy. The most rapid onset of action is achieved with intravenous injection. Intravenous injection is recommended for the emergency symptomatic medical management of acute opiate analgesic overdosage. In emergency situations where injectable pharmacotherapy was not feasible, naloxone has been successfully administered by endotracheal tube.

Repeated doses of naloxone at periodic intervals for up to 48 hours may be required because of the relatively long duration of action of some opiate analgesics (e.g., methadone [Dolophine®]). Medical monitoring of respiratory rate is necessary to evaluate the need for repeated doses of naloxone (i.e., respiratory rate less than 10 respirations/minute) because of its relatively short half-life of elimination and, thus, short duration of action.

AVAILABLE DOSAGE FORMS, STORAGE, AND COMPATIBILITY

Injectables, intramuscular, intravenous, or subcutaneous: 0.02, 0.4 mg/ml (neonatal formulations); 1 mg/ml (child and adult formulation)

Notes

Visually inspect injectable formulations for particulate matter and discoloration prior to use whenever solution and packaging permit. Do not mix naloxone injectable with injectable formulations that contain bisulfite, metabisulfite, long-chain or high-molecular-weight anions, or any solution that has an alkaline pH. Do not add any other drug to naloxone injectable unless its chemical and physical compatibility with naloxone is known.

Safely store the injectable at controlled room temperature (15 ° to 30 °C; 59 ° to 86 °F).

PROPOSED MECHANISM OF ACTION

Naloxone exhibits essentially no direct pharmacologic action other than antagonizing the actions of opiate analgesics by competitively blocking the endogenous endorphin receptors in the CNS. This action reverses analgesia and the signs and symptoms of opiate analgesic overdosage, particularly respiratory depression. It also produces the acute opiate analgesic withdrawal syndrome among patients who are addicted to opiate analgesics.

PHARMACOKINETICS/PHARMACODYNAMICS

Naloxone is well absorbed ($\sim$90%) following oral ingestion. However, bioavailability is low (i.e., $F = 0.02$) because of significant first-pass hepatic metabolism. The onset of action for naloxone is usually within 2 minutes of intravenous injection. Its onset of action is only slightly less rapid when injected intramuscularly or subcutaneously. The duration of naloxone's action is 1 to 4 hours and depends on the dose and method of administration. Intramuscular injection produces a more prolonged action than does intravenous injection. The requirement for repeat doses of naloxone depends on the opiate analgesic being antagonized (i.e., short- or long-acting opiate) for the symptomatic management of opiate analgesic overdosage and the severity of the overdosage. Following intramuscular, intravenous, or subcutaneous injection, naloxone is distributed rapidly in the body. Its mean apparent volume of distribution is $\sim$2 liters/kg. Naloxone is metabolized in the liver and excreted in the urine. Total body clearance is $\sim$1.5 liters/minute. The mean half-life of elimination is $\sim$1 hour (range: 30 to 90 minutes). Due to immature mechanisms of liver metabolism and urinary excretion among neonates, the mean half-life of elimination is prolonged to $\sim$3 hours for this age group.

RELATIVE CONTRAINDICATIONS

Hypersensitivity to naloxone

CAUTIONS AND COMMENTS

Prescribe naloxone pharmacotherapy cautiously to patients who

- are known or suspected to be addicted to opiate analgesics. Abrupt and complete reversal of opiate analgesic action may produce the opiate analgesic withdrawal syndrome among these patients. The severity of the syndrome depends on the degree of addiction (i.e., opiate analgesic used, dosage, and duration of use), the naloxone dose, and its method of administration, and individual patient factors (e.g., personality and concomitant medical and psychological disorders). Lower dosages of naloxone (i.e., 10 to 20% of the usual recommended dosage) generally are recommended initially for these patients. The dosage is then adjusted (increased) according to individual patient response.
- have respiratory depression (severe). These patients require higher dosages than usually recommended and close medical monitoring, even after satisfactory response has been achieved. Repeated doses may be required because the duration of action of some opiate analgesics (e.g., methadone [Dolophine®]) may exceed that of naloxone.

CLINICALLY SIGNIFICANT DRUG INTERACTIONS

There have been no reports of drug interactions involving naloxone other than its expected antagonism of opiate analgesics.

ADVERSE DRUG REACTIONS

Although naloxone exhibits essentially no direct pharmacologic action, other than its expected antagonism of opiate analgesics, abrupt reversal of opiate analgesic overdosage may result in nausea, vomiting, sweating, tachycardia, increased blood pressure, tremulousness, and cardiac arrest.

OVERDOSAGE

There have been no reports of naloxone overdosage.

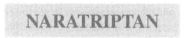

NARATRIPTAN

(nar′ a trip tan)

TRADE NAME

Amerge®

CLASSIFICATION

Antimigraine (vascular serotonin receptor agonist)

APPROVED INDICATIONS FOR NEUROPSYCHOLOGICAL DISORDERS

Pharmacotherapy for the symptomatic management of:

- vascular headaches: migraine headaches, with or without aura. *Note*: Naratriptan pharmacotherapy is *not* indicated for the prevention of migraine (i.e., as prophylactic pharmacotherapy) *nor* is it indicated for the treatment of basilar or hemiplegic migraine.

USUAL DOSAGE AND ADMINISTRATION

Vascular Headaches: Migraine Headaches, With or Without Aura

Adults: Initially, 1 or 2.5 mg orally. If the migraine headache returns, or if only partial response has been obtained, the initial dose may be repeated once after a *minimum* of four hours.

MAXIMUM: 5 mg orally during any 24-hour period

Women who are, or who may become, pregnant: FDA Pregnancy Category C. Safety and efficacy of naratriptan pharmacotherapy for women who are pregnant have not been established. Avoid prescribing naratriptan pharmacotherapy to women who are pregnant. If naratriptan pharmacotherapy is required, advise patients of potential benefits and possible risk to themselves and the embryo, fetus, or neonate. Collaboration with the patient's obstetrician is indicated.

Women who are breast-feeding: Safety and efficacy of naratriptan pharmacotherapy for women who are breast-feeding and their neonates and infants have not been established. However, naratriptan is thought (based on animal studies) to be excreted in breast milk. Avoid prescribing naratriptan pharmacotherapy to women who are breast-feeding. If naratriptan pharmacotherapy is required, breast-feeding probably should be discontinued. If desired, lactation may be maintained and breast-feeding resumed following the discontinuation of short-term naratriptan pharmacotherapy.

For details and discussion regarding related basic principles of clinical pharmacology, readers are referred to the first text in this series, *The Pharmacologic Basis of Psychotherapeutics: An Introduction for Psychologists.*

Elderly adults: Safety and efficacy of naratriptan pharmacotherapy for elderly adults who are 65 years of age and older have not been established. However, a higher incidence and greater severity of ADRs is expected because of a greater frequency of coronary artery disease, hepatic dysfunction, and renal dysfunction among patients in this age group. Naratriptan pharmacotherapy is *not* recommended for this age group.

Adults who have mild to moderate liver dysfunction: 1 mg orally per migraine attack. Subsequent migraine attacks may be treated with a similar dose provided that a *minimum* of four hours has elapsed since the previous dose.

MAXIMUM: 2.5 mg orally during any 24-hour period

Children and adolescents younger than 18 years of age: Safety and efficacy of naratriptan pharmacotherapy for children and adolescents who are younger than 18 years of age have not been established. Naratriptan pharmacotherapy is *not* recommended for this age group.

Notes, Vascular Headaches: Migraine Headaches, With or Without Aura

Generally, the safety and efficacy of naratriptan pharmacotherapy for the symptomatic management of more than four migraine headaches in a 30-day period have not been established.

AVAILABLE DOSAGE FORMS, STORAGE, AND COMPATIBILITY

Tablets, oral: 1, 2.5 mg

Notes

General instructions for patients: Instruct patients who are receiving naratriptan pharmacotherapy, as appropriate, to

- ingest each dose of the naratriptan oral tablets whole with adequate liquid chaser (i.e., 60 to 120 ml of water). The naratriptan oral tablets should *not* be broken, chewed, or crushed.
- safely store naratriptan dosage forms out of the reach of children in tightly closed, light- and child-resistant containers at controlled room temperature (20 ° to 25 °C, 68 ° to 77 °F).
- obtain an available patient information sheet regarding naratriptan pharmacotherapy from their pharmacist at the time that their prescription is dispensed. Encourage patients to clarify any questions that they may have regarding naratriptan pharmacotherapy with their pharmacist or, if needed, to consult their prescribing psychologist.

PROPOSED MECHANISM OF ACTION

Naratriptan is an agonist for the vascular serotonin receptor subtypes 5-HT_{1B} and 5-HT_{1D}. Activation of these receptors, which are present on cranial arteries, on the basilar artery, and in the vasculature of the dura mater, produce vasoconstriction. The vasoconstriction of these arteries, which are dilated and edematous during a migraine attack, appears to be correlated with migraine relief. The activation of the 5-HT_{1B} and 5-HT_{1D} receptors, which are located on sensory nerve endings in the trigeminal system, also inhibits the release of pro-inflammatory neuropeptides.

PHARMACOKINETICS/PHARMACODYNAMICS

Naratriptan is well absorbed following oral ingestion, with a bioavailability of ~70%. Peak blood concentrations are obtained in 2 to 3 hours. Food does not affect the bioavailability of naratriptan. Naratriptan is ~30% bound to plasma proteins and has a mean apparent volume of distribution of 170 liters. Naratriptan is metabolized by several different cytochrome P450 isoenzymes in the liver to a number of inactive metabolites. The renal clearance of naratriptan (~220 ml/minute) exceeds the glomerular filtration rate, indicating that it is subject to active tubular secretion. Approximately 50% of naratriptan is excreted in unchanged form in the urine. The mean half-life of elimination is 6 hours, and the mean total body clearance is 6.6 ml/kg/hour.

Significant migraine relief generally is noted within 1 to 3 hours following oral ingestion. Naratriptan is efficacious in providing symptomatic relief to ~66% of patients who have moderate to severe migraine headache. Although its onset of action generally is slower than other available "triptans," its duration of action reportedly is significantly longer.

RELATIVE CONTRAINDICATIONS

Angina pectoris
Basilar migraine
Cardiac dysrhythmias, particularly tachycardias
Cerebrovascular accident, recent history of
Coronary artery disease
Coronary vasospasm (Prinzmetal's angina)
Ergot pharmacotherapy, concurrent or within the previous 24 hours because of possible additive vasoconstriction
Hemiplegic migraine
Hepatic dysfunction, severe
Hypersensitivity to naratriptan
Hypertension, uncontrolled
Ischemic bowel disease
Ischemic heart disease
Myocardial infarction, history of
Myocardial ischemia
Renal dysfunction, severe
Transient ischemic attacks
Zolmitriptan, or other vascular serotonin receptor agonist pharmacotherapy, concurrent or within the previous 24 hours because of possible additive vasoconstriction

CAUTIONS AND COMMENTS

Patients who require intermittent, long-term naratriptan pharmacotherapy and who possess noted risk factors for coronary artery disease (CAD) (e.g., diabetes, hypercholesterolemia, hypertension, obesity, tobacco smoking) are advised to undergo periodic medical evaluation of cardiovascular status in order to reduce the risks associated with naratriptan pharmacotherapy among patients with unrecognized cardiovascular disease.

Caution patients who are receiving naratriptan pharmacotherapy against

- performing activities that require alertness, judgment, or physical coordination (e.g., driving an automobile, operating dangerous equipment, supervising children) until their response to naratriptan pharmacotherapy is known. Naratriptan may affect these mental and physical functions adversely.

CLINICALLY SIGNIFICANT DRUG INTERACTIONS

Concurrent naratriptan pharmacotherapy and the following may result in clinically significant drug interactions:

Dihydroergotamine and Related Ergot Pharmacotherapy

See "Relative Contraindications."

Pharmacotherapy With Oral Contraceptives

Concurrent oral contraceptive pharmacotherapy reduces both the total body clearance (~30%) and the apparent volume of distribution (~20%) of naratriptan resulting in a corresponding increase in naratriptan blood concentrations.

Tobacco Smoking

Tobacco smoking may increase the total body clearance of naratriptan by ~30%.

ADVERSE DRUG REACTIONS

Adverse drug reactions associated with naratriptan pharmacotherapy generally are transient and self-limiting. Naratriptan pharmacotherapy commonly has been associated with: dizziness, drowsiness, fatigue, malaise, nausea, and neck stiffness. Naratriptan pharmacotherapy also has been associated with the following ADRs, listed according to body system:

Cardiovascular: angina (rare), cardiac dysrhythmias (rare), coronary vasospasm (rare), and hypertension (transient)
CNS: drowsiness
Cutaneous: flushing
GI: hyposalivation, nausea, and vomiting
Ocular: photophobia
Respiratory: shortness of breath (dyspnea)
Miscellaneous: sensations of numbness, prickling, or tingling (paresthesias)

OVERDOSAGE

Clinical data concerning naratriptan overdosage are not available. In the absence of such data, naratriptan overdosage should be treated as a medical emergency requiring symptomatic support of body systems with attention to increasing naratriptan elimination. There is no known antidote.

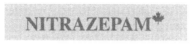

NITRAZEPAM

(nye tra′ ze pam)

TRADE NAME

Mogadon®

CLASSIFICATION

Anticonvulsant (benzodiazepine)

APPROVED INDICATIONS FOR NEUROPSYCHOLOGICAL DISORDERS

Pharmacotherapy for the prophylactic and symptomatic management of:

• seizure disorders: myoclonic seizures among children

USUAL DOSAGE AND ADMINISTRATION

Seizure Disorders: Myoclonic Seizures Among Children

Children (up to 30 kg body weight):   0.3 to 1 mg/kg daily orally in three divided doses

Notes, Seizure Disorders: Myoclonic Seizures Among Children

Initially, prescribe lower dosages (i.e., 0.2 mg/kg daily orally) and evaluate individual patient response. Higher dosages may be required for children who are refractory to anticonvulsant pharmacotherapy. However, higher dosages are commonly associated with excessive drowsiness.

AVAILABLE DOSAGE FORMS, STORAGE, AND COMPATIBILITY

Tablets, oral: 5, 10 mg

Notes

General instructions for patients: Instruct patients who are receiving nitrazepam pharmacotherapy, or their parents or legal guardians in regard to the patient, to

---

For details and discussion regarding related basic principles of clinical pharmacology, readers are referred to the first text in this series, *The Pharmacologic Basis of Psychotherapeutics: An Introduction for Psychologists.*

- safely store nitrazepam oral tablets out of the reach of children in tightly closed, light- and child-resistant containers at controlled room temperature (15° to 30°C; 59° to 86°F).
- obtain an available patient information sheet regarding nitrazepam pharmacotherapy from their pharmacist at the time that their prescription is dispensed. Encourage patients, or their parents or legal guardians in regard to the patient, to clarify any questions that they may have regarding nitrazepam pharmacotherapy with their pharmacist or, if needed, to consult their prescribing psychologist.

PROPOSED MECHANISM OF ACTION

Nitrazepam is a benzodiazepine with anticonvulsant actions. The exact mechanism of its anticonvulsant action has not yet been fully determined. However, it appears to be related to nitrazepam's ability to raise the seizure threshold.

See also "Benzodiazepines, General Monograph."

PHARMACOKINETICS/PHARMACODYNAMICS

Nitrazepam is well absorbed from the GI tract following oral ingestion (i.e., $F = 0.8$). Generally, peak blood concentrations are achieved within 3 hours. Nitrazepam is distributed widely in body tissues. It is ~90% bound to plasma proteins and has an apparent volume of distribution of ~2 to 3 liters/kg. Nitrazepam is metabolized extensively in the liver and, together with its metabolites, is excreted primarily in the urine. Only 1% of nitrazepam is excreted in unchanged form in the urine. The mean half-life of elimination is 30 hours (range: 18 to 57 hours) and the mean total body clearance is ~6 liters/minute.

RELATIVE CONTRAINDICATIONS

Hypersensitivity to nitrazepam or other benzodiazepines
Myasthenia gravis
Narrow-angle glaucoma, acute. However, nitrazepam can be prescribed for patients who have open-angle glaucoma and are receiving appropriate pharmacotherapy for its management. Collaboration with the patient's ophthalmologist is indicated. (See also "Benzodiazepines, General Monograph.")
Problematic patterns of alcohol or other abusable psychotropic use, history of
Sleep apnea syndrome

CAUTIONS AND COMMENTS

Long-term nitrazepam pharmacotherapy, or regular personal use, may result in addiction and habituation. Abrupt discontinuation of long-term pharmacotherapy or regular personal use has been associated with a benzodiazepine withdrawal syndrome similar to the alcohol withdrawal syndrome. Severe benzodiazepine withdrawal signs and symptoms, including abdominal and muscle cramps, convulsions, tremor, vomiting, and sweating, have been associated with the discontinuation of long-term high-dosage pharmacotherapy, or regular personal use. Avoid the abrupt discontinuation of nitrazepam pharmacotherapy, particularly when pharmacotherapy has been extended over several months. A gradual reduction of dosage is recommended before nitrazepam pharmacotherapy is completely discontinued.

Prescribe nitrazepam pharmacotherapy cautiously to patients who

- have histories of problematic patterns of alcohol or other abusable psychotropic use. These patients may be at particular risk for the development of problematic patterns of nitrazepam use. Monitor these patients closely for signs and symptoms of problematic patterns of use.
- have kidney or liver dysfunction. Nitrazepam's half-life of elimination may by significantly increased among these patients.
- have latent depression. Benzodiazepine pharmacotherapy may exacerbate depression. Monitor these patients carefully for increased suicide risk. Suicide precautions may be indicated.

Caution patients who are receiving nitrazepam pharmacotherapy, or their parents or legal guardians in regard to the patient, against

- drinking alcohol or using other drugs that produce CNS depression. Concurrent use may result in severe CNS depression.
- increasing their prescribed dosage, using their nitrazepam more often than prescribed, or abruptly discontinuing their nitrazepam pharmacotherapy without first consulting with their prescribing psychologist. Nitrazepam is addicting and habituating. Abrupt discontinuation of pharmacotherapy, or regular personal use, may result in the benzodiazepine withdrawal syndrome.
- performing activities that require alertness, judgment, or physical coordination (e.g., playing sports, taking tests at school) until their response to nitrazepam pharmacotherapy is known. Nitrazepam may affect these mental and physical functions adversely.

In addition to these general precautions, caution patients, or their parents or legal guardians in regard to the patient, to

- inform their prescribing psychologist if they begin or discontinue any other pharmacotherapy while receiving nitrazepam pharmacotherapy.

CLINICALLY SIGNIFICANT DRUG INTERACTIONS

Concurrent nitrazepam pharmacotherapy and the following may result in clinically significant drug interactions:

Alcohol Use

Concurrent alcohol use may increase the CNS depressant action of nitrazepam. Advise patients or their parents or legal guardians in regard to the patient to avoid, or limit, their use of alcohol while receiving nitrazepam pharmacotherapy.

Pharmacotherapy With CNS Depressants and Other Drugs That Produce CNS Depression

Concurrent nitrazepam pharmacotherapy and pharmacotherapy with opiate analgesics, sedative-hypnotics, or other drugs that produce CNS depression (e.g., antihistamines, phenothiazines, TCAs) may result in additive CNS depression.

Pharmacotherapy With Drugs That Inhibit Cytochrome P450-Mediated Hepatic Metabolism

Concurrent nitrazepam pharmacotherapy with drugs that inhibit cytochrome P450-mediated hepatic metabolism (e.g., cimetidine [Tagamet®], erythromycin [E-Mycin®]) may result in the delayed or decreased elimination of nitrazepam. This interaction may result in significant increases in nitrazepam blood concentrations and associated effects.

See also "Benzodiazepines, General Monograph."

ADVERSE DRUG REACTIONS

Nitrazepam pharmacotherapy commonly has been associated with dizziness, drowsiness, falling, fatigue, incoordination (ataxia), lethargy, lightheadedness, mental confusion, and a staggering gait. Nitrazepam pharmacotherapy also has been associated with the following ADRs, listed according to body system:

Cardiovascular: hypotension
CNS: depression, disorientation, headache, memory impairment, and nightmares. Paradoxical reactions, including agitation, anxiety (acute), and violent behavior, have been reported. If these ADRs are observed, discontinue nitrazepam pharmacotherapy.
GI: constipation, diarrhea, heartburn, and nausea
Hematologic: rarely, granulocytopenia and leukopenia
Ophthalmic: blurred vision

See also "Benzodiazepines, General Monograph."

OVERDOSAGE

Signs and symptoms of nitrazepam overdosage resemble those associated with other benzodiazepine overdosage (see "Benzodiazepines, General Monograph"). Initial signs and symptoms include confusion, drowsiness, increasing sedation leading to coma, and reduced reflexes. Nitrazepam overdosage requires emergency symptomatic medical support of body systems with attention to increasing nitrazepam elimination. Flumazenil (Anexate®, Romazicon®), the benzodiazepine antagonist, may be required. However, flumazenil pharmacotherapy may induce seizure disorders among patients whose seizures are being managed with nitrazepam or other benzodiazepine pharmacotherapy. *Extreme care is warranted.* The use of flumazenil in this clinical situation generally is *not* recommended. See the flumazenil monograph.

OPIATE ANALGESICS
[General Monograph]

(oh′ pee ate)

GENERIC NAMES

For trade names, see individual drug monographs.

Anileridine✱ (phenylpiperidine derivative)
Buprenorphine★ (phenanthrene derivative) (mixed agonist/antagonist)
Butorphanol (phenanthrene derivative) (mixed agonist/antagonist)
Codeine (methylmorphine) (phenanthrene derivative)
Dezocine★ (aminotetralin derivative) (mixed agonist/antagonist)
Fentanyl (phenylpiperidine derivative)
Heroin (diacetylmorphine, diamorphine) (phenanthrene derivative)
Hydromorphone (phenanthrene derivative)
Levorphanol (phenanthrene derivative)
Meperidine (pethidine) (phenylpiperidine derivative)
Methadone (diphenylheptane derivative)
Morphine (phenanthrene derivative)
Nalbuphine (phenanthrene derivative) (mixed agonist/antagonist)
Oxycodone (phenanthrene derivative)
Oxymorphone (phenanthrene derivative)
Pentazocine (phenanthrene derivative) (mixed agonist/antagonist)
Propoxyphene (dextropropoxyphene) (diphenylheptane derivative)

CLASSIFICATION

Opiate analgesic (C-II)

See also individual opiate analgesic monographs.

APPROVED INDICATIONS FOR NEUROPSYCHOLOGICAL DISORDERS

Adjunctive pharmacotherapy for the symptomatic management of:

- pain disorders: acute pain, mild to severe, and chronic cancer pain, moderate to severe

---

For details and discussion regarding related basic principles of clinical pharmacology, readers are referred to the first text in this series, *The Pharmacologic Basis of Psychotherapeutics: An Introduction for Psychologists.*

Opiate analgesic	Pain
Codeine (methylmorphine)	Mild to moderate
Propoxyphene	Mild to moderate
Anileridine	Moderate to severe
Butorphanol	Moderate to severe
Fentanyl	Moderate to severe
Hydromorphone	Moderate to severe
Meperidine (pethidine)	Moderate to severe
Methadone	Moderate to severe
Nalbuphine	Moderate to severe
Oxycodone	Moderate to severe
Oxymorphone	Moderate to severe
Pentazocine	Moderate to severe
Heroin (diacetylmorphine, diamorphine)	Severe
Levorphanol	Severe
Morphine	Severe

USUAL DOSAGE AND ADMINISTRATION

Pain Disorders

Adults: See table "Opiate Analgesics: Approximate Dosage Equivalents" and individual opiate analgesic monographs. *Note:* Buprenorphine, butorphanol, dezocine, nalbuphine, and pentazocine are mixed opiate agonist/antagonist analgesics. Mixed opiate agonist/antagonist analgesics may precipitate the opiate analgesic withdrawal syndrome among patients who are addicted to pure opiate agonist analgesics (e.g., heroin, morphine).

Opiate analgesics: approximate dosage equivalents.

Opiate analgesic	Intramuscular or subcutaneous formulation (mg)	Oral formulation (mg)
Anileridine	25	75
Butorphanol	2	2 (intranasal)
Codeine	120	200
Fentanyl	0.2	—
Heroin	5	20
Hydromorphone	1.5	7.5
Levorphanol	2	4
Meperidine	75	300
Methadone	10	20
Morphine	**10**	**30**
Nalbuphine	10	—
Oxycodone	15	30
Oxymorphone	1.5	10 (rectal)
Pentazocine	60	180
Propoxyphene	50	100

Women who are, or who may become, pregnant: FDA Pregnancy Category C. Safety and efficacy of opiate analgesic pharmacotherapy for women who are pregnant have not been established. Some opiate analgesics may be used to relieve pain during labor and delivery. Opiate analgesics cross the placental barrier. Thus, their use during labor and delivery may result in drowsiness, lethargy, or other expected pharmacologic actions (e.g., respiratory depression, constipation) among neonates. Although opiate analgesic pharmacotherapy during pregnancy has not been associated with congenital malformations (i.e., birth defects), long-term maternal opiate analgesic pharmacotherapy, or regular personal use, may result in the opiate analgesic withdrawal syndrome among neonates as their opiate analgesic blood concentrations decrease following birth.

The signs and symptoms of the neonatal opiate analgesic withdrawal syndrome include excessive crying and irritability, fever, hyperactive reflexes, increased respiratory rate, increased number of stools, sneezing, tremors, vomiting, and yawning. The intensity of these signs and symptoms does not always reflect the amount or duration of maternal opiate analgesic pharmacotherapy, or regular personal use. There is no general consensus regarding the best approach for the medical management of the neonatal opiate analgesic withdrawal syndrome.

Avoid prescribing opiate analgesic pharmacotherapy to women who are pregnant. If opiate analgesic pharmacotherapy is required, advise patients of potential benefits and possible risks to themselves and the embryo, fetus, or neonate. Collaboration with the patient's obstetrician is required. Opiate analgesic pharmacotherapy is *not* recommended for women prior to labor unless potential benefits outweigh possible risks to the fetus or neonate. Opiate analgesic pharmacotherapy during labor may result in drowsiness, lethargy, and other expected pharmacologic actions (e.g., constipation, lethargy, poor sucking, respiratory depression) among neonates.

Women who are breast-feeding: Safety and efficacy of opiate analgesic pharmacotherapy for women who are breast-feeding and their neonates and infants have not been established. Opiate analgesics have been detected in breast milk in amounts that can result in expected pharmacologic actions (e.g., CNS or respiratory depression, constipation) and addiction among breast-fed neonates and infants. These neonates and infants will experience the opiate analgesic withdrawal syndrome when maternal opiate analgesic use or breast-feeding is discontinued. Avoid prescribing opiate analgesic pharmacotherapy to women who are breast-feeding. If opiate analgesic pharmacotherapy is required, breast-feeding probably should be discontinued. If desired, lactation may be maintained and breast-feeding resumed following the discontinuation of short-term opiate analgesic pharmacotherapy. Collaboration with the patient's pediatrician is indicated.

Elderly, frail, or debilitated patients and those who have kidney or liver dysfunction: Initially prescribe lower dosages of opiate analgesics, or longer dosing intervals, for elderly, frail, or debilitated patients. Gradually increase the dosage according to individual patient response. These patients may be more sensitive to the pharmacologic actions of opiate analgesics, especially CNS depression, respiratory depression, and constipation, than are younger or healthier adult patients. The metabolism and elimination of opiate analgesics also may be slowed among these patients. Also initially prescribe lower dosages and gradually increase the dosage, according to individual patient response, for patients who have liver or kidney dysfunction. See individual opiate analgesic monographs.

Children younger than 2 years of age: The safety and efficacy of opiate analgesic pharmacotherapy for children younger than 2 years of age have not been established. Children younger than 2 years of age may be sensitive to the pharmacologic actions of opiate analgesics, particularly CNS depression, respiratory depression, and constipation. Paradoxical excitement also is particularly likely to occur among young children. Thus, opiate analgesic pharmacotherapy generally is *not* recommended for this age group.

Children 2 years of age and older: See individual opiate analgesic monographs.

Notes, Pain Disorders: Acute Pain, Mild to Severe, and Chronic Cancer Pain, Moderate to Severe

Initiating and maintaining opiate analgesic pharmacotherapy: The prescription of opiate analgesics for the symptomatic management of acute pain, moderate to severe, and chronic cancer pain, moderate to severe, requires a thorough psychological assessment and diagnosis of the pain disorder, its cause, and its effects on the mental health of the patient. Collaboration with the patient's advanced practice nurse, family physician, or other specialist (e.g., oncologist) may be required in order to evaluate other aspects of the pain experience (effects on activities of daily living) as relevant to the provision of optimal adjunctive pharmacotherapy with a minimum of adverse effects. Generally prescribe the lowest effective dosage as infrequently as possible, with the therapeutic goal of optimal pain management with a minimum of ADRs. Individualize the daily dosage and method of administration for each patient according to such factors as the nature and severity of the pain; heart, kidney, and liver function; daily dosage of other pharmacotherapy, including opiate analgesic pharmacotherapy prescribed previously or concurrently; and history of addiction and habituation to opiate analgesics, or other abusable psychotropics, with attention to the associated degree of tolerance. Adjust the initial dosage to individual patient response. It may be occasionally necessary to exceed the usual recommended dosage for patients who have severe pain or who have developed tolerance to the analgesic action of opiate analgesics.

INTRAVENOUS OPIATE ANALGESIC PHARMACOTHERAPY: Opiate analgesics should *not* be injected intravenously unless the opiate antagonist, naloxone (Narcan®), and medical personnel and equipment, including that needed for assisted or controlled respiration, are immediately available for the emergency management of the serious and potentially fatal ADRs associated with intravenous opiate analgesic pharmacotherapy. The incidence and severity of ADRs, including severe respiratory depression, apnea, hypotension, peripheral circulatory collapse, and cardiac arrest, may increase with the rapid intravenous injection of opiate analgesics. Patients should be lying down during intravenous injection and individual response to intravenous pharmacotherapy should be closely monitored.

During the first 2 to 3 days of effective pain management, patients may sleep for several hours. This somnolence may be incorrectly attributed to excessive CNS depression rather than effective pain management among exhausted patients who previously had ineffective pain management. Following the relief of severe pain, periodically attempt to reduce the dosage of the opiate analgesic or to replace injectable pharmacotherapy with oral, transdermal, or other appropriate opiate analgesic pharmacotherapy (see "Available Dosage Forms, Storage, and Compatibility"). The prescription of lower dosages and alternate dosage forms and methods of administration, or the complete discontinuation of opiate analgesic pharmacotherapy, may become possible as a result of optimal pain management, physiological change, or associated improved psychological health among patients who have pain disorders that require adjunctive opiate analgesic pharmacotherapy.

AVAILABLE DOSAGE FORMS, STORAGE, AND COMPATIBILITY

A wide variety of dosage forms are available to individualize opiate analgesic pharmacotherapy. These dosage forms include oral tablets (both regular and extended-release tablets); injectables for intramuscular, intravenous, and subcutaneous use; rectal suppositories; nasal sprays; and transdermal delivery systems.

See individual opiate analgesic monographs.

Notes

General instructions for patients: Instruct patients who are receiving opiate analgesic pharmacotherapy to

- safely store opiate analgesic dosage forms out of the reach of children. See individual opiate analgesic monographs for additional storage requirements.
- obtain an available patient information sheet regarding opiate analgesic pharmacotherapy from their pharmacist at the time that their prescription is dispensed. Encourage patients to clarify any questions that they may have regarding opiate analgesic pharmacotherapy with their pharmacist or, if needed, to consult their prescribing psychologist.

PROPOSED MECHANISM OF ACTION

The opiate analgesics act primarily on the CNS. The perception of and emotional response to pain is modified when opiate analgesics bind with stereospecific receptors in the CNS. Five major groups of opiate receptors have been identified: delta, epsilon, kappa, mu, and sigma. Opiate analgesic activity occurs at the mu, kappa, and sigma receptors. These receptors are found in the highest concentrations in the hypothalamus, limbic system, midbrain, spinal cord, and thalamus. Pure opiate agonist analgesics (e.g., morphine) exert their activity mainly at the mu receptor. In addition to analgesia, opiate analgesic agonists suppress the cough reflex, alter mood (e.g., produce euphoria or dysphoria), and cause mental clouding, nausea, vomiting, and respiratory depression. Nausea and vomiting probably are caused by the stimulation of the chemoreceptor trigger zone. Mixed opiate analgesic agonists/antagonists (e.g., butorphanol, nalbuphine, pentazocine) act primarily at the kappa receptors.

Peripheral vasodilation, reduced peripheral resistance, and the inhibition of baroreceptors can result in postural (orthostatic) hypotension and fainting (syncope). The inhibition of GI peristalsis can result in constipation. Increased bladder sphincter tone may cause urinary retention. High dosages have been associated with excitation or seizures. Morphine and its congeners cause abnormal contraction of the pupils or "pin-point" pupils (miosis). Therapeutic dosages also increase accommodation and sensitivity to light and may decrease intraocular pressure.

PHARMACOKINETICS/PHARMACODYNAMICS

Opiate analgesics are absorbed rapidly after oral, rectal, intramuscular, intranasal, subcutaneous, or transdermal administration. Following oral ingestion, most opiate analgesics undergo significant first-pass hepatic metabolism. They are metabolized by the liver and excreted primarily in the urine after conjugation with glucuronic acid in the kidneys. Morphine is generally the proto-type to which all other opiate analgesics are compared. See the morphine monograph. See also the other individual opiate analgesic monographs.

RELATIVE CONTRAINDICATIONS

CNS depression, severe
Coma
Diarrhea associated with poisoning. Opiate analgesics may slow GI tract motility and, thus, slow the elimination of the toxic substance involved in the poisoning. Opiate analgesic pharmacotherapy is contraindicated for these patients until the toxic substance has been eliminated from the GI tract.
Hypersensitivity to opiate analgesics, history of. Patients who report a history of a hyper-sensitivity reaction to morphine (e.g., generalized rash, shortness of breath) should *not* be prescribed codeine, hydromorphone, oxycodone, or oxymorphone because of the risk for cross-sensitivity.
MAOI pharmacotherapy, concurrent or within 14 days. Fentanyl, heroin, meperidine, or morphine pharmacotherapy and MAOI pharmacotherapy, concurrent or within 14 days, is relatively contraindicated. Concurrent pharmacotherapy may result in toxic reactions with varied signs and symptoms. These signs and symptoms include coma, cyanosis, hy-perexcitability, hypertension, hypotension, and severe respiratory depression. See "Drug Interactions."
Respiratory dysfunction, including any condition where there is a significant decrease in res-piratory reserve (e.g., bronchial asthma, cor pulmonale, emphysema, or kyphoscoliosis). Opiate analgesic pharmacotherapy may further compromise respiratory function among these patients.
Upper airway obstruction

CAUTIONS AND COMMENTS

Opiate analgesics are addicting and habituating. Long-term opiate analgesic pharmacotherapy, or regular personal use, is associated with addiction and habituation. Abrupt discontinuation of long-term opiate analgesic pharmacotherapy, or regular personal use, may result in the opi-ate analgesic withdrawal syndrome. The opiate analgesic withdrawal syndrome also may oc-cur among patients who are addicted to pure opiate analgesic agonists (e.g., morphine) when an opiate analgesic antagonist (e.g., naloxone [Narcan®]) or a mixed opiate analgesic ago-nist/antagonist (e.g., pentazocine [Talwin®] is administered.

Signs and symptoms of the acute opiate analgesic withdrawal syndrome include abdominal pain, body aches, chills, diarrhea, difficulty sleeping, gooseflesh (piloerection), loss of appetite (anorexia), nervousness, restlessness, runny nose (rhinitis), shivering, sneezing, stomach cramps, sweating (excessive), tachycardia, tremors, unexplained fever, weakness, and yawning. Although the opiate analgesic withdrawal syndrome is not generally life-threatening, the appropriate pre-scription and monitoring of opiate analgesic pharmacotherapy and the gradual discontinuation of long-term pharmacotherapy will prevent or minimize these signs and symptoms.

Prescribe opiate analgesic pharmacotherapy cautiously to patients who

- have abdominal disorders (e.g., acute appendicitis). Opiate analgesics may obscure the diagnosis or clinical management of these medical disorders.
- have Addison's disease or adrenocortical insufficiency. Opiate analgesics inhibit the re-lease of corticotropin.

- are elderly, frail, or debilitated. These patients may be at risk for CNS or respiratory depression. See information on patients with respiratory dysfunction, below.
- have CNS depression, including that associated with acute alcohol intoxication.
- have gallbladder disease. Opiate analgesics increase biliary tract pressure and cause smooth muscle spasms. These actions may result in biliary spasm or colic.
- have head injuries or other medical disorders associated with increased intracranial pressure. The respiratory depressant action of the opiate analgesics and their ability to elevate cerebrospinal fluid pressure may be markedly exaggerated among these patients. Opiate analgesic pharmacotherapy also may obscure the clinical course of these conditions.
- have histories of problematic patterns of opiate analgesic or other abusable psychotropic use. These patients may be at increased risk for the development of problematic patterns of opiate analgesic use, including addiction and habituation.
- have hypertrophy of the prostate or urethral stricture. Opiate analgesics may increase vesical sphincter tone. This action may exacerbate these conditions and make urination difficult for these patients.
- have hypotension, including that associated with blood loss, shock, antihypertensive or other pharmacotherapy, or other conditions that interfere with the maintenance of normal blood pressure. The action of opiate analgesics on the smooth muscles of the blood vessels may cause severe hypotension among these patients. Opiate analgesic pharmacotherapy also has been associated with postural (orthostatic) hypotension among elderly and other susceptible patients.
- have liver dysfunction (severe).
- have myxedema or hypothyroidism. Opiate analgesic pharmacotherapy may place these patients at increased risk for CNS and respiratory depression.
- have respiratory dysfunction, including chronic obstructive pulmonary disease, cor pulmonale, hypoxia or hypercapnia, pre-existing respiratory depression, substantially decreased respiratory reserve, or other conditions that may compromise respiratory function (e.g., kyphoscoliosis).

Caution patients who are receiving opiate analgesic pharmacotherapy against

- performing activities that require alertness, judgment, or physical coordination (e.g., driving an automobile, operating dangerous equipment, supervising children) until their response to opiate analgesics is known. Opiate analgesic pharmacotherapy may affect these mental and physical functions adversely.

In addition to this general precaution, caution patients to

- avoid or limit the concurrent use of other CNS depressants, including alcohol, other opiate analgesics, sedative-hypnotics, or other drugs that depress the CNS (e.g., cough and cold products containing antihistamines, such as diphenhydramine [Benadryl®] or triprolidine, found in combination with other active ingredients in Actifed® cough and cold products). Concurrent use may result in severe CNS and respiratory depression. Family members or others involved with the patient's care should be cautioned to observe for over-sedation and other CNS depressant actions. They also should be advised to implement safety precautions, as needed (e.g., supervised ambulation or tobacco smoking). Hospitalization or supervised home care may be required for patients who require opiate analgesic pharmacotherapy. (Also see information on monitoring respiratory rate, below.)
- be aware of the addiction potential of opiate analgesics. Instruct patients, family members, and others involved with their care regarding the safe storage of opiate analgesics in the home to prevent possible misuse or accidental poisoning, which may be fatal.
- inform their prescribing psychologist if they begin or discontinue any other pharmacotherapy while receiving opiate analgesic pharmacotherapy.

- monitor respiratory rate. An emergency protocol, including the placement by the telephone of emergency telephone numbers, should be in place in the event of significant respiratory depression or overdosage. Family members or others involved with the patient's care should be cautioned to observe for changes in respiratory function. Hospitalization or supervised home care may be required for patients who require opiate analgesic pharmacotherapy. (Also see previous information on avoiding or limiting the concurrent use of other CNS depressants.)

CLINICALLY SIGNIFICANT DRUG INTERACTIONS

Concurrent opiate analgesic pharmacotherapy and the following may result in clinically significant drug interactions:

Alcohol Use

Concurrent use of alcohol among patients who are receiving opiate analgesic pharmacotherapy may result in additive CNS depression. Advise patients to avoid, or limit, their use of alcohol while receiving opiate analgesic pharmacotherapy.

Anticholinergic Pharmacotherapy and Pharmacotherapy With Other Drugs That Produce Anticholinergic Actions

Concurrent opiate analgesic and anticholinergic (e.g., atropine) pharmacotherapy, or pharmacotherapy with other drugs that produce anticholinergic actions (e.g., phenothiazines, TCAs), may increase constipation, drowsiness, and urinary retention among susceptible patients (e.g., elderly, frail, or debilitated patients).

Cimetidine Pharmacotherapy

Concurrent opiate analgesic and cimetidine (Tagamet®) pharmacotherapy may result in opiate analgesic toxicity (e.g., respiratory depression). The mechanism for this interaction has not been established clearly. However, most likely it is associated with a decrease in the metabolism of the opiate analgesics by cimetidine.

MAOI Pharmacotherapy

Concurrent opiate analgesic pharmacotherapy with fentanyl (Sublimaze®), meperidine (pethidine, Demerol®), or morphine (M.O.S.®) and MAOI pharmacotherapy (including selegiline) has been associated with serious ADRs. The mechanism of this interaction has not been established clearly. Fentanyl, meperidine, or morphine pharmacotherapy should be prescribed with extreme caution, if at all, to patients who are receiving MAOI pharmacotherapy (including selegiline) or within 14 days of such pharmacotherapy. See "Relative Contraindications."

Pharmacotherapy With Other Opiate Analgesics, Including Opiate Analgesic Agonists and Mixed Opiate Analgesic Agonists/Antagonists

Concurrent pharmacotherapy with two or more opiate analgesic agonists may produce additive actions. These actions may result in severe CNS depression, respiratory depression, and hypotension. Avoid prescribing concurrent opiate analgesic agonist pharmacotherapy. Concurrent pharmacotherapy with a mixed opiate analgesic agonist/antagonist (e.g., butorphanol [Stadol NS®], nalbuphine [Nubain®], pentazocine [Talwin®]) and a pure opiate analgesic agonist may reduce the analgesic action of both drugs. This combination of pharmacotherapy also may precipitate the opiate analgesic withdrawal syndrome among patients who are addicted to opiate analgesic agonists. Avoid concurrent opiate analgesic agonist and opiate analgesic agonist/antagonist pharmacotherapy. See also "Pharmacotherapy With CNS Depressants and Other Drugs That Produce CNS Depression," immediately following.

Pharmacotherapy With CNS Depressants and Other Drugs That Produce CNS Depression

Concurrent opiate analgesic pharmacotherapy with other opiate analgesics, sedative-hypnotics, or other drugs that produce CNS depression (e.g., antihistamines, phenothiazines, TCAs) may result in additive CNS depression. If concurrent pharmacotherapy is required, reduce the dosages of one or both drugs accordingly. See also "Pharmacotherapy With Other Opiate Analgesic Agonists, Including Opiate Analgesic Agonists and Mixed Opiate Analgesic Agonists/Antagonists," previous.

TCA Pharmacotherapy

Concurrent opiate analgesic and TCA pharmacotherapy may potentiate the respiratory depressant action of the opiate analgesic. See also "Pharmacotherapy with CNS Depressants and Other Drugs That Produce CNS Depression," above.

ADVERSE DRUG REACTIONS

The major ADRs associated with opiate analgesic pharmacotherapy are respiratory depression and respiratory arrest. To a lesser extent, circulatory depression, shock, and cardiac arrest also may occur. Other ADRs associated with opiate analgesic pharmacotherapy, listed according to body system, include:

Cardiovascular: bradycardia, fainting (syncope), hypertension, palpitations, phlebitis following intravenous injection, postural hypotension, and supraventricular tachycardia

CNS: agitation, alterations of mood, disorientation, dreams, drowsiness, euphoria, dysphoria, headache, hallucinations, insomnia, sedation, seizures, and toxic psychosis. Reportedly, patients who have migraine headaches may be more susceptible to the ADRs associated with butorphanol pharmacotherapy. (See the butorphanol monograph.)

Cutaneous: edema; excessive sweating; flushing or feelings of warmth; hives (urticaria); local tissue irritation and induration following subcutaneous injection, particularly when repeated injections are required; pain at the injection site; severe itching (pruritus); skin rashes; and wheal and flare over the vein following intravenous injection.

Genitourinary: impotence, reduced sex drive, and urinary hesitancy or retention
GI: biliary tract spasm, constipation, cramps, diarrhea, dry mouth, dyspepsia, loss of appetite (anorexia), nausea, taste alterations, and vomiting. Constipation, nausea, and vomiting seem to be more prominent among non-hospitalized patients and those who are not experiencing severe pain.

Constipation Lower dosages are recommended for elderly, frail, or debilitated patients. These patients, particularly those who are bedridden, may become impacted. Caution patients to maintain a balanced diet and an adequate intake of water. An appropriate regimen of bowel management and exercise may be required, particularly when initiating long-term opiate analgesic pharmacotherapy. Collaboration with the patient's advanced practice nurse, physician, oncologist, or community health nurse may be indicated.

Nausea and vomiting Nausea and vomiting often occur following a single dose of an opiate analgesic. Nausea and vomiting also may be troublesome when long-term opiate analgesic pharmacotherapy is initiated. When initiating long-term pharmacotherapy for the symptomatic management of chronic cancer pain, also consider the prescription of an antiemetic. Collaboration with the patient's advanced practice nurse, family physician, or a specialist (e.g., oncologist) may be required.

Musculoskeletal: incoordinated muscle movements and weakness
Ocular: abnormal contraction of the pupils (miosis) and visual disturbances
Miscellaneous: spasm of the larynx (laryngospasm)

OVERDOSAGE

Signs and symptoms of opiate overdosage include respiratory depression with reduced respiratory rate and tidal volume; Cheyne–Stokes respirations; cyanosis, extreme somnolence progressing to stupor or coma, skeletal muscle flaccidity, cold clammy skin, and sometimes hypotension and bradycardia. Severe overdosage may result in apnea, circulatory collapse, cardiac arrest, and death. Abnormal dilation of the pupils (mydriasis) may occur with terminal narcosis, severe hypoxia, or as a toxic reaction associated with meperidine or its congeners. The signs and symptoms of severe propoxyphene overdosage include focal and generalized seizures. Nephrogenic diabetes insipidus and electrocardiogram abnormalities also may occur.

Opiate analgesic overdosage requires emergency symptomatic medical support of body systems, particularly respiratory function, with attention to increasing opiate analgesic elimination. Naloxone (Narcan®), a pure opiate analgesic antagonist, is a specific antidote against the respiratory depression associated with opiate analgesic agonist and mixed opiate analgesic agonist/antagonist overdosages. However, the usual dosage of the opiate analgesic antagonist will precipitate the opiate analgesic withdrawal syndrome among patients who are addicted to opiate analgesics. The severity of the withdrawal syndrome depends on the severity of the patient's addiction and the dose of the antagonist administered. The use of opiate analgesic antagonists among patients who are addicted to opiates should be avoided if possible. If an opiate analgesic antagonist is required for the medical management of serious respiratory depression and other signs and symptoms of overdosage among these patients, lower dosages and cautious dosage titration are recommended. (See also the naloxone monograph.)

OXYCODONE
[Dihydrohydroxycodeinone]

(ox i koe′ done)

TRADE NAMES

OxyContin®
OxyFAST®
OxyIR®
Roxicodone®
Supeudol®

CLASSIFICATION

Opiate analgesic (C-II)

See also "Opiate Analgesics, General Monograph."

APPROVED INDICATIONS FOR NEUROPSYCHOLOGICAL DISORDERS

Adjunctive pharmacotherapy for the symptomatic management of:

- pain disorders: acute pain, moderate to severe, and chronic cancer pain, moderate to severe

USUAL DOSAGE AND ADMINISTRATION

Pain Disorders: Acute Pain, Moderate to Severe, and Chronic Cancer Pain, Moderate to Severe

Adults: 5 to 10 mg (regular capsules or tablets) orally every six hours, as needed; *or* 10 to 20 mg (rectal suppositories) rectally every six to eight hours, as needed; *or* 10 to 80 mg (extended-release tablets) orally every twelve hours, as needed (see "Notes, Pain Disorders: Acute Pain, Moderate to Severe, and Chronic Cancer Pain, Moderate to Severe").

Women who are, or who may become, pregnant: FDA Pregnancy Category B. Safety and efficacy of oxycodone pharmacotherapy for women who are pregnant have not been established. Long-term oxycodone pharmacotherapy, or regular personal use, during pregnancy may result in the neonatal opiate analgesic withdrawal syndrome (see "Opiate Analgesics, General Monograph"). Avoid prescribing oxycodone pharmacotherapy to women who are pregnant. If oxycodone pharmacotherapy is required, advise patients of potential benefits and possible risks to themselves and the embryo, fetus, or neonate. Collaboration with the patient's obstetrician is indicated.

For details and discussion regarding related basic principles of clinical pharmacology, readers are referred to the first text in this series, *The Pharmacologic Basis of Psychotherapeutics: An Introduction for Psychologists.*

Women who are breast-feeding: Safety and efficacy of oxycodone pharmacotherapy for women who are breast-feeding and their neonates and infants have not been established. Oxycodone is excreted in breast milk in concentrations higher than maternal blood concentrations. Expected pharmacologic actions (e.g., drowsiness, lethargy) may be observed among breast-fed neonates and infants, who also may become addicted. Avoid prescribing oxycodone pharmacotherapy to women who are breast-feeding. If oxycodone pharmacotherapy is required, breast-feeding probably should be discontinued. If desired, lactation may be maintained and breast-feeding resumed following the discontinuation of short-term oxycodone pharmacotherapy. Collaboration with the patient's pediatrician may be indicated.

Elderly, frail, or debilitated patients: Generally prescribe lower dosages for elderly, frail, or debilitated patients. Gradually increase the dosage, if needed, according to individual patient response. These patients may be more sensitive to the pharmacologic actions of oxycodone than are younger or healthier adult patients.

Children and adolescents younger than 18 years of age: Safety and efficacy of oxycodone pharmacotherapy for children and adolescents have not been established. Oxycodone pharmacotherapy is *not* recommended for this age group.

Notes, Pain Disorders: Acute Pain, Moderate to Severe, and Chronic Cancer Pain, Moderate to Severe

The difference in the recommended dosages for oral oxycodone and rectal oxycodone pharmacotherapy is due to the effects of first-pass hepatic metabolism on the oxycodone oral dosage forms. Adjust the dosage to the type and severity of pain and individual patient response. It may be necessary to occasionally exceed the usual recommended dosage for patients who have severe pain or who have developed tolerance to oxycodone's analgesic action. Adjunctive oral oxycodone pharmacotherapy usually is adequate for the symptomatic management of acute moderate to severe pain or for chronic, severe, cancer pain. However, oral oxycodone pharmacotherapy should *not* be prescribed for the symptomatic management of chronic benign pain.

Oral oxycodone extended-release tablet pharmacotherapy for the symptomatic management of chronic severe cancer pain: Clinical experience with oral oxycodone extended-release tablet pharmacotherapy for the initial management of chronic severe cancer pain is limited and generally is not recommended. The oral oxycodone extended-release tablets are formulated in high dosages (i.e., 10, 20, 40, 80 mg). They also are formulated to have a prolonged duration of action (i.e., ~12 hours). Although these features contraindicate their use for the initial management of severe chronic cancer pain because of the associated difficulty establishing adequate analgesia, these same features can be used to provide effective and convenient oral opiate analgesic pharmacotherapy once adequate analgesia with the regular oral formulations has been achieved. In this regard, only prescribe oxycodone oral extended-release tablet pharmacotherapy for patients whose moderate to severe cancer pain has been managed adequately with regular oral dosage forms of oxycodone or other opiate analgesics. For these patients, calculate their total current daily opiate analgesic requirement to determine the equivalent oral oxycodone daily dosage. (See the "Usual Dosage and Administration" section of "Opiate Analgesics, General Monograph.")

Initially prescribe the equivalent oral oxycodone daily dosage in two equally divided doses at 12-hour intervals using the oral oxycodone extended-release tablets. This initial recommended equivalent daily dosage is generally a conservative estimate of the required daily dosage. Most patients will need an adjustment (i.e., increase) in their dosage. For these patients, increase the dosage at 24-hour intervals, as needed, according to individual patient response. Breakthrough pain during the 24 hours following the initiation of oral oxycodone extended-release tablet pharmacotherapy generally requires an increase in dosage rather than a decrease in dosing interval. Once therapeutic benefit has been achieved, maintain oxycodone oral extended-release tablet pharmacotherapy with the lowest effective dosage. Periodically attempt to reduce the dosage or discontinue pharmacotherapy. (See also "Opiate Analgesics, General Monograph.")

AVAILABLE DOSAGE FORMS, STORAGE, AND COMPATIBILITY

Capsules, oral: 5 mg
Solution, concentrated oral (OxyFAST®; Roxicodone Intensol®): 20 mg/ml
Solution, oral (unit dose Patient Cups®): 5 mg/5 ml (contains 0.4% to 8% alcohol, depending upon the manufacturer)
Suppositories, rectal: 10, 20 mg
Tablets, oral: 5, 10 mg
Tablets, oral extended-release: 10, 20, 40, 80 mg

Notes

Caution is required when prescribing oxycodone oral formulations. Do *not* confuse the oxycodone concentrated oral solution (Intensol®, 20 mg/ml) with the regular oral solution (1 mg/ml). Do *not* confuse the oral oxycodone extended-release tablets (10, 20, 40, 80 mg) with the regular oral oxycodone tablets (5, 10 mg).

General instructions for patients: Instruct patients who are receiving oxycodone pharmacotherapy to

- measure each dose of the oral oxycodone concentrated solution (Roxicodone Intensol® [20 mg/ml]) with the calibrated dropper supplied with the product by the manufacturer to help to assure that an accurate dose is measured and ingested.
- swallow each dose of the oral oxycodone extended-release tablets whole without breaking, chewing, or crushing. Breaking, chewing, or crushing the oral oxycodone extended-release tablets may result in the absorption of a potentially toxic dose of oxycodone. Also instruct patients to ingest each dose with an adequate amount of liquid chaser (i.e., 60 to 120 ml of water).
- safely store the oxycodone oral capsules, tablets, or solutions out of the reach of children. Oral capsules and tablets also should be stored in tightly closed, child- and light-resistant containers at controlled room temperature (15° to 30°C; 59° to 86°F) out of the reach of children.
- safely store oxycodone rectal suppositories under refrigeration (2° to 8°C; 36° to 46°F) out of the reach of children.
- obtain an available patient information sheet regarding oxycodone pharmacotherapy from their pharmacist at the time that their prescription is dispensed. Encourage patients to clarify any questions that they may have regarding oxycodone pharmacotherapy with their pharmacist or, if needed, to consult their prescribing psychologist.

PROPOSED MECHANISM OF ACTION

Oxycodone is a semi-synthetic opiate with several actions qualitatively similar to morphine. It appears to elicit its analgesic and CNS depressant actions primarily by binding to the endorphin receptors in the CNS. However, the exact mechanism of action has not yet been fully determined. See "Opiate Analgesics, General Monograph."

PHARMACOKINETICS/PHARMACODYNAMICS

Approximately 60% to 90% of oxycodone is absorbed following oral ingestion. Although oxycodone undergoes extensive first-pass hepatic metabolism, it is similar to codeine and methadone in that it retains at least half of its analgesic action when orally ingested. Oxycodone's apparent volume of distribution is ~2.6 liters/kg. Its plasma protein binding is low (~45%) and its duration of analgesic action is generally 4 to 5 hours. Oxycodone is metabolized extensively, primarily to inactive metabolites. However, low concentrations of an active metabolite, oxymorphone, have been identified. Oxycodone and its metabolites are excreted primarily by the kidneys, with up to 20% being eliminated in unchanged form. The total plasma clearance of oxycodone among adults is ~0.8 liters/minute. The mean half-life of elimination is ~4 hours.

RELATIVE CONTRAINDICATIONS

Head injury or any other medical disorder associated with increased intracranial or cerebrospinal fluid pressure

Hypersensitivity to oxycodone or morphine

Respiratory dysfunction, including any medical disorder where there is a significant decrease in respiratory reserve (e.g., bronchial asthma, cor pulmonale, emphysema, or kyphosis)

CAUTIONS AND COMMENTS

Oxycodone is addicting and habituating. It has a high addiction potential and is a commonly abused oral opiate analgesic. Prescribe oxycodone pharmacotherapy cautiously to patients who have histories of substance-use disorders or any of the conditions listed in the "Cautions and Comments" section of the "Opiate Analgesics, General Monograph."

Caution patients who are receiving oxycodone pharmacotherapy against

- drinking alcohol or using other drugs that can produce CNS depression. Concurrent use with oxycodone can result in excessive CNS depression.
- performing activities that require alertness, judgment, and physical coordination (e.g., driving an automobile, operating dangerous equipment, supervising children) until their response to oxycodone pharmacotherapy is known. Oxycodone may affect these mental and physical functions adversely.

In addition to these general precautions, caution patients who are receiving oxycodone pharmacotherapy to

- inform their prescribing psychologist if they begin or discontinue any other pharmacotherapy while receiving oxycodone pharmacotherapy.

CLINICALLY SIGNIFICANT DRUG INTERACTIONS

Concurrent oxycodone pharmacotherapy and the following may result in clinically significant drug interactions:

Alcohol Use

Concurrent alcohol use may increase the CNS depressant action of oxycodone. Advise patients to avoid, or limit, their use of alcohol while receiving oxycodone pharmacotherapy.

Pharmacotherapy With CNS Depressants and Other Drugs That Produce CNS Depression

Concurrent oxycodone pharmacotherapy and pharmacotherapy with other opiate analgesics, sedative-hypnotics, or other drugs that produce CNS depression (e.g., antihistamines, phenothiazines, TCAs) may result in additive CNS depression.

ADVERSE DRUG REACTIONS

Oxycodone pharmacotherapy has been commonly associated with dizziness, lightheadedness, nausea, and vomiting. It also has been associated with constipation, dry mouth, euphoria or dysphoria, severe itching (pruritus), and skin rash.

See also "Opiate Analgesics, General Monograph."

OVERDOSAGE

The signs and symptoms of oxycodone overdosage resemble those associated with other opiate analgesic overdosage (see "Opiate Analgesics, General Monograph"). Oxycodone overdosage requires emergency symptomatic medical support of body systems with attention to increasing oxycodone elimination. The opiate antagonist, naloxone (Narcan®), usually is required to reverse the respiratory depression associated with oxycodone and other opiate analgesic overdosage.

OXYMORPHONE

(ox i mor' fone)

TRADE NAME

Numorphan®

CLASSIFICATION

Opiate analgesic (C-II)

See also "Opiate Analgesics, General Monograph."

APPROVED INDICATIONS FOR NEUROPSYCHOLOGICAL DISORDERS

Adjunctive pharmacotherapy for the symptomatic management of:

• pain disorders: acute pain, moderate to severe

USUAL DOSAGE AND ADMINISTRATION

Pain Disorders, Acute Pain, Moderate to Severe

Adults: Initially, 1 to 1.5 mg intramuscularly or subcutaneously; *or* 5 mg rectally; or 0.5 mg intravenously slowly every 4 to 6 hours, as needed

Women who are, or who may become, pregnant: FDA Pregnancy Category C. Safety and efficacy of oxymorphone pharmacotherapy for women who are pregnant have not been established. Long-term oxymorphone pharmacotherapy during pregnancy, or regular personal use, may result in the neonatal opiate withdrawal syndrome (see "Opiate Analgesics, General Monograph"). Avoid prescribing oxymorphone pharmacotherapy to women who are pregnant. If oxymorphone pharmacotherapy is required, advise patients of potential benefits and possible risks to themselves and the embryo, fetus, or neonate. Collaboration with the patient's obstetrician is indicated.

Women who are breast-feeding: Safety and efficacy of oxymorphone pharmacotherapy for women who are breast-feeding and their neonates and infants have not been established (see "Opiate Analgesics, General Monograph"). Avoid prescribing oxymorphone pharmacotherapy to women who are breast-feeding. If oxymorphone pharmacotherapy is required, breast-feeding probably should be discontinued. If desired, lactation may be maintained and breast-feeding resumed following the discontinuation of short-term oxymorphone pharmacotherapy. Collaboration with the patient's pediatrician may be indicated.

For details and discussion regarding related basic principles of clinical pharmacology, readers are referred to the first text in this series, *The Pharmacologic Basis of Psychotherapeutics: An Introduction for Psychologists.*

Elderly, frail, or debilitated patients: Generally prescribe lower dosages of oxymorphone for elderly, frail, or debilitated patients. Gradually increase the dosage according to individual patient response. These patients may be more sensitive to the pharmacologic actions of oxymorphone than are younger or healthier adult patients.

Children younger than 12 years of age: The safety and efficacy of oxymorphone pharmacotherapy for children younger than 12 years of age have not been established. Oxymorphone pharmacotherapy is *not* recommended for this age group.

Notes, Acute Pain, Moderate to Severe

Initiate oxymorphone pharmacotherapy with lower dosages. Gradually increase the dosage according to individual patient response until the pain is managed adequately. Oxymorphone pharmacotherapy with the rectal suppositories may be prescribed when oral opiate analgesic pharmacotherapy is not feasible (e.g., patients are nauseated or vomiting) and injectable pharmacotherapy is not desired. Oxymorphone rectal suppositories also may be of benefit for elderly, frail, or debilitated patients who may require a potent, rapid-acting analgesic and generally are unable to tolerate oral or injectable opiate analgesic pharmacotherapy.

AVAILABLE DOSAGE FORMS, STORAGE, AND COMPATIBILITY

Injectables, intramuscular, intravenous, or subcutaneous: 1, 1.5 mg/ml
Suppository, rectal: 5 mg

Notes

The oxymorphone injectable formulation contains sodium dithionite, a sulfite. Sulfites may cause hypersensitivity reactions, including anaphylactic reactions, among susceptible patients. Although relatively uncommon, these reactions appear to occur with a higher incidence among patients who have asthma.

General instructions for patients: Instruct patients who are receiving oxymorphone pharmacotherapy, or those assisting them with their pharmacotherapy, to

- safely store oxymorphone injectables protected from light at controlled room temperature (15° to 30°C; 59° to 86°F).
- safely store oxymorphone rectal suppositories under refrigeration (2° to 8°C; 36° to 46°F) and out of the reach of children.
- obtain an available patient information sheet regarding oxymorphone pharmacotherapy from their pharmacist at the time that their prescription is dispensed. Encourage patients to clarify any questions that they may have regarding oxymorphone pharmacotherapy with their pharmacist or, if needed, to consult their prescribing psychologist.

PROPOSED MECHANISM OF ACTION

Oxymorphone is a potent opiate analgesic that appears to elicit its analgesic action primarily by binding to the endorphin receptors in the CNS. However, the exact mechanism of action has not yet been fully determined. See also "Opiate Analgesics, General Monograph."

PHARMACOKINETICS/PHARMACODYNAMICS

When injected, 1 mg of oxymorphone is equivalent to 10 mg of morphine. When compared to morphine, oxymorphone reportedly produces equal analgesia with less respiratory depression. The onset of action is rapid and generally occurs within 5 to 10 minutes after intravenous injection, 10 to 15 minutes after intramuscular or subcutaneous injection, and 15 to 30 minutes after rectal insertion. Analgesia persists for 3 to 6 hours. Oxymorphone is conjugated with glucuronic acid in the liver and is excreted in the urine. Additional data are not available.

RELATIVE CONTRAINDICATIONS

Hypersensitivity to oxymorphone, morphine, or other opiate analgesics
Respiratory depression
Seizure disorders

CAUTIONS AND COMMENTS

Addiction and habituation are associated with long-term oxymorphone pharmacotherapy, or regular personal use. Prescribe oxymorphone pharmacotherapy cautiously for patients who have histories of substance-use disorders or who

- are receiving concurrent pharmacotherapy with other opiate analgesics or other drugs that can depress CNS or respiratory function. Concurrent pharmacotherapy may result in additive CNS and respiratory depression.

Caution patients who are receiving oxymorphone pharmacotherapy against

- performing activities that require alertness, judgment, and physical coordination (e.g., driving an automobile, operating dangerous equipment, supervising children) until their response to oxymorphone is known. The CNS depressant action of oxymorphone may affect these mental and physical functions adversely.

In addition to this general precaution, caution patients who are receiving oxymorphone pharmacotherapy to

- inform their prescribing psychologist if they begin or discontinue any other pharmacotherapy while receiving oxymorphone pharmacotherapy.

CLINICALLY SIGNIFICANT DRUG INTERACTIONS

Concurrent oxymorphone pharmacotherapy and the following may result in clinically significant drug interactions:

Alcohol Use

Concurrent alcohol use may increase the CNS depressant action of oxymorphone. Advise patients to avoid, or limit, their use of alcohol while receiving oxymorphone pharmacotherapy.

Pharmacotherapy With CNS Depressants and Other Drugs That Produce CNS Depression

Concurrent oxymorphone pharmacotherapy and pharmacotherapy with other opiate analgesics, sedative-hypnotics, or other drugs that produce CNS depression (e.g., antihistamines, phenothiazines, TCAs) may result in additive CNS depression.

ADVERSE DRUG REACTIONS

Oxymorphone pharmacotherapy has been associated with abnormal contraction of the pupils or "pin-point pupils" (miosis), drowsiness, dysphoria, GI complaints, headache, itching, lightheadedness, nausea, respiratory depression, and vomiting.

See also "Opiate Analgesics, General Monograph."

OVERDOSAGE

The signs and symptoms of oxymorphone overdosage resemble those associated with other opiate analgesic overdosage (see "Opiate Analgesics, General Monograph"). Oxymorphone overdosage requires emergency symptomatic medical support of body systems with attention to increasing oxymorphone elimination. The opiate analgesic antagonist, naloxone (Narcan®), usually is required to reverse the respiratory depression associated with oxymorphone and other opiate analgesic overdosage.

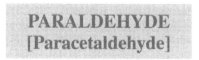

PARALDEHYDE
[Paracetaldehyde]

(par al′ de hyde)

TRADE NAME

Paral®

Generally available under the generic name

CLASSIFICATION

Anticonvulsant (acetaldehyde polymer) (C-IV)

APPROVED INDICATIONS FOR NEUROPSYCHOLOGICAL DISORDERS

Pharmacotherapy for the short-term symptomatic management of:

- seizure disorders. Paraldehyde pharmacotherapy is indicated for the symptomatic management of status epilepticus and seizures associated with eclampsia, poisoning, tetanus, and the alcohol withdrawal syndrome. *Note*: It is recommended that paraldehyde be prescribed for this approved indication *only* when other anticonvulsant pharmacotherapy is ineffective or contraindicated.

USUAL DOSAGE AND ADMINISTRATION

Seizure Disorders

Adults: The usual dosage depends on the indication for paraldehyde pharmacotherapy.

SEIZURES *NOT* ASSOCIATED WITH THE ALCOHOL WITHDRAWAL SYNDROME: 5 to 15 ml of paraldehyde oral solution (diluted 1:10) via nasogastric tube every four hours as needed according to individual patient response

SEIZURES ASSOCIATED WITH THE ALCOHOL WITHDRAWAL SYNDROME: 5 to 10 ml of paraldehyde solution (diluted 1:10) orally every four to six hours for the first 24 hours, then every two hours for the next 24 hours.

MAXIMUM: 60 ml of paraldehyde solution orally on day 1; subsequent days, 40 ml of paraldehyde solution daily orally

For details and discussion regarding related basic principles of clinical pharmacology, readers are referred to the first text in this series, *The Pharmacologic Basis of Psychotherapeutics: An Introduction for Psychologists.*

Women who are, or who may become, pregnant: FDA Pregnancy Category "not established." Safety and efficacy of paraldehyde pharmacotherapy for women who are pregnant have not been established. Paraldehyde readily crosses the placenta and appears in the fetal circulation. Avoid prescribing paraldehyde pharmacotherapy to women who are pregnant. If paraldehyde pharmacotherapy is required for the management of seizures related to eclampsia, advise patients of potential benefits and possible risks to themselves and the embryo, fetus, or neonate. Neonates born to mothers who received paraldehyde during labor may exhibit significant respiratory depression. Collaboration with the patient's obstetrician is indicated.

Women who are breast-feeding: Safety and efficacy of paraldehyde pharmacotherapy for women who are breast-feeding and their neonates and infants have not been established. Avoid prescribing paraldehyde pharmacotherapy to women who are breast-feeding. If paraldehyde pharmacotherapy is required, breast-feeding probably should be discontinued. If desired, lactation may be maintained and breast-feeding resumed following the discontinuation of short-term pharmacotherapy.

Elderly, frail, or debilitated patients: Initially, generally prescribe lower dosages of paraldehyde for elderly, frail, or debilitated patients. These patients may be more sensitive to the pharmacologic actions of paraldehyde than are younger or healthier adult patients.

Neonates: For the symptomatic management of status epilepticus: 0.15 to 0.3 ml/kg orally or rectally every six hours as required to control seizures; *or* 150 mg/kg/hour (i.e., 3 ml of 5% solution/kg/hour) intravenously over two hours *once daily*

Children: For the symptomatic management of seizures: 200 to 400 mg/kg (i.e., 0.2 to 0.4 ml undiluted paraldehyde/kg) prepared as a 30% to 50% solution in cotton seed oil, olive oil, or normal saline and administered rectally every four to eight hours as needed; *or* 100 to 150 mg/kg (i.e., 2 to 3 ml of 5% paraldehyde solution/kg) intravenously over 15 to 20 minutes, followed by 20 mg/kg/hour (i.e., 0.4 ml of 5% paraldehyde solution/kg/hour) as a continuous intravenous infusion. (See "Notes, Seizure Disorders.")

Notes, Seizure Disorders

Injectable paraldehyde pharmacotherapy

INTRAMUSCULAR PHARMACOTHERAPY: Paraldehyde can be administered intramuscularly. However, intramuscular injection is *not* recommended because of the associated high incidence of sterile abscesses.

INTRAVENOUS PHARMACOTHERAPY: Intravenous pharmacotherapy is recommended only in emergency situations, where patients have been proven to be refractory to more conventional anticonvulsant pharmacotherapy (e.g., diazepam pharmacotherapy).

Oral paraldehyde pharmacotherapy: Dilute the paraldehyde solution in 100 to 200 ml of milk or iced fruit juice *prior* to administration in order to disguise the unpleasant odor and taste of paraldehyde. Diluting the oral solution also prevents or minimizes associated GI irritation.

Rectal paraldehyde pharmacotherapy: Dilute the paraldehyde rectal solution (1:10) with cotton seed oil, olive oil, or normal saline *prior* to administration in order to prevent or minimize associated irritation of the rectal mucosa.

AVAILABLE DOSAGE FORMS, STORAGE, AND COMPATIBILITY

Injectable, intravenous: 1 gram/ml[*]
Solution, oral, rectal: 1 gram/ml

Notes

The paraldehyde injectable formulation is not commercially available in the United States and must be prepared freshly under sterile conditions in the pharmacy department of a hospital prior to use. Advise medical staff to:

- safely store paraldehyde formulations out of the reach of children in tightly closed, light- and child-resistant containers at controlled room temperature (15 ° to 25 °C; 59 ° to 77 °F).
- avoid getting the paraldehyde solution on clothing, eyes, or skin. Paraldehyde has been associated with contact dermatitis.

General instructions for patients: Instruct patients who are receiving paraldehyde pharmacotherapy to

- clarify any questions that they may have regarding paraldehyde pharmacotherapy with their prescribing psychologist.

PROPOSED MECHANISM OF ACTION

The exact mechanism of anticonvulsant action of paraldehyde has not yet been fully determined. However, it is believed to be due to a general depressant action upon several areas of the CNS including the reticular activating system. The margin between anticonvulsant and hypnotic dosages is narrow.

PHARMACOKINETICS/PHARMACODYNAMICS

Paraldehyde solution is absorbed rapidly and well from the GI tract following oral ingestion. Peak blood concentrations are achieved within 30 to 60 minutes. Paraldehyde is widely distributed in the body. It is extensively metabolized ($\sim$90%) within the liver. Paraldehyde is depolymerized to acetaldehyde, which is oxidized by acetaldehyde dehydrogenase to acetic acid and, subsequently, carbon dioxide and water. Approximately 7% of an oral dose is excreted in unchanged form through the lungs. The half-life of elimination ranges from 3.5 to 9.5 hours (mean = 7.5 hours). Additional data are not available.

RELATIVE CONTRAINDICATIONS

Chronic obstructive lung disease (e.g., asthma)
Disulfiram pharmacotherapy
Gastroenteritis
Hepatic insufficiency, severe

CAUTIONS AND COMMENTS

Prolonged use of paraldehyde may result in addiction and habituation.

CLINICALLY SIGNIFICANT DRUG INTERACTIONS

Concurrent paraldehyde pharmacotherapy and the following may result in clinically significant drug interactions:

Alcohol Use

Concurrent alcohol use may increase the CNS depressant action of paraldehyde.

Disulfiram Pharmacotherapy

Disulfiram (Antabuse®) inhibits the enzyme acetaldehyde dehydrogenase. Thus, acetaldehyde, a toxic product of paraldehyde decomposition, accumulates in the body. Avoid the concurrent use of disulfiram and paraldehyde.

Pharmacotherapy With CNS Depressants and Other Drugs That Produce CNS Depression

Concurrent paraldehyde pharmacotherapy and pharmacotherapy with opiate analgesics, sedative-hypnotics, or other drugs that produce CNS depression (e.g., antihistamines, phenothiazines, TCAs) may result in additive CNS depression.

ADVERSE DRUG REACTIONS

Paraldehyde pharmacotherapy commonly has been associated with erythematous rash and gastric irritation. Paraldehyde pharmacotherapy also has been associated with metabolic acidosis.

OVERDOSAGE

Signs and symptoms of paraldehyde overdosage include pulmonary edema and respiratory depression. Metabolic acidosis also may occur. A characteristic odor of paraldehyde on the breath facilitates diagnosis. Paraldehyde overdosage requires emergency symptomatic medical support of body systems with attention to increasing paraldehyde elimination. There is no known antidote.

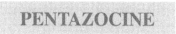

PENTAZOCINE

(pen taz' oh seen)

TRADE NAMES

Talwin®
Talwin Nx® (See "Available Dosage Forms, Storage, and Compatibility," and "Notes, Pain Disorders: Acute Pain, Moderate to Severe, and Chronic Cancer Pain, Moderate to Severe.")

CLASSIFICATION

Opiate analgesic (mixed agonist/antagonist) (C-IV)

See also "Opiate Analgesics, General Monograph."

APPROVED INDICATIONS FOR NEUROPSYCHOLOGICAL DISORDERS

Adjunctive pharmacotherapy for the symptomatic management of:

- pain disorders: acute pain, moderate to severe, and chronic cancer pain, moderate to severe

USUAL DOSAGE AND ADMINISTRATION

Acute Pain, Moderate to Severe, and Chronic Cancer Pain, Moderate to Severe

Adults: 30 to 60 mg intramuscularly, intravenously, or subcutaneously every three to four hours, as needed; *or* 50 to 100 mg orally every three to four hours with meals, as needed

MAXIMUM: 360 mg daily intramuscularly or intravenously; *or* 600 mg daily orally

Women who are, or who may become, pregnant: FDA Pregnancy Category C. Safety and efficacy of pentazocine pharmacotherapy for women who are pregnant have not been established. Pentazocine crosses the placenta. Blood concentrations among neonates at delivery are equal to ~65% of maternal blood concentrations. Neonates born to women who have received pentazocine pharmacotherapy, or regularly used pentazocine, during pregnancy or near term may display expected pharmacologic actions (e.g., drowsiness, lethargy, respiratory depression). They also may display signs and symptoms of the neonatal opiate analgesic withdrawal syndrome. See "Opiate Analgesics, General Monograph." Avoid prescribing pentazocine pharmacotherapy to women who are pregnant. If pentazocine pharmacotherapy is required, advise patients of potential benefits and possible risks to themselves and the embryo, fetus, or neonate. Collaboration with the patient's obstetrician is indicated.

Women who are breast-feeding: Safety and efficacy of pentazocine pharmacotherapy for women who are breast-feeding and their neonates and infants have not been established (see "Opiate Analgesics, General Monograph"). Avoid prescribing pentazocine pharmacotherapy to women who are breast-feeding. If pentazocine pharmacotherapy is required, breast-feeding probably should be discontinued. If desired, lactation may be maintained and breast-feeding resumed following the discontinuation of short-term pentazocine pharmacotherapy.

Elderly, frail, or debilitated patients and those who have liver dysfunction: Generally prescribe lower dosages of pentazocine for elderly, frail, or debilitated patients and those who have liver dysfunction. Gradually increase the dosage according to individual patient response. These patients may be more sensitive to the pharmacologic actions of pentazocine than are younger or healthier adult patients. Pentazocine pharmacotherapy may produce marked sedation among these patients. Also avoid injectable pentazocine pharmacotherapy among these patients because of the potential for serious CNS and respiratory depression.

Children younger than 12 years of age: Safety and efficacy of pentazocine pharmacotherapy for children younger than 12 years of age have not been established. Pentazocine pharmacotherapy is *not* recommended for this age group.

Notes, Pain Disorders: Acute Pain, Moderate to Severe, and Chronic Cancer Pain, Moderate to Severe

Note the differences in recommended dosages for oral and injectable pentazocine pharmacotherapy. An oral dosage of pentazocine is about one-quarter to one-third as effective as an equal injectable dosage.

Multiple intramuscular injections of the pentazocine lactate injectable formulation have been associated with severe sclerosis of the skin, subcutaneous tissues, and underlying muscle at injection sites. When more than one injection is required, carefully rotate injection sites. When long-term pharmacotherapy is required, replace injectable pentazocine pharmacotherapy as soon as possible with oral pharmacotherapy. Avoid subcutaneous injection because of pentazocine's potential to seriously damage subcutaneous tissues.

AVAILABLE DOSAGE FORMS, STORAGE, AND COMPATIBILITY

Injectable, intramuscular or intravenous: 30 mg/ml
Tablets, oral: 50 mg (see "Notes")

Notes

Injectable pentazocine formulations: Pentazocine injectable formulations are available in both single-unit dose ampules and cartridge-needle injection delivery systems (Carpuject®). Do *not* mix the pentazocine injectable in the same syringe with injectable formulations of barbiturates, chlordiazepoxide, or diazepam, because a precipitate will form. The Carpuject® system contains sodium bisulfite, which may cause hypersensitivity reactions, including anaphylactic reactions, among susceptible patients. Although relatively uncommon, these reactions appear to occur with a higher incidence among patients who have asthma.

Oral pentazocine formulations: The pentazocine oral tablet formulations are different for the United States and Canada. The Talwin Nx® tablets are available in the United States, whereas the Talwin® tablets are available in Canada.

TALWIN NX® ORAL TABLETS: In the United States, the oral pentazocine tablets (i.e., Talwin Nx®) have been formulated with 0.5 mg of naloxone, an opiate analgesic antagonist (see the naloxone monograph). The naloxone was added to the pentazocine oral tablet formulation to prevent its illicit intravenous use as "poor man's heroin." The naloxone is poorly absorbed from the GI tract following oral ingestion and, thus, has virtually no effect on the analgesic action of pentazocine. However, if the Talwin Nx® tablet is illicitly crushed, dissolved, and injected intravenously, the naloxone is absorbed immediately, blocking the desired action of the pentazocine.

TALWIN® ORAL TABLETS: In Canada, Talwin® oral tablets contain sodium metabisulfite. Sulfites may cause hypersensitivity reactions, including anaphylactic reactions, among susceptible patients. Although relatively uncommon, these reactions appear to occur with a higher incidence among patients who have asthma. These tablets are illicitly used by intravenous drug users for their opiate agonist/antagonist actions. The Talwin® tablets available in Canada do *not* contain naloxone.

General instructions for patients: Instruct patients who are receiving pentazocine pharmacotherapy to

- safely store pentazocine oral tablets out of the reach of children in tightly closed, light- and child-resistant containers at controlled room temperature (15° to 30 °C; 59° to 86 °F).
- obtain an available patient information sheet regarding pentazocine pharmacotherapy from their pharmacist at the time that their prescription is dispensed. Encourage patients to clarify any questions that they may have regarding pentazocine pharmacotherapy with their pharmacist or, if needed, to consult their prescribing psychologist.

PROPOSED MECHANISM OF ACTION

Pentazocine primarily elicits its analgesic, CNS depressant, and respiratory depressant actions by binding to the endorphin receptors in the CNS. However, its exact mechanism of action has not yet been fully determined. See also "Opiate Analgesics, General Monograph."

PHARMACOKINETICS/PHARMACODYNAMICS

The pharmacokinetics and pharmacodynamics of pentazocine depend upon its formulation for injectable or oral pharmacotherapy.

Injectable Pentazocine Formulations

Pentazocine's analgesic action occurs within 3 minutes after intravenous injection and within 30 minutes after intramuscular or subcutaneous injection. The duration of analgesia lasts for 3 to 4 hours. A dose of 30 mg by injection is approximately equal in analgesic action to 10 mg of morphine or 75 to 100 mg of meperidine (pethidine, Demerol®). Pentazocine weakly antagonizes the analgesic action of morphine and meperidine. It also produces incomplete reversal of the cardiovascular, respiratory, and CNS depression induced by morphine and meperidine. Pentazocine has approximately one-fiftieth the antagonistic action of naloxone. The respiratory depressant action of pentazocine is equal to, or less than, that observed after a single dose of other opiate analgesics. Pentazocine's associated respiratory depression appears to have a ceiling effect with repeated doses of 30 to 60 mg.

Oral Pentazocine Formulations

The analgesic action of 50 mg of orally ingested pentazocine is equivalent to ~60 mg of orally ingested codeine. Pentazocine is well absorbed following oral ingestion. However, only ~20% of the oral dose reaches the systemic circulation because of extensive first-pass hepatic metabolism. The onset of action following oral ingestion is within 30 minutes. The duration of action is 3 hours or longer. The onset and duration of action are, in part, related to the dose ingested and the severity of the patient's pain. Peak blood concentrations of orally ingested pentazocine generally are achieved within 1 to 3 hours. Pentazocine is ~60% bound to plasma proteins. Less than 20% of pentazocine is excreted in unchanged form in the urine. The half-life of elimination is ~2 to 3 hours and the total body clearance is ~1.4 liters/minute. The half-life of elimination may be significantly prolonged among patients who have liver dysfunction.

RELATIVE CONTRAINDICATIONS

Addiction and habituation to opiate analgesics, history of
Hypersensitivity to pentazocine
Opiate analgesic agonist pharmacotherapy (i.e., morphine pharmacotherapy), concurrent

CAUTIONS AND COMMENTS

Pentazocine is addicting and habituating. Long-term pentazocine pharmacotherapy, or regular personal use, may result in addiction and habituation. Pentazocine has mixed opiate agonist/antagonist actions. Abrupt discontinuation after long-term pharmacotherapy, or regular personal use, may result in a reportedly mild form of the opiate analgesic withdrawal syndrome. Signs and symptoms of this withdrawal syndrome include abdominal cramps, anxiety, fever, restlessness, runny nose (rhinorrhea), and tears. Pentazocine also may cause signs and symptoms of the opiate analgesic withdrawal syndrome among patients who are receiving long-term opiate analgesic pharmacotherapy with pure opiate analgesic agonists (e.g., morphine). The oral tablet formulation of pentazocine (Talwin Nx®) contains both pentazocine and naloxone in an attempt to discourage the widespread illicit intravenous injection of pentazocine.

Although further study is needed, pentazocine reportedly does not generally produce addiction among patients who require long-term (300 days) pentazocine pharmacotherapy for the symptomatic management of chronic pain. Signs and symptoms of the opiate analgesic withdrawal syndrome were not observed among a sample of patients, even upon abrupt discontinuation of pentazocine pharmacotherapy. However, a pentazocine withdrawal syndrome has been reported for a few patients after the discontinuation of regular long-term use. To avoid the possibility of precipitating the signs and symptoms of the opiate analgesic withdrawal syndrome, reduce the dosage gradually when discontinuing long-term pentazocine pharmacotherapy.

Prescribe pentazocine pharmacotherapy cautiously to patients who

- have acute inflammation of the gall bladder (cholecystitis) or pancreas (pancreatitis) or who will be undergoing surgery of the biliary tract. Opiate analgesics generally increase biliary tract pressure. Although pentazocine reportedly causes little or no elevation of biliary pressure, caution is advised.
- have head injuries, intracranial lesions, or other conditions associated with increased intracranial pressure. The respiratory depressant action associated with pentazocine and its potential for elevating cerebrospinal fluid pressure may markedly increase intracranial pressure among these patients. Pentazocine's analgesic and sedative actions also may obscure the clinical course of these patients.
- have histories of problematic patterns of opiate or other abusable psychotropic use. Prescribe the least quantity of pentazocine feasible to help to avoid the development of problematic patterns of use, including unadvised patient increases in dosage or frequency of use. Pentazocine, a mixed opiate analgesic agonist/antagonist, has weak opiate analgesic antagonist action. Patients who are addicted to pure opiate analgesic agonists (e.g., morphine) may experience signs and symptoms of the opiate analgesic withdrawal syndrome.
- have kidney dysfunction, including obstructive uropathy. Urinary retention has been rarely associated with pentazocine pharmacotherapy.
- have liver dysfunction. Serious liver dysfunction appears to predispose patients to a higher incidence of ADRs (e.g., anxiety, apprehension [marked], dizziness, drowsiness), even when usual recommended dosages of pentazocine are prescribed. These ADRs may be related to the accumulation of pentazocine, which is associated with its decreased metabolism by the liver.
- have respiratory depression, limited respiratory function (e.g., severely limited respiratory reserve, severe bronchial asthma, other obstructive respiratory conditions), or cyanosis. The respiratory depressant action of pentazocine may further compromise respiratory function among these patients.

Caution patients who are receiving pentazocine pharmacotherapy against

- performing activities that require alertness, judgment, and physical coordination (e.g., driving an automobile, operating dangerous equipment, supervising children) until their response to pentazocine pharmacotherapy is known. The CNS depressant action of pentazocine may affect these mental and physical functions adversely.

In addition to this general precaution, caution patients who are receiving pentazocine pharmacotherapy to

- inform their prescribing psychologist if they begin or discontinue any other pharmacotherapy while receiving pentazocine pharmacotherapy.

CLINICALLY SIGNIFICANT DRUG INTERACTIONS

Concurrent pentazocine pharmacotherapy and the following may result in clinically significant drug interactions:

Alcohol Use

Concurrent alcohol use may increase the CNS depressant action of pentazocine. Advise patients to avoid, or limit, their use of alcohol while receiving pentazocine pharmacotherapy.

Pharmacotherapy With CNS Depressants and Other Drugs That Produce CNS Depression

Concurrent pentazocine pharmacotherapy and pharmacotherapy with other opiate analgesics, sedative-hypnotics, or other drugs that produce CNS depression (e.g., antihistamines, phenothiazines, TCAs) may result in additive CNS depression.

Tobacco Smoking

Concurrent tobacco smoking may increase the metabolism of pentazocine. Higher dosages of pentazocine may be required for patients who smoke tobacco.

See also "Opiate Analgesics, General Monograph."

ADVERSE DRUG REACTIONS

Acute onset of confusion, disorientation, and hallucinations (usually visual) have been reported among some patients who were receiving recommended dosages of pentazocine. These ADRs usually have resolved spontaneously within hours of the discontinuation of pentazocine pharmacotherapy. The cause of these ADRs is unknown. Resume pentazocine pharmacotherapy cautiously among patients who experience these ADRs. Monitor them carefully for the recurrence of these ADRs, and if they recur, discontinue pentazocine pharmacotherapy. Further pentazocine pharmacotherapy is not advised.

Oral pentazocine pharmacotherapy commonly has been associated with nausea, sedation, somnolence, vertigo, and vomiting. Sedation may be more marked among elderly, frail, or debilitated patients. Injectable pentazocine pharmacotherapy has been commonly associated with dizziness, euphoria, lightheadedness, nausea, stinging upon injection, and vomiting. Ulceration (sloughing) and severe sclerosis of the skin and subcutaneous tissues, and, rarely, underlying muscles, have been reported with repeated multiple injections at one site. Avoid prescribing injectable pharmacotherapy whenever possible. If required, rotate injection sites carefully. In addition to these ADRs, pentazocine pharmacotherapy has been associated with the following ADRs, listed according to body system:

Cardiovascular: circulatory depression and shock, hypertension, syncope (fainting), and tachycardia
CNS: confusion, depression, disorientation, disturbed dreams, excitement, hallucinations, headache, insomnia, irritability, and sedation
Cutaneous: dermatitis, including severe itching (pruritus); edema of the face; flushed skin, including congestion and distention of blood vessels (plethora); nodules and soft tissue induration or cutaneous depression at injection sites; and toxic epidermal necrolysis
GI: constipation, cramps, diarrhea, dry mouth, and taste alterations
Hematologic: depression of white blood cells, particularly granulocytes (reversible), and eosinophilia (moderate, transient)
Musculoskeletal: weakness, and, rarely, tremor
Ocular: abnormal contraction of the pupils (miosis); blurred vision; constant, involuntary cyclical movement of the eyeballs (nystagmus); double vision (diplopia); and focusing difficulty
Otic: ringing in the ears (tinnitus)
Miscellaneous: chills

See also "Opiate Analgesics, General Monograph."

OVERDOSAGE

Signs and symptoms of pentazocine overdosage are similar to the signs and symptoms associated with other opiate analgesic overdosage (see "Opiate Analgesics, General Monograph"). However, pentazocine does not appear to produce the severe respiratory depression usually associated with opiate analgesic agonist overdosage. Regardless, pentazocine overdosage requires emergency symptomatic medical support of body systems with attention to increasing pentazocine elimination. Naloxone (Narcan®) is the specific and effective antagonist for the respiratory depression associated with pentazocine overdosage.

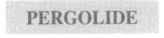

PERGOLIDE

(per' go lide)

TRADE NAME

Permax®

CLASSIFICATION

Antiparkinsonian (synthetic ergot derivative; dopamine agonist)

APPROVED INDICATIONS FOR NEUROPSYCHOLOGICAL DISORDERS

Adjunctive pharmacotherapy for the symptomatic management of:

- Parkinson's disease. Pergolide pharmacotherapy is prescribed in combination with levodopa pharmacotherapy (generally in combination with a peripheral decarboxylase inhibitor).

USUAL DOSAGE AND ADMINISTRATION

Parkinson's Disease

Adults: Initially, 0.05 mg daily orally in a single dose for two days. Increase the dosage by 0.1 to 0.15 mg every third day over the next 12 days. Commencing on day 15 of pergolide pharmacotherapy, increase the dosage by 0.25 mg every third day until an optimal dosage is achieved. The *mean* therapeutic dosage of pergolide is 3 mg daily orally in three divided doses.

MAXIMUM: 6 mg daily orally

Women who are, or who may become, pregnant: FDA Pregnancy Category B. Safety and efficacy of pergolide pharmacotherapy for women who are pregnant have not been established. Avoid prescribing pergolide pharmacotherapy to women who are pregnant. If pergolide pharmacotherapy is required, advise patients of potential benefits and possible risks to themselves and the embryo, fetus, or neonate. Collaboration with the patient's obstetrician is indicated.

Women who are breast-feeding: Safety and efficacy of pergolide pharmacotherapy for women who are breast-feeding and their neonates and infants have not been established. Avoid prescribing pergolide pharmacotherapy to women who are breast-feeding. If pergolide pharmacotherapy is required, breast-feeding probably should be discontinued.

For details and discussion regarding related basic principles of clinical pharmacology, readers are referred to the first text in this series, *The Pharmacologic Basis of Psychotherapeutics: An Introduction for Psychologists.*

Elderly, frail, or debilitated patients: Generally prescribe lower dosages for elderly, frail, or debilitated patients. These patients may be more sensitive to the pharmacologic actions of pergolide than are younger or healthier adult patients.

Children and adolescents younger than 18 years of age: Safety and efficacy of pergolide pharmacotherapy for children and adolescents who are younger than 18 years of age have not been established. Pergolide pharmacotherapy is *not* recommended for this age group.

Notes, Parkinson's Disease

Initiating pergolide pharmacotherapy: The optimal dosage of pergolide is generally achieved by means of a gradual increase in dosage and slow titration over approximately two weeks. This approach has been found to be of benefit in regard to minimizing the occurrence of associated ADRs. At the same time, as indicated by individual patient response, the levodopa dosage (generally in combination with a peripheral decarboxylase inhibitor) may be decreased cautiously.

Discontinuing pergolide pharmacotherapy: The abrupt discontinuation of pergolide pharmacotherapy has been associated with confusion and hallucinations that may persist for several days. Discontinue pergolide pharmacotherapy gradually over a period of one to two weeks to avoid these ADRs.

AVAILABLE DOSAGE FORMS, STORAGE, AND COMPATIBILITY

Tablets, oral: 0.05, 0.25, 1 mg

Notes

General instructions for patients: Instruct patients who are receiving pergolide pharmacotherapy to

- safely store pergolide oral tablets out of the reach of children in child-resistant containers at controlled room temperature (15° to 30°C; 59° to 86°F).
- obtain an available patient information sheet regarding pergolide pharmacotherapy from their pharmacist at the time that their prescription is dispensed. Encourage patients to clarify any questions that they may have regarding pergolide pharmacotherapy with their pharmacist or, if needed, to consult their prescribing psychologist.

PROPOSED MECHANISM OF ACTION

The exact mechanism of pergolide's antiparkinsonian action has not yet been fully determined. Pergolide appears to act primarily by stimulating postsynaptic dopamine (i.e., D1 and D2) receptors in the corpus striatum.

PHARMACOKINETICS/PHARMACODYNAMICS

Pergolide appears to be adequately absorbed from the GI tract following oral ingestion. Peak blood concentrations are generally achieved after 1 to 2 hours. Pergolide is ~90% bound to plasma proteins. It is completely metabolized to several active and inactive metabolites, which are excreted in the urine (55%), feces (40%), and breath (5%). Additional data are not available.

RELATIVE CONTRAINDICATIONS

Hypersensitivity to pergolide or other ergot derivatives

CAUTIONS AND COMMENTS

Caution patients who are receiving pergolide pharmacotherapy against

- performing activities that require alertness, judgment, or physical coordination (e.g., driving an automobile, operating dangerous equipment, supervising children) until their response to pergolide pharmacotherapy is known. Pergolide may affect these mental and physical functions adversely.

CLINICALLY SIGNIFICANT DRUG INTERACTIONS

Concurrent pergolide pharmacotherapy and the following may result in clinically significant drug interactions:

Antipsychotic Pharmacotherapy

Concurrent pergolide and antipsychotic pharmacotherapy may result in the decreased therapeutic efficacy of both drugs. Pergolide is a dopamine agonist, whereas antipsychotics are generally dopamine antagonists.

ADVERSE DRUG REACTIONS

Pergolide pharmacotherapy commonly has been associated with confusion, constipation, diarrhea, dizziness, dyskinesia, dyspepsia, hallucinations, hypotension (postural), insomnia, nausea, runny nose (rhinitis), and somnolence. Pergolide pharmacotherapy also has been associated with the following ADRs, listed according to body system:

Cardiovascular: congestive heart failure, palpitations, sinus tachycardia, syncope (fainting), and vasodilation
CNS: anxiety, depression, feelings of restlessness and an inability to sit (akathisia), paranoid reactions, and psychosis
Cutaneous: facial edema, peripheral edema, rash, and weight gain
GI: dry mouth, loss of appetite (anorexia), taste alterations, and vomiting
Musculoskeletal: twitching
Ophthalmic: double vision (diplopia)
Respiratory: hiccups and shortness of breath (dyspnea)
Miscellaneous: pain

OVERDOSAGE

Signs and symptoms of pergolide overdosage include agitation, hallucinations, hypotension, nausea, and vomiting. Pergolide overdosage requires emergency symptomatic medical support of body systems with attention to increasing pergolide elimination. Antipsychotic pharmacotherapy may be indicated for the symptomatic management of associated CNS stimulation. There is no known antidote.

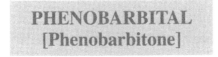

PHENOBARBITAL
[Phenobarbitone]

(fee noe bar' bi tal)

TRADE NAMES

Barbilixir®
Luminal®
Solfoton®

CLASSIFICATION

Sedative-hypnotic (barbiturate) (C-IV)

See "Barbiturates, General Monograph."

APPROVED INDICATIONS FOR NEUROPSYCHOLOGICAL DISORDERS

Pharmacotherapy for the prophylactic and symptomatic management of:

- seizure disorders: partial and tonic-clonic seizures

USUAL DOSAGE AND ADMINISTRATION

Seizure Disorders: Partial and Tonic-Clonic Seizures

Adults: 100 to 300 mg daily orally 30 minutes before retiring for bed in the evening

Women who are, or who may become, pregnant: FDA Pregnancy Category D. Safety and efficacy of phenobarbital pharmacotherapy for women who are pregnant have not been established. Numerous reports in the published literature have associated the use of phenobarbital with various fetal and congenital malformations (i.e., birth defects), including cleft lip and palate, congenital dislocated hip, microcephaly, and wide fontanelle. In addition, the neonatal barbiturate withdrawal syndrome, developmental delay, and psychomotor retardation have been noted among neonates and infants born to mothers who had used phenobarbital regularly during pregnancy. See "Barbiturates, General Monograph." Do *not* prescribe phenobarbital pharmacotherapy to women who are pregnant.

Women who are breast-feeding: Safety and efficacy of phenobarbital pharmacotherapy for women who are breast-feeding and their neonates and infants have not been established. Phenobarbital is excreted in sufficient quantities in breast milk to cause drowsiness and lethargy among nursing neonates and infants. These neonates and infants also may become addicted.

For details and discussion regarding related basic principles of clinical pharmacology, readers are referred to the first text in this series, *The Pharmacologic Basis of Psychotherapeutics: An Introduction for Psychologists.*

See "Barbiturates, General Monograph." Avoid prescribing phenobarbital pharmacotherapy to women who are breast-feeding. If phenobarbital pharmacotherapy is required, breast-feeding should be discontinued.

Elderly, frail, or debilitated patients: Generally prescribe lower dosages of phenobarbital for elderly, frail, or debilitated patients. These patients may be more sensitive to the pharmacologic actions of phenobarbital, particularly its respiratory depressant action, than are younger or healthier adult patients. Phenobarbital pharmacotherapy also has been associated with increased excitability among these patients.

Children: 3 to 6 mg/kg daily orally 30 minutes before bedtime. See also "Notes, Seizure Disorders."

Notes, Seizure Disorders

Phenobarbital pharmacotherapy has been associated with deficits on neuropsychologic test scores, primarily as a result of impaired short-term memory and memory concentration tasks among children. It also has been associated with problematic behavior (e.g., disobedience, hyperactivity, irritability, stubbornness) among children.

See "Barbiturates, General Monograph."

AVAILABLE DOSAGE FORMS, STORAGE, AND COMPATIBILITY

Capsules, oral: 16, 65 mg
Drops, oral: 16 mg/ml
Elixir, oral: 3, 4 mg/ml (contains 10% to 13.5% alcohol)
Injectables, intramuscular or intravenous: 30, 60, 65, 120, 130 mg/ml (contains 10% alcohol). Injectables generally are indicated for use among hospitalized patients who require phenobarbital pharmacotherapy for the immediate control of seizures.
Suppositories, rectal: 8, 15, 30, 60, 100, 120 mg
Tablets, oral: 8.5, 15, 16, 30, 32, 50, 60, 65, 100 mg

Notes

Phenobarbital is available in a variety of injectable, oral, and rectal formulations that can be prescribed to meet the individual needs of patients who require phenobarbital pharmacotherapy for the prophylactic or symptomatic management of seizure disorders.

Phenobarbital injectable formulations: Some injectable formulations of phenobarbital contain sodium bisulfite. Sulfites may cause hypersensitivity reactions, including anaphylactic reactions, among susceptible patients. Although relatively uncommon, these reactions appear to occur with a higher incidence among patients who have asthma.

Phenobarbital oral formulations: The phenobarbital oral drops (i.e., Sedadrops®) contain tartrazine. Tartrazine may cause hypersensitivity reactions, including bronchial asthma, among susceptible patients, particularly those who have a hypersensitivity to aspirin.

General instructions for patients: Instruct patients who are receiving phenobarbital pharmacotherapy to

- safely store phenobarbital oral dosage forms out of the reach of children in tightly closed child- and light-resistant containers.
- obtain an available patient information sheet regarding phenobarbital pharmacotherapy from their pharmacist at the time that their prescription is dispensed. Encourage patients to clarify any questions that they may have regarding phenobarbital pharmacotherapy with their pharmacist or, if needed, to consult their prescribing psychologist.

PROPOSED MECHANISM OF ACTION

The exact mechanism of phenobarbital's anticonvulsant action has not been fully determined. Phenobarbital appears to act primarily at the level of the thalamus, where it interferes with impulse transmission to the cortex. See also "Barbiturates, General Monograph."

PHARMACOKINETICS/PHARMACODYNAMICS

Phenobarbital is slowly but well absorbed (90% to 100%) following oral ingestion. Peak blood concentrations are generally achieved within 12 hours. Onset of action depends on the method of administration, but is generally within 60 minutes. After intravenous injection, onset of action occurs within 5 minutes. The onset of action following intramuscular injection is slightly slower than that following oral ingestion or rectal insertion.

The duration of action is 6 to 12 hours. Phenobarbital is ~50% plasma protein bound and has an apparent volume of distribution of 0.5 liters/kg. Of the barbiturates, phenobarbital is the least soluble and has the slowest distribution. Phenobarbital is not as extensively metabolized as other barbiturates because of its low lipid solubility. Almost 25% is excreted unchanged in the urine. The half-life of elimination is ~4 days (range: 80 to 120 hours). The total body clearance ranges from 4 to 5 ml/minute and the half-life of elimination ranges from ~2 to 6 days.

Therapeutic Drug Monitoring

Blood samples for periodic therapeutic drug monitoring should be obtained from trough blood concentrations (i.e., just before the next dose). In cases of suspected toxicity, blood samples may be obtained at any time. Generally, phenobarbital blood concentrations of 10 μg/ml produce sedation; 40 μg/ml produce sleep; 50 μg/ml (215 mmol/liter), or higher, are toxic and may produce coma; and 80 μg/ml, or higher, may be fatal.

RELATIVE CONTRAINDICATIONS

Liver dysfunction, severe
Hypersensitivity to phenobarbital or other barbiturates
Kidney dysfunction, severe
Porphyria
Pregnancy
Respiratory depression, severe

CAUTIONS AND COMMENTS

Long-term phenobarbital pharmacotherapy, or regular personal use, may lead to addiction and habituation. Sudden discontinuation of long-term phenobarbital pharmacotherapy, or regular personal use, can result in the barbiturate withdrawal syndrome. This withdrawal syndrome is considered to be a medical emergency that can be fatal if not appropriately treated.

Prescribe phenobarbital pharmacotherapy cautiously to patients who

- are concurrently receiving oral anticoagulant pharmacotherapy because of the associated difficulty in stabilizing prothrombin times.
- have CNS or respiratory depression. Phenobarbital may increase both CNS and respiratory depression among these patients.
- have kidney or liver dysfunction. The metabolism and elimination of phenobarbital may be prolonged among these patients.

Caution patients who are receiving phenobarbital pharmacotherapy against

- performing activities that require alertness, judgment, and physical coordination (e.g., driving an automobile, operating dangerous equipment, supervising children) until their response to phenobarbital pharmacotherapy is known. Phenobarbital may affect these mental and physical functions adversely.

In addition to this general precaution, caution patients who are receiving phenobarbital pharmacotherapy to

- inform their prescribing psychologist if they begin or discontinue any other pharmacotherapy while receiving phenobarbital pharmacotherapy.

CLINICALLY SIGNIFICANT DRUG INTERACTIONS

Concurrent phenobarbital pharmacotherapy and the following may result in clinically significant drug interactions:

Alcohol Use

Concurrent alcohol use may increase the CNS depressant action of phenobarbital. Advise patients to avoid, or limit, their use of alcohol while receiving phenobarbital pharmacotherapy.

Pharmacotherapy With CNS Depressants and Other Drugs That Produce CNS Depression

Concurrent phenobarbital pharmacotherapy and pharmacotherapy with opiate analgesics, other sedative-hypnotics, and other drugs that produce CNS depression (e.g., antihistamines, phenothiazines, TCAs) may result in additive CNS depression.

Pharmacotherapy With Drugs That Are Primarily Metabolized by the Liver

Phenobarbital may stimulate the production of hepatic microsomal enzymes that are responsible for the metabolism of many different drugs, resulting in decreased therapeutic efficacy of these drugs. Whenever phenobarbital is prescribed or discontinued, attention must be given to the effect on the patient's other pharmacotherapy (e.g., corticosteroid, oral anticoagulant, oral contraceptive, or quinidine [Biquin®] pharmacotherapy). Collaboration with other prescribers may be required so that dosages can be appropriately adjusted (i.e., increased or decreased), if necessary.

See also "Barbiturates, General Monograph."

ADVERSE DRUG REACTIONS

Phenobarbital pharmacotherapy has been associated with mental changes and reduced performance on neuropsychologic tests, osteomalacia, respiratory depression, sedation, and skin rash.

See also "Barbiturates, General Monograph."

OVERDOSAGE

See "Barbiturates, General Monograph."

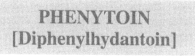

PHENYTOIN
[Diphenylhydantoin]

(fen′ i toyn)

TRADE NAME

Dilantin®

CLASSIFICATION

Anticonvulsant (hydantoin derivative)

APPROVED INDICATIONS FOR NEUROPSYCHOLOGICAL DISORDERS

Pharmacotherapy for the prophylactic and symptomatic management of:

- seizure disorders: partial seizures with complex symptomatology and tonic-clonic seizures. Also, injectable phenytoin pharmacotherapy is indicated for the symptomatic management of status epilepticus and for the prevention and treatment of seizures occurring during or following neurosurgery.

USUAL DOSAGE AND ADMINISTRATION

Seizure Disorders: Partial Seizures and Tonic-Clonic Seizures

Adults: 300 mg daily orally in three divided doses

MAXIMUM: 600 mg daily orally

Women who are, or who may become, pregnant: FDA Pregnancy Category D. Safety and efficacy of phenytoin pharmacotherapy for women who are pregnant have not been established. However, published clinical reports and studies have implicated maternal phenytoin pharmacotherapy with an increased incidence of congenital malformations (i.e., birth defects). These teratogenic effects have been characterized as the fetal hydantoin syndrome and include cardiac malformations, cleft lip and palate, CNS malformations, and developmental delay. Phenytoin use during pregnancy also has been associated with neonatal coagulation defects, which have resulted in hemorrhage. Vitamin K_1 (phytonadione) pharmacotherapy for the mother, one month prior to and during delivery, and for the neonate, upon delivery, is recommended in order to prevent or treat this coagulation defect. Avoid prescribing phenytoin pharmacotherapy to women

For details and discussion regarding related basic principles of clinical pharmacology, readers are referred to the first text in this series, *The Pharmacologic Basis of Psychotherapeutics: An Introduction for Psychologists.*

who are pregnant. If phenytoin pharmacotherapy is required, advise patients of potential bene-fits and possible risks to themselves and the embryo, fetus, or neonate. Collaboration with the patient's obstetrician is indicated.

Women who are breast-feeding: Safety and efficacy of phenytoin pharmacotherapy for women who are breast-feeding and their neonates and infants have not been established. Al-though small amounts of phenytoin generally are excreted in breast milk, idiosyncratic reactions (e.g., cyanosis, methemoglobinemia) have been reported among breast-fed neonates and infants. Avoid prescribing phenytoin pharmacotherapy to women who are breast-feeding. If phenytoin pharmacotherapy is required, breast-feeding probably should be discontinued. Collaboration with the patient's pediatrician may be indicated.

Elderly adults: See "Usual Dosage and Administration" for adults. Generally prescribe lower dosages for elderly, frail, or debilitated patients. These patients may be more sensitive to the pharmacologic actions of phenytoin than are younger or healthier adult patients.

Children and adolescents: Initially, phenytoin pharmacotherapy is prescribed for chil-dren and adolescents, depending on age, according to the following table:

Age	Usual phenytoin dosage
6 months to 3 years	7 to 9 mg/kg/day orally in two or three divided doses
4 to 6 years	6.5 mg/kg/day orally in two or three divided doses
7 to 9 years	6 mg/kg/day orally in two or three divided doses
10 to 16 years	3 to 5 mg/kg/day orally in two or three divided doses

MAXIMUM: 300 mg daily orally

Notes, Seizure Disorders: Partial Seizures and Tonic-Clonic Seizures

Phenytoin pharmacotherapy should be guided by appropriate TDM.

Initiating and maintaining phenytoin pharmacotherapy: Phenytoin usually can be pre-scribed as a single daily dose for most adults. Adjust phenytoin oral maintenance dosages, when-ever possible, at intervals of at least 7 days. Waiting for 7 days will allow steady-state levels to be achieved and better evaluation of patient response.

Discontinuing phenytoin pharmacotherapy: Abrupt discontinuation of phenytoin phar-macotherapy among patients who have seizure disorders may result in withdrawal seizures and status epilepticus. Discontinue phenytoin pharmacotherapy by gradually reducing the dosage, unless therapeutically contraindicated, over a period of at least 1 week. This gradual reduction of dosage will help to reduce the risk for withdrawal seizures, including status epilepticus.

Seizure Disorders: Status Epilepticus

Adults: 10 to 15 mg/kg intravenously. Slowly inject phenytoin intravenously at a rate *not* exceeding 50 mg/minute. Note that this will require, for example, ~20 minutes for the intra-venous injection of phenytoin to a 70-kg adult patient.

Children: 15 to 20 mg/kg intravenously. Slowly inject phenytoin intravenously at a rate *not* exceeding 3 mg/kg/minute or 50 mg/minute, whichever is *less.*

Notes, Seizure Disorders: Status Epilepticus

Other appropriate adjunctive pharmacotherapy (e.g., intravenous barbiturate or benzodiazepine pharmacotherapy) may be required for the rapid control of status epilepticus because of the required slow rate of intravenous phenytoin administration. See also the fosphenytoin monograph.

Seizure Disorders: Prophylaxis for Neurosurgery

Adults: 100 to 200 mg intramuscularly every four hours during neurosurgery and every four hours during the postoperative period

AVAILABLE DOSAGE FORMS, STORAGE, AND COMPATIBILITY

Capsules, oral: 30, 100 mg
Capsules, oral extended-release: 30, 100 mg
Suspensions, oral: 6, 25 mg/ml (orange-vanilla flavored) (contains 0.6% alcohol)
Tablets, oral chewable: 50 mg
Injectable, intravenous: 50 mg/ml (contains 10% alcohol and 40% propylene glycol)

Notes

Phenytoin sodium 100 mg is approximately equivalent to phenytoin acid 92 mg.

General instructions for patients: Instruct patients who are receiving phenytoin pharmacotherapy, as appropriate, to

- safely store phenytoin oral capsules and tablets out of the reach of children in tightly closed, light- and child-resistant containers at controlled room temperature (15° to 25°C; 59° to 77°F). Discard discolored capsules safely and appropriately.
- obtain an available patient information sheet regarding phenytoin pharmacotherapy from their pharmacist at the time that their prescription is dispensed. Encourage patients to clarify any questions that they may have regarding phenytoin pharmacotherapy with their pharmacist or, if needed, to consult their prescribing psychologist.

PROPOSED MECHANISM OF ACTION

The exact mechanism of action of phenytoin for the prophylactic and symptomatic management of seizure disorders has not yet been fully determined. However, a major component of phenytoin's anticonvulsant action appears to be related to the reduction of post-tetanic potentiation (PTP) of synaptic transmission and associated limitation of seizure discharge and spread from its focus within the motor cortex. This mechanism appears to be mediated by the prevention of the accumulation of intracellular sodium by either reducing the passive influx of sodium or increasing the efficiency of the sodium pump during tetanic stimulation. Phenytoin also reduces the maximal activity of the brainstem centers that are responsible for the tonic phase of tonic-clonic (grand mal) seizures.

PHARMACOKINETICS/PHARMACODYNAMICS

Phenytoin is slowly but generally well absorbed (~90%) following oral ingestion. Peak blood concentrations are achieved in 3 to 12 hours. Phenytoin is ~90% bound to plasma proteins and has a mean apparent volume of distribution of 45 liters. It is metabolized extensively in the liver with ~1% excreted in unchanged form in the urine. Phenytoin displays dose-dependent kinetics. Its mean Vmax = 6 mg/kg/day and Kmax = 6 mg/liter. The mean half-life of elimination of phenytoin ranges from 6 to 24 hours, depending upon blood concentration (i.e., dosage). Therefore, a small dosage increase may result in a large increase in phenytoin blood concentration, particularly as the elimination process becomes saturated. Phenytoin pharmacokinetics also is subject to wide interpatient variability.

Therapeutic Drug Monitoring

Effective blood concentrations of phenytoin for the suppression of tonic-clonic seizures is 10 µg/ml. Initial signs and symptoms of toxicity (e.g., nystagmus) are generally not observed until phenytoin blood concentrations equal or exceed 20 µg/ml. More serious ADRs (e.g., incoordination [ataxia]) generally are not observed until phenytoin blood concentrations equal or exceed 30 µg/ml.

RELATIVE CONTRAINDICATIONS

Hypersensitivity to phenytoin or other hydantoin derivatives. *Note*: In addition to this general contraindication, intravenous phenytoin pharmacotherapy is contraindicated for patients who have the following: Adams–Stokes syndrome; second- and third-degree AV block; SA block; and sinus bradycardia. Phenytoin decreases the automaticity of cardiac tissue.

CAUTIONS AND COMMENTS

Prescribe phenytoin pharmacotherapy cautiously for patients who

- have diabetes. Phenytoin pharmacotherapy may raise blood glucose concentrations among patients who have diabetes. This effect appears to occur as a result of phenytoin's inhibitory effects on insulin release.
- have osteoporosis. Phenytoin pharmacotherapy has been associated with osteomalacia. This effect appears to be due to phenytoin's interference with vitamin D metabolism.
- are undergoing neuropsychological testing. Phenytoin pharmacotherapy has been associated with deficits on neuropsychological tests among children. This effect appears to occur primarily as a result of associated impairment of attention, problem solving, and visuomotor task performance.

Caution patients who are receiving phenytoin pharmacotherapy against

- performing activities that require alertness, judgment, or physical coordination (e.g., driving an automobile, operating dangerous equipment, supervising children) until their response to phenytoin pharmacotherapy is known. Phenytoin may affect these mental and physical functions adversely.

In addition to this general precaution, caution patients who are receiving phenytoin pharmacotherapy to

- inform their prescribing psychologist if they begin or discontinue any other pharmacotherapy while receiving phenytoin pharmacotherapy.
- inform their prescribing psychologist if they develop a skin rash. Phenytoin pharmacotherapy should be discontinued immediately if a skin rash develops. The development of a skin rash may be symptomatic of such serious ADRs as lupus erythematosus, Stevens–Johnson syndrome, or toxic epidermal necrolysis. Collaboration with the patient's family physician or a specialist (e.g., dermatologist) is indicated for the medical diagnosis and management of these serious ADRs.

CLINICALLY SIGNIFICANT DRUG INTERACTIONS

Concurrent phenytoin pharmacotherapy and the following may result in clinically significant drug interactions:

Alcohol Use

Concurrent alcohol use may increase the CNS depressant action of phenytoin. Advise patients to avoid, or limit, their use of alcohol while receiving phenytoin pharmacotherapy. (See also other listed interactions.)

Pharmacotherapy With CNS Depressants and Other Drugs That Produce CNS Depression

Concurrent phenytoin pharmacotherapy and pharmacotherapy with opiate analgesics, sedative-hypnotics, or other drugs that produce CNS depression (e.g., antihistamines, phenothiazines, TCAs) may result in additive CNS depression.

Pharmacotherapy With Drugs That May Increase Phenytoin Blood Concentrations

Several different drugs, including alcohol (acute intoxication), amiodarone (Cardarone®), chloramphenicol (Chloromycetin®), cimetidine (Tagamet®), dicumarol, disulfiram (Antabuse®), erythromycin (E-Mycin®), ethosuximide (Zarontin®), fluconazole (Diflucan®), fluoxetine (Prozac®), isoniazid (INH®), ketoconazole (Nizoral®), methylphenidate (Ritalin®), omeprazole (Prilosec®), phenothiazines, phenylbutazone (Novo-Butazone®), salicylates, sulfonamides, ticlopidine (Ticlid®), topiramate (Topamax®), trazodone (Desyrel®), valproic acid (Depakene®), and warfarin (Coumadin®), can *increase* phenytoin blood concentrations, primarily by means of inhibition of phenytoin's hepatic metabolism. Phenytoin blood concentrations should be monitored carefully whenever pharmacotherapy with these drugs is either initiated or discontinued. If necessary, appropriate modifications should be made to the phenytoin dosage. Collaboration with the prescribers of these potentially interacting drugs may be indicated.

Pharmacotherapy With Drugs That Decrease Phenytoin Blood Concentrations

Several drugs, including alcohol (chronic use), carbamazepine (Tegretol®), ciprofloxacin (Cipro®), diazoxide (Hyperstat®), phenobarbital (Luminal®), reserpine (Serpasil®), rifampin (Rimactane®), sucralfate (Sulcrate®), theophylline (Theo-Dur®), and vigabatrin (Sabril®), can *decrease* phenytoin blood concentrations, primarily by means of induction of phenytoin's hepatic metabolism. Phenytoin blood concentrations should be monitored carefully whenever pharmacotherapy with these drugs is either initiated or discontinued. If necessary, appropriate modifications should be made to the phenytoin dosage. Collaboration with the prescribers of these potentially interacting drugs may be indicated.

Pharmacotherapy With Drugs for Which Therapeutic Efficacy May Be Reduced by Concurrent Phenytoin Pharmacotherapy

Several different drugs, including corticosteroids, diazoxide (Hyperstat®), digoxin (Lanoxin®), doxycycline (Doxycin®), estrogens, furosemide (Lasix®), levodopa (Dopar®), methadone, oral contraceptives, quinidine (Biquin®), theophylline (Theo-Dur®), vitamin D, and warfarin (Coumadin®), may have their therapeutic efficacy diminished by concurrent phenytoin pharmacotherapy. These potential interactions appear to occur primarily by means of the induction by phenytoin of their hepatic metabolism. Patients who are receiving concurrent pharmacotherapy should be monitored carefully for possible therapeutic failure. Appropriate changes to their prescribed pharmacotherapy should be made, if required. Collaboration with the prescribers of these potentially interacting drugs is indicated.

ADVERSE DRUG REACTIONS

Phenytoin pharmacotherapy has been commonly associated with decreased coordination, mental confusion, and slurred speech. Phenytoin pharmacotherapy also has been associated with the following ADRs, listed according to body system:

Cardiovascular: rarely, decreased systolic blood pressure
CNS: depression, dizziness, drowsiness, fatigue, headache, insomnia, irritability, nervousness (transient), unsteadiness, and reduced performance on neuropsychological tests
Cutaneous: transient skin rashes of the morbilliform, or measles-like, type. Rarely, rashes indicative of potentially fatal cutaneous reactions, including lupus erythematosus, Stevens–Johnson syndrome, and toxic epidermal necrolysis, may occur. (See "Cautions and Comments.")
GI: constipation, gingival hyperplasia, nausea, and vomiting
Hematologic: rarely, agranulocytosis and thrombocytopenia
Hepatic: abnormal liver function tests, liver damage, and toxic hepatitis
Musculoskeletal: incoordination (ataxia), motor twitching, and tremor
Ophthalmic: blurred vision and double vision (diplopia)

Peripheral Nervous System: sensory peripheral neuropathy, particularly among patients who are receiving long-term phenytoin pharmacotherapy
Renal: rarely, abnormal kidney function tests
Miscellaneous: hypertrichosis and Peyronie's disease

OVERDOSAGE

Defective voluntary muscular coordination (ataxia), difficult and defective speech with intact mental function (dysarthria), and constant, cyclical, involuntary movement of the eyeball (nystagmus) are generally the cardinal initial signs and symptoms of phenytoin overdosage. Signs and symptoms of phenytoin overdosage also include circulatory depression, coma, hyperflexia, hypotension, lethargy, nausea, respiratory depression, slurred speech, and vomiting. Phenytoin overdosage is potentially fatal and should be treated as a medical emergency requiring symptomatic medical support of body systems with attention to increasing phenytoin elimination. There is no known antidote.

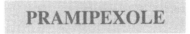

PRAMIPEXOLE

(pram i pex' ole)

TRADE NAME

Mirapex®

CLASSIFICATION

Antiparkinsonian (benzothiazolamine derivative, non-ergot dopamine D2 receptor agonist)

APPROVED INDICATIONS FOR NEUROPSYCHOLOGICAL DISORDERS

Pharmacotherapy for the symptomatic management of:

• Parkinson's disease: idiopathic

USUAL DOSAGE AND ADMINISTRATION

Parkinson's Disease: Idiopathic

Adults: Initially, 0.375 mg daily orally in three divided doses for seven days. Then 0.75 mg daily orally in three divided doses for an additional seven days. Increase the daily oral dosage by 0.75 mg at weekly intervals until maximal therapeutic benefit is achieved with a minimum of ADRs.

MAXIMUM: 4.5 mg daily orally

Women who are, or who may become, pregnant: FDA Pregnancy Category C. Safety and efficacy of pramipexole pharmacotherapy for women who are pregnant have not been established. Avoid prescribing pramipexole pharmacotherapy to women who are pregnant.

Women who are breast-feeding: Safety and efficacy of pramipexole pharmacotherapy for women who are breast-feeding and their neonates and infants have not been established. However, pramipexole is known to inhibit prolactin secretion and is believed to be excreted in breast milk. Avoid prescribing pramipexole pharmacotherapy to women who are breast-feeding.

Elderly patients and those who have liver or kidney dysfunction: No special adjustments to the usual recommended adult dosage are required for elderly patients. Although the effect of severe liver dysfunction has not been clinically evaluated, it is not expected that dosage

For details and discussion regarding related basic principles of clinical pharmacology, readers are referred to the first text in this series, *The Pharmacologic Basis of Psychotherapeutics: An Introduction for Psychologists.*

adjustments are required for patients who have liver dysfunction. Pramipexole undergoes very little hepatic metabolism (see "Pharmacokinetics/Pharmacodynamics"). However, the pramipexole dosage must be reduced appropriately for patients who have severe kidney dysfunction. See the table "Pramipexole Dosing for Adult Patients Who Have Kidney Dysfunction."

Pramipexole dosing for adult patients who have kidney dysfunction.

Creatinine clearance	Initial dosage	Maximal dosage
$\geqslant$ 60 ml/minute	0.375 mg daily orally in three divided doses	4.5 mg daily orally in three divided doses
35 to 59 ml/minute	0.25 mg daily orally in two divided doses	3 mg daily orally in two divided doses
15 to 34 ml/minute	0.25 mg daily orally in a single dose	1.5 mg daily orally in a single dose
< 15 ml/minute	Safety and efficacy of pramipexole pharmacotherapy have not been established for patients who have a creatinine clearance of less than 15 ml/minute. Pramipexole pharmacotherapy is *not* recommended for these patients.	Safety and efficacy of pramipexole pharmacotherapy have not been established for patients who have a creatinine clearance of less than 15 ml/minute. Pramipexole pharmacotherapy is *not* recommended for these patients.

Children and adolescents younger than 18 years of age: Safety and efficacy of pramipexole pharmacotherapy for children and adolescents who are younger than 18 years of age have not been established. Pramipexole pharmacotherapy is *not* recommended for this age group.

Notes, Parkinson's Disease: Idiopathic

Pramipexole pharmacotherapy may be prescribed for the symptomatic management of Parkinson's disease alone or in combination with levodopa pharmacotherapy. Generally, combination pramipexole and levodopa pharmacotherapy can effect a reduction in the previous dosage of levodopa. Pramipexole also may elicit a reduced "off" time among a significant minority of patients who have idiopathic Parkinson's disease and who are experiencing a deteriorating response to levodopa pharmacotherapy (i.e., the "on–off" phenomenon).

AVAILABLE DOSAGE FORMS, STORAGE, AND COMPATIBILITY

Tablets, oral: 0.125, 0.25, 0.5, 1, 1.5 mg

Notes

General instructions for patients: Instruct patients who are receiving pramipexole pharmacotherapy to

- safely store pramipexole oral tablets out of the reach of children in child-resistant containers at controlled room temperature (15° to 30°C; 59° to 86°F).
- ingest each dose of their pramipexole tablets with food to prevent or minimize associated nausea.
- obtain an available patient information sheet regarding pramipexole pharmacotherapy from their pharmacist at the time that their prescription is dispensed. Encourage patients to clarify any questions that they may have regarding pramipexole pharmacotherapy with their pharmacist or, if needed, to consult their prescribing psychologist.

PROPOSED MECHANISM OF ACTION

The exact mechanism of antiparkinsonian action of pramipexole has not yet been fully determined. However, pramipexole is a dopamine receptor agonist with a demonstrated high affinity for D2 receptors and a particularly high affinity for the D3 receptor subtype. Thus, it is thought that pramipexole elicits its action by directly stimulating post-synaptic dopamine receptors within the corpus striatum.

PHARMACOKINETICS/PHARMACODYNAMICS

Pramipexole is rapidly and well absorbed following oral ingestion ($F = 0.9$). Peak blood concentrations are generally achieved in ~2 hours. The ingestion of food does not affect absorption. Pramipexole is ~15% bound to plasma proteins and has an apparent volume of distribution of ~500 liters. Pramipexole is excreted in the urine primarily in unchanged form (~90%). The half-life of elimination is ~12 hours (range: 8 to 16 hours) and the mean total body clearance is ~6 ml/kg/minute.

RELATIVE CONTRAINDICATIONS

Hypersensitivity to pramipexole

CAUTIONS AND COMMENTS

Prescribe pramipexole pharmacotherapy cautiously to patients who

- have kidney dysfunction. See "Usual Dosage and Administration" for "Elderly Patients and Those Who Have Liver or Kidney Dysfunction."

Caution patients who are receiving pramipexole pharmacotherapy against

- performing activities that require alertness, judgment, or physical coordination (e.g., driving an automobile, operating dangerous equipment, supervising children) until their response to pramipexole pharmacotherapy is known. Pramipexole may affect these mental and physical functions adversely.

CLINICALLY SIGNIFICANT DRUG INTERACTIONS

Concurrent pramipexole pharmacotherapy and the following may result in clinically significant drug interactions:

Alcohol Use

Concurrent alcohol use may increase the CNS depressant action of pramipexole. Advise patients to avoid, or limit, their use of alcohol while receiving pramipexole pharmacotherapy.

Cimetidine Pharmacotherapy

The renal tubular secretion of pramipexole may be significantly reduced by concurrent cimetidine (Tagamet®) pharmacotherapy. This interaction may result in an ~40% increase in the half-life of elimination of pramipexole.

Pharmacotherapy With CNS Depressants and Other Drugs That Produce CNS Depression

Concurrent pramipexole pharmacotherapy and pharmacotherapy with opiate analgesics, sedative-hypnotics, or other drugs that produce CNS depression (e.g., antihistamines, phenothiazines, TCAs) may result in additive CNS depression.

ADVERSE DRUG REACTIONS

Pramipexole pharmacotherapy commonly has been associated with the following ADRs: a reduction or loss of strength generally associated with muscular or cerebellar disease (asthenia), constipation, dizziness, dyspepsia, hallucinations, insomnia, malaise, nausea, and somnolence. Elderly patients, in particular, appear to be at increased risk for pramipexole-induced hallucinations and should be informed of the possible occurrence of this ADR prior to the initiation of pramipexole pharmacotherapy. Pramipexole pharmacotherapy also has been associated with confusion and dyskinesia, particularly among patients who have advanced Parkinson's disease.

OVERDOSAGE

In the absence of reported clinical experience with pramipexole overdosage, it should be treated as a medical emergency requiring symptomatic medical support of body systems with attention to increasing pramipexole elimination. There is no known antidote.

PRIMIDONE
[Desoxyphenobarbital; Primaclone]

(pri′ mi done)

TRADE NAME

Mysoline®

CLASSIFICATION

Anticonvulsant (phenobarbital structural analogue)

APPROVED INDICATIONS FOR NEUROPSYCHOLOGICAL DISORDERS

Pharmacotherapy for the prophylactic and symptomatic management of:

- seizure disorders: partial seizures with complex symptomatology (i.e., psychomotor seizures) and tonic-clonic (grand mal) seizures

USUAL DOSAGE AND ADMINISTRATION

Seizure Disorders: Partial and Tonic-Clonic Seizures

Adults: Initially, 100 to 125 mg daily orally, 30 minutes before retiring for bed in the evening for days 1 to 3 of primidone pharmacotherapy. Then, 200 to 250 mg daily orally in two divided doses for days 4 to 6. Then, 300 to 375 mg daily orally in three divided doses for days 7 to 9. Continue with maintenance pharmacotherapy (see "Maintenance," below).

MAINTENANCE: The usual maintenance dosage is 750 to 1000 mg daily orally in three or four divided doses

MAXIMUM: 2000 mg daily orally

Women who are, or who may become, pregnant: FDA Pregnancy Category D. Safety and efficacy of primidone pharmacotherapy for women who are pregnant have not been established. Primidone pharmacotherapy during pregnancy has been associated with various congenital malformations (i.e., birth defects). It also has been associated with neonatal coagulation defects and resultant neonatal hemorrhage. Vitamin K_1 (phytonadione) administration both to the mother, for 1 month prior to and during delivery, and to the neonate at delivery is recommended in order to prevent or treat this coagulation defect. Avoid prescribing primidone pharmacotherapy

For details and discussion regarding related basic principles of clinical pharmacology, readers are referred to the first text in this series, *The Pharmacologic Basis of Psychotherapeutics: An Introduction for Psychologists.*

to women who are pregnant. If primidone pharmacotherapy is required, advise patients of potential benefits and possible risks to themselves and the embryo, fetus, or neonate. Collaboration with the patient's obstetrician is indicated.

Women who are breast-feeding: Safety and efficacy of primidone pharmacotherapy for women who are breast-feeding and their neonates and infants have not been established. Primidone, and its active metabolites phenobarbital and phenylethylmalonamide, are excreted in breast milk. Avoid prescribing primidone pharmacotherapy to women who are breast-feeding. If primidone pharmacotherapy is required, breast-feeding probably should be discontinued.

Elderly, frail, or debilitated patients: Generally prescribe lower dosages for elderly, frail, or debilitated patients. These patients may be more sensitive to the pharmacologic actions of primidone than are younger or healthier adult patients.

Children 8 years of age and older: Initially, 50 mg daily orally at bedtime for days 1 to 3 of primidone pharmacotherapy. Then 100 mg daily orally in two divided doses for days 4 to 6. Then, 200 mg daily orally in two divided doses for days 7 to 9. Continue with maintenance pharmacotherapy according to individual patient response (see "Maintenance," below).

MAINTENANCE: The usual maintenance dosage is 375 to 750 mg daily orally in three divided doses; *or* 12 to 25 mg/kg daily orally in 2 or 3 divided doses.

Notes, Seizure Disorders: Partial and Tonic-Clonic Seizures

Initiating and maintaining primidone pharmacotherapy: See "Usual Dosage and Administration."

Discontinuing primidone pharmacotherapy: Abrupt discontinuation of primidone pharmacotherapy may result in status epilepticus. The primidone dosage should be reduced gradually, unless therapeutically contraindicated, over a period of 2 weeks, until it is completely discontinued in order to reduce the risk for withdrawal seizures, including status epilepticus.

See the phenobarbital monograph.

AVAILABLE DOSAGE FORMS, STORAGE, AND COMPATIBILITY

Suspension, oral: 250 mg/5 ml
Tablets, oral: 50, 250 mg
Tablets, oral chewable: 125 mg✳

Notes

General instructions for patients: Instruct patients who are receiving primidone pharmacotherapy to

- shake the primidone oral suspension well before measuring each dose to help to assure that an accurate dose is measured and ingested.

- safely store the primidone oral suspension and oral tablets out of the reach of children in tightly closed, light- and child-resistant containers at controlled room temperature (15° to 25°C; 59° to 77°F).
- obtain an available patient information sheet regarding primidone pharmacotherapy from their pharmacist at the time that their prescription is dispensed. Encourage patients to clarify any questions that they may have regarding primidone pharmacotherapy with their pharmacist or, if needed, to consult their prescribing psychologist.

PROPOSED MECHANISM OF ACTION

The exact mechanism of primidone's anticonvulsant action has not yet been fully established. Primidone and two of its metabolites possess anticonvulsant activity. Primidone is metabolized to the active metabolites, phenobarbital and phenylethylmalonamide (PEMA). See the phenobarbital monograph for additional information regarding the mechanism of action of these metabolites.

PHARMACOKINETICS/PHARMACODYNAMICS

Primidone is well absorbed from the GI tract (~90%) following oral ingestion. Peak blood concentrations are achieved in ~4 hours. Primidone is ~20% bound to plasma proteins and has a mean apparent volume of distribution of 0.7 liters/kg. Approximately 50% of primidone is excreted in unchanged form in the urine. The mean half-life of elimination is ~15 hours. The mean total body clearance is ~2 liters/kg/hour.

Therapeutic Drug Monitoring

Primidone is metabolized to phenobarbital and PEMA. PEMA is more toxic than primidone and possesses relatively weak anticonvulsant activity. See the phenobarbital monograph for TDM guidelines for phenobarbital.

RELATIVE CONTRAINDICATIONS

Hypersensitivity to primidone or phenobarbital
Porphyria

CAUTIONS AND COMMENTS

Prescribe primidone pharmacotherapy cautiously to patients who have the conditions listed in the "Cautions and Comments" section of the phenobarbital monograph.
Caution patients who are receiving primidone pharmacotherapy against

- performing activities that require alertness, judgment, or physical coordination (e.g., driving an automobile, operating dangerous equipment, supervising children) until their response to primidone pharmacotherapy is known. Primidone may affect these mental and physical functions adversely.

In addition to this general precaution, caution patients who are receiving primidone pharmacotherapy to

- inform their prescribing psychologist if they begin or discontinue any other pharmacotherapy while receiving primidone pharmacotherapy.

CLINICALLY SIGNIFICANT DRUG INTERACTIONS

Concurrent primidone pharmacotherapy and the following may result in clinically significant drug interactions:

Alcohol Use

Concurrent alcohol use may increase the CNS depressant action of primidone. Advise patients to avoid, or limit, their use of alcohol while receiving primidone pharmacotherapy.

Pharmacotherapy With CNS Depressants and Other Drugs That Produce CNS Depression

Concurrent primidone pharmacotherapy and pharmacotherapy with opiate analgesics, sedative-hypnotics, or other drugs that produce CNS depression (e.g., antihistamines, phenothiazines, TCAs) may result in additive CNS depression.

See also the phenobarbital monograph.

ADVERSE DRUG REACTIONS

Primidone pharmacotherapy has been commonly associated with dizziness, incoordination (ataxia), lethargy, loss of appetite (anorexia), nausea, vertigo, and vomiting. Primidone pharmacotherapy also has been associated with the following ADRs, listed according to body system:

CNS: drowsiness, fatigue, hyperexcitability (among children), and psychosis (rare).
Cutaneous: loss of hair (alopecia), lupus-like syndrome, and morbilliform (measles-like) rash.
Hematologic: agranulocytosis (rare), eosinophilia, leukopenia, and megaloblastic anemia (rare and usually responsive to folic acid pharmacotherapy. Generally, the discontinuation of primidone pharmacotherapy is not required.).
Ophthalmic: diplopia and nystagmus.
Miscellaneous: edema of the eyeballs, leg edema, and malignant lymphoma-like syndrome.

See also "Adverse Drug Reactions" section of the phenobarbital monograph.

OVERDOSAGE

See "Overdosage" section of the phenobarbital monograph.

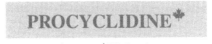

PROCYCLIDINE

(proe sye′ kli deen)

TRADE NAME

Kemadrin®

CLASSIFICATION

Antiparkinsonian (synthetic tertiary amine antimuscarinic)

APPROVED INDICATIONS FOR NEUROPSYCHOLOGICAL DISORDERS

Pharmacotherapy for the symptomatic management of:

- Parkinson's disease: arteriosclerotic, drug-induced, idiopathic, and post-encephalitic

USUAL DOSAGE AND ADMINISTRATION

Parkinson's Disease: Arteriosclerotic, Drug-Induced, Idiopathic, and Post-Encephalitic

Adults: 7.5 mg daily orally in three divided doses. If this dosage is well tolerated and additional therapeutic effect is required, the dosage may gradually be increased to 15 mg daily orally in three divided doses.

MAXIMUM: 30 mg daily orally

Women who are, or who may become, pregnant: FDA Pregnancy Category "not established." Safety and efficacy of procyclidine pharmacotherapy for women who are pregnant have not been established. Avoid prescribing procyclidine pharmacotherapy to women who are pregnant. If procyclidine pharmacotherapy is required, advise patients of potential benefits and possible risks to themselves and the embryo, fetus, or neonate. Collaboration with the patient's obstetrician is indicated.

Women who are breast-feeding: Safety and efficacy of procyclidine pharmacotherapy for women who are breast-feeding and their neonates and infants have not been established. Avoid prescribing procyclidine pharmacotherapy to women who are breast-feeding. If procyclidine pharmacotherapy is required, breast-feeding probably should be discontinued.

For details and discussion regarding related basic principles of clinical pharmacology, readers are referred to the first text in this series, *The Pharmacologic Basis of Psychotherapeutics: An Introduction for Psychologists.*

Elderly, frail, or debilitated patients: Generally prescribe lower dosages for elderly, frail, or debilitated patients. These patients may be more sensitive to the pharmacologic actions of procyclidine than are younger or healthier adult patients.

Children and adolescents younger than 18 years of age: Safety and efficacy of procyclidine pharmacotherapy for children and adolescents who are younger than 18 years of age have not been established. Procyclidine pharmacotherapy is *not* recommended for this age group.

Notes, Parkinson's Disease: Arteriosclerotic, Drug-Induced, Idiopathic, and Post-Encephalitic

Ingestion of each dose of procyclidine after meals or with food may minimize associated epigastric irritation. Usually, procyclidine pharmacotherapy is of greater efficacy for the symptomatic management of rigidity rather than tremor. For patients who require additional therapeutic effect, prescribe one additional dose of 2.5 to 5 mg daily orally 30 minutes before retiring for bed in the evening.

AVAILABLE DOSAGE FORMS, STORAGE, AND COMPATIBILITY

Elixir, oral: 2.5 mg/5 ml (vanilla peppermint–flavored, contains alcohol)
Tablets, oral: 5 mg

Notes

General instructions for patients: Instruct patients who are receiving procyclidine pharmacotherapy to

- ingest each dose of the procyclidine oral elixir or oral tablets after meals or with food to minimize associated epigastric distress.
- safely store procyclidine oral tablets out of the reach of children in tightly closed, child-resistant containers at controlled room temperature (15° to 30°C; 59° to 86°F).
- obtain an available patient information sheet regarding procyclidine pharmacotherapy from their pharmacist at the time that their prescription is dispensed. Encourage patients to clarify any questions that they may have regarding procyclidine pharmacotherapy with their pharmacist or, if needed, to consult their prescribing psychologist.

PROPOSED MECHANISM OF ACTION

The exact mechanism of procyclidine's antiparkinsonian action has not yet been fully determined. Procyclidine is chemically related to trihexyphenidyl and elicits an atropine-like antispasmodic effect on smooth muscle.

PHARMACOKINETICS/PHARMACODYNAMICS

Data are not available.

RELATIVE CONTRAINDICATIONS

Angle-closure (narrow-angle) glaucoma
Hypersensitivity to procyclidine
Myasthenia gravis
Tachycardia, secondary to cardiac insufficiency or thyrotoxicosis

CAUTIONS AND COMMENTS

Prescribe procyclidine pharmacotherapy cautiously to patients who

- have cardiac dysrhythmias. Procyclidine pharmacotherapy may cause tachycardia among these patients.
- have histories of mental disorders. Procyclidine pharmacotherapy may aggravate or cause several mental disorders. Adverse drug reactions related to procyclidine include agitation, confusion, disorientation, hallucinations, inability to concentrate, memory impairment, psychosis, and restlessness. These ADRs appear to occur with the greatest incidence and severity among the elderly.
- have urinary retention. Procyclidine pharmacotherapy may significantly aggravate or cause urinary retention as a direct result of its antimuscarinic activity. This effect may be most pronounced and problematic among elderly men who have prostatic hypertrophy.

Caution patients who are receiving procyclidine pharmacotherapy against

- performing activities that require alertness, judgment, or physical coordination (e.g., driving an automobile, operating dangerous equipment, supervising children) until their response to procyclidine pharmacotherapy is known. Procyclidine may affect these mental and physical functions adversely.

CLINICALLY SIGNIFICANT DRUG INTERACTIONS

Concurrent procyclidine pharmacotherapy and the following may result in clinically significant drug interactions:

Alcohol Use

Concurrent alcohol use may increase the CNS depressant action of procyclidine. Advise patients to avoid, or limit, their use of alcohol while receiving procyclidine pharmacotherapy.

Pharmacotherapy With CNS Depressants and Other Drugs That Produce CNS Depression

Concurrent procyclidine pharmacotherapy and pharmacotherapy with opiate analgesics, sedative-hypnotics, or other drugs that produce CNS depression (e.g., antihistamines, phenothiazines, TCAs) may result in additive CNS depression.

ADVERSE DRUG REACTIONS

Generally, procyclidine pharmacotherapy is well tolerated. However, it commonly has been associated with ADRs related to its anticholinergic actions, particularly dry mouth. Procyclidine pharmacotherapy also has been associated with the following ADRs, listed according to body system:

Cardiovascular: increased heart rate (tachycardia)
CNS: confusion, disorientation, hallucinations, lightheadedness, memory impairment, slurred speech, and toxic psychosis. (See also "Cautions and Comments.")
Cutaneous: rash
Genitourinary: painful or difficult urination (dysuria)
GI: constipation and epigastric distress
Musculoskeletal: muscular weakness
Ophthalmic: blurred vision and dilated pupils (mydriasis)

OVERDOSAGE

Signs and symptoms of procyclidine overdosage include convulsions, drowsiness, dry mouth, excitement, giddiness, mental confusion, nausea, and vomiting. Procyclidine overdosage should be treated as a medical emergency requiring symptomatic medical support of body systems with attention to increasing procyclidine elimination. Physostigmine (Antilirium®) is an antidote. However, the use of physostigmine generally is not recommended because of 1) the ADRs associated with its use (e.g., asystole, seizures); and 2) its relative contraindication for use among patients who have asthma, cardiovascular disease, gangrene, and mechanical obstruction of the GI or genitourinary tracts.

PROPOXYPHENE

(proe pox′ i feen)

TRADE NAMES

Darvon®
Darvon-N®
Novo-Propoxyn®

CLASSIFICATION

Opiate analgesic (C-IV)

See also "Opiate Analgesics, General Monograph."

APPROVED INDICATIONS FOR NEUROPSYCHOLOGICAL DISORDERS

Adjunctive pharmacotherapy for the symptomatic management of:

- pain disorders: acute pain, mild to moderate, and chronic cancer pain, mild to moderate

USUAL DOSAGE AND ADMINISTRATION

Acute Pain, Mild to Moderate, and Chronic Cancer Pain, Mild to Moderate

Adults: 65 mg (chloride salt) *or* 100 mg (napsylate salt) orally every four hours, as required for symptomatic relief of pain

MAXIMUM: 390 mg (chloride salt) *or* 600 mg (napsylate salt) daily orally

Women who are, or who may become, pregnant: FDA Pregnancy Category C. Safety and efficacy of propoxyphene pharmacotherapy for women who are pregnant have not been established. Various physical malformations (e.g., beaked nose, congenital hip dislocation, micrognathia) and the signs and symptoms of the neonatal opiate analgesic withdrawal syndrome (e.g., irritability, seizures, tremors) have been reported. However, the data are inconclusive. See also "Opiate Analgesics, General Monograph." Avoid prescribing propoxyphene pharmacotherapy to women who are pregnant. If propoxyphene pharmacotherapy is required, advise patients of potential benefits and possible risks to themselves and the embryo, fetus, or neonate. Collaboration with the patient's obstetrician is indicated.

For details and discussion regarding related basic principles of clinical pharmacology, readers are referred to the first text in this series, *The Pharmacologic Basis of Psychotherapeutics: An Introduction for Psychologists.*

Women who are breast-feeding: Safety and efficacy of propoxyphene pharmacotherapy for women who are breast-feeding and their neonates and infants have not been established. Low concentrations of propoxyphene are excreted in breast milk and would appear to be unlikely to affect breast-fed neonates or infants. However, ADRs have been noted among breast-fed neonates of mothers who were prescribed propoxyphene during the postpartum period. See also "Opiate Analgesics, General Monograph." Avoid prescribing propoxyphene pharmacotherapy to women who are breast-feeding. If propoxyphene pharmacotherapy is required, breast-feeding probably should be discontinued. If desired, lactation may be maintained and breast-feeding resumed following the discontinuation of short-term propoxyphene pharmacotherapy. Collaboration with the patient's pediatrician is indicated.

Elderly adults: See "Usual Dosage and Administration" for adults. Note that the rate of propoxyphene metabolism may be reduced among some elderly patients.

Children: Safety and efficacy of propoxyphene pharmacotherapy for children have not been established. Propoxyphene pharmacotherapy is *not* recommended for this age group.

AVAILABLE DOSAGE FORMS, STORAGE, AND COMPATIBILITY

Capsules, oral (chloride salt): 32, 65 mg
Suspension, oral (napsylate salt): 10 mg/ml
Tablets, oral (napsylate salt): 50, 100 mg

Notes

General instructions for patients: Instruct patients who are receiving propoxyphene pharmacotherapy to

- shake the propoxyphene oral suspension well prior to measuring each dose to help to assure that an accurate dose is measured and ingested.
- safely store propoxyphene oral dosage forms out of the reach of children in tightly closed, child-resistant containers.
- obtain an available patient information sheet regarding propoxyphene pharmacotherapy from their pharmacist at the time that their prescription is dispensed. Encourage patients to clarify any questions that they may have regarding propoxyphene pharmacotherapy with their pharmacist or, if needed, to consult their prescribing psychologist.

PROPOSED MECHANISM OF ACTION

Propoxyphene elicits its analgesic, CNS depressant, and respiratory depressant actions primarily by binding to the endorphin receptors in the CNS. The exact mechanism of action has not yet been fully determined. See also "Opiate Analgesics, General Monograph."

PHARMACOKINETICS/PHARMACODYNAMICS

Propoxyphene is well absorbed following oral ingestion. Peak blood concentrations are achieved within 3 hours. Propoxyphene is extensively metabolized in the liver and excreted almost entirely as metabolites in the urine. The half-life of elimination ranges from 6 to 12 hours. Generally, the duration of action is 4 to 6 hours. Additional data are not available.

RELATIVE CONTRAINDICATIONS

Addiction and habituation to propoxyphene or other abusable psychotropics, history of
Hypersensitivity to propoxyphene
Ritonavir (Norvir®) pharmacotherapy, concurrent (see "Clinically Significant Drug Interactions")
Suicidal ideation

CAUTIONS AND COMMENTS

Long-term propoxyphene pharmacotherapy, or regular personal use, has been associated with the development of addiction and, particularly, habituation. Propoxyphene will only partially suppress the opiate analgesic withdrawal syndrome among people who are addicted to opiate analgesics. Therefore, the sudden replacement of other opiate analgesics with propoxyphene among patients who are addicted to the opiate analgesics may result in the opiate analgesic withdrawal syndrome. To avoid precipitating the opiate analgesic withdrawal syndrome among these patients, gradually reduce the dosage of the other opiate analgesics before initiating propoxyphene pharmacotherapy.

Despite its reputation as being much less addictive than other opiate analgesics (i.e., the abuse liability of propoxyphene is similar to that of codeine, although lower), propoxyphene is an abusable psychotropic. Frequent requests for repeat prescriptions require careful investigation. Propoxyphene has no real advantage over acetaminophen or aspirin for the symptomatic management of mild to moderate pain. Avoid prescribing propoxyphene when pain disorders can be managed by these or other nonopiate analgesics.

Prescribe propoxyphene pharmacotherapy cautiously to patients who

- are receiving pharmacotherapy with other CNS depressants (e.g., opiate analgesics, sedative-hypnotics) or other drugs that produce CNS depression (e.g., antihistamines, phenothiazines, TCAs). Concurrent pharmacotherapy may result in additive CNS depression.
- have depression, suicidal ideation or histories of suicide attempts, or histories of problematic patterns of abusable psychotropic use. Whenever possible, avoid prescribing opiate analgesics to these patients. While some overdosage deaths have been associated with accidental ingestion, many deaths associated with propoxyphene overdosage reportedly involved patients who had previous histories of psychological problems, suicidal ideation or suicide attempts, and problematic patterns of abusable psychotropic use. Prescribe for dispensing only small quantities of propoxyphene and closely monitor patient response. Carefully reevaluate the need for continued propoxyphene pharmacotherapy.

Caution patients who are receiving propoxyphene pharmacotherapy against

- drinking alcohol while receiving propoxyphene pharmacotherapy. Alcohol can potentiate the CNS depressant actions of propoxyphene and may result in serious CNS depression.
- performing activities that require alertness, judgment, and physical coordination (e.g., driving an automobile, operating dangerous equipment, supervising children) until their response to propoxyphene pharmacotherapy is known. Propoxyphene pharmacotherapy may affect these mental and physical functions adversely.

In addition to these general precautions, caution patients who are receiving propoxyphene pharmacotherapy to

• inform their prescribing psychologist if they begin or discontinue any other pharmacotherapy while receiving propoxyphene pharmacotherapy.

CLINICALLY SIGNIFICANT DRUG INTERACTIONS

Concurrent propoxyphene pharmacotherapy and the following may result in clinically significant drug interactions:

Alcohol Use

Concurrent alcohol use may increase the CNS depressant action of propoxyphene. Alcohol reportedly enhances the bioavailability of propoxyphene by ~25%, probably by reducing its first-pass hepatic metabolism. Advise patients to avoid, or limit, their use of alcohol while receiving propoxyphene pharmacotherapy.

Pharmacotherapy With CNS Depressants and Other Drugs That Produce CNS Depression

Concurrent propoxyphene pharmacotherapy and pharmacotherapy with other opiate analgesics, sedative-hypnotics, or other drugs that produce CNS depression (e.g., antihistamines, phenothiazines, TCAs) may result in additive CNS depression.

Ritonavir Pharmacotherapy

Ritonavir (Norvir®), an antiretroviral drug indicated for the pharmacologic management of HIV infection, may significantly inhibit the hepatic microsomal enzyme metabolism of propoxyphene. This interaction may result in severe toxicity, including cardiotoxicity and respiratory depression. Concurrent propoxyphene and ritonavir pharmacotherapy is *contraindicated*.

Tobacco Smoking

Concurrent tobacco smoking may increase the metabolism of propoxyphene. Thus, tobacco smokers may experience less pain relief than nonsmokers when equal dosages are prescribed. Higher dosages of propoxyphene may be required for patients who smoke tobacco.

See also "Opiate Analgesics, General Monograph."

ADVERSE DRUG REACTIONS

Propoxyphene pharmacotherapy has been associated with dizziness; drowsiness; dysphoria or euphoria; GI complaints, including abdominal pain, constipation, nausea, and vomiting; headache; insomnia; lightheadedness; paradoxical excitement; sedation; skin rash; and visual disturbances (usually minor). Long-term pharmacotherapy with dosages exceeding 800 mg daily has been associated with convulsions and toxic psychosis.

See also "Opiate Analgesics, General Monograph."

OVERDOSAGE

Signs and symptoms of propoxyphene overdosage resemble those associated with other opiate analgesic overdosage and include respiratory depression (e.g., decrease in respiratory rate and tidal volume, Cheyne–Stokes respirations), extreme somnolence progressing to stupor or coma, initial contraction of the pupils followed by dilation of the pupils as hypoxia increases, and circulatory collapse (see also "Opiate Analgesics, General Monograph"). In addition to the signs and symptoms of general opiate analgesic overdosage, local and generalized seizures occur in most cases of severe propoxyphene overdosage. Propoxyphene overdosage, alone or in combination with alcohol or other CNS depressants, has resulted in a significant number of overdosage deaths. Fatalities within the first hour of overdosage are common.

Propoxyphene overdosage requires emergency symptomatic medical support of body systems with attention to increasing propoxyphene elimination. The opiate antagonist, naloxone (Narcan®), is a specific antidote against the respiratory depression produced by propoxyphene.

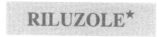

RILUZOLE*

(ri′ loo zole)

TRADE NAME

Rilutek®

CLASSIFICATION

Centrally-acting antiglutamatic (benzothiazolamine derivative)

APPROVED INDICATIONS FOR NEUROPSYCHOLOGICAL DISORDERS

Pharmacotherapy for the symptomatic management of:

- amyotrophic lateral sclerosis (ALS, Lou Gehrig disease, dejerine-type Charcot syndrome): familial or sporadic

USUAL DOSAGE AND ADMINISTRATION

ALS: *Familial or Sporadic*

Adults: 100 mg daily orally in two divided doses at 12-hour intervals

MAXIMUM: 100 mg daily orally

Women who are, or who may become, pregnant: FDA Pregnancy Category C. Safety and efficacy of riluzole pharmacotherapy for women who are pregnant have not been established. Avoid prescribing riluzole pharmacotherapy to women who are pregnant. If riluzole pharmacotherapy is required, advise patients of potential benefits and possible risk to themselves and the embryo, fetus, or neonate. Collaboration with the patient's obstetrician is indicated.

Women who are breast-feeding: Safety and efficacy of riluzole pharmacotherapy for women who are breast-feeding and their neonates and infants have not been established. Avoid prescribing riluzole pharmacotherapy to women who are breast-feeding. If riluzole pharmacotherapy is required, breast-feeding probably should be discontinued.

Elderly adults: See "Usual Dosage and Administration" for adults.

Children and adolescents younger than 18 years of age: Safety and efficacy of riluzole pharmacotherapy for children and adolescents who are younger than 18 years of age have not been established. Riluzole pharmacotherapy is *not* recommended for this age group.

For details and discussion regarding related basic principles of clinical pharmacology, readers are referred to the first text in this series, *The Pharmacologic Basis of Psychotherapeutics: An Introduction for Psychologists.*

Notes, ALS: Familial or Sporadic

Exceeding the maximum recommended daily dosage of riluzole provides no additional therapeutic benefit and may increase the incidence and severity of associated ADRs.

AVAILABLE DOSAGE FORMS, STORAGE, AND COMPATIBILITY

Tablets, oral: 50 mg

Notes

General instructions for patients: Instruct patients who are receiving riluzole pharmacotherapy to

- ingest each dose of riluzole oral tablets on an empty stomach (i.e., 1 hour before or 2 hours after meals) in order to provide maximum absorption and therapeutic benefit.
- safely store riluzole oral tablets out of the reach of children in tightly closed, light- and child-resistant containers at controlled room temperature (20° to 25 °C; 68° to 77 °F).
- obtain an available patient information sheet regarding riluzole pharmacotherapy from their pharmacist at the time that their prescription is dispensed. Encourage patients to clarify any questions that they may have regarding riluzole pharmacotherapy with their pharmacist or, if needed, to consult their prescribing psychologist.

PROPOSED MECHANISM OF ACTION

The exact mechanism of action of riluzole for the treatment of ALS has not yet been determined. However, the following mechanisms of action appear to be involved: 1) inhibition of glutamic acid release; 2) inactivation of voltage-dependent sodium ion channels; and 3) activation of a G-protein-dependent signal transduction pathway. These mechanisms of action appear to provide neuroprotection by means of preventing the accumulation and resultant activity of excitatory amino acids (EAAs), such as glutamate, at CNS synapses and resultant excitotoxicity and cell death.

Riluzole pharmacotherapy can prolong survival time and forestall the need for tracheotomy among patients who have ALS. However, muscle strength and neurologic function generally do not improve. The ultimate course of the disease remains undeterred.

PHARMACOKINETICS/PHARMACODYNAMICS

Riluzole is well absorbed from the GI tract following oral ingestion (~90%). Oral bioavailability is reduced because of first-pass hepatic metabolism ($F = 0.6$). A high-fat meal decreases bioavailability by ~20%. Riluzole is highly plasma protein bound (~96%). It is metabolized extensively in the liver, principally by cytochrome P450-dependent hydroxylation and glucuronidation. CYP1A2 is the principal isoenzyme involved in N-hydroxylation reactions. Approximately 22% is excreted in unchanged form in the urine. The mean half-life of elimination is 12 hours.

The pharmacokinetics of riluzole are reportedly unaffected by age or gender. However, some studies have reported genetic effects. In comparative studies, native Japanese subjects have been found to have total body clearance rates that were 50% lower than those found for Caucasian subjects even when adjustments were made for average body weight. The mechanism of this reduced clearance has not yet been determined.

RELATIVE CONTRAINDICATIONS

Hypersensitivity to riluzole

CAUTIONS AND COMMENTS

It is recommended that serum aminotransferases, including serum transaminase (ALT/SGPT, AST/SGOT), be measured before initiating riluzole pharmacotherapy because of the potential for riluzole-induced liver damage. Subsequently, liver enzymes should be monitored monthly for the first 3 months of therapy. Thereafter, they should be monitored every 3 months for the remainder of the first year of pharmacotherapy, and then monitored periodically.

Riluzole-induced increases in serum ALT/SGOT levels usually occur within the first 3 months of pharmacotherapy and are transient. Riluzole pharmacotherapy should be discontinued in the event of prolonged severalfold increases in ALT/SGOT levels or if the patient develops clinical jaundice. Collaboration with the patient's physician is indicated.

In rare cases, marked neutropenia (i.e., absolute neutrophil count less than $500/mm^3$) has been associated with riluzole pharmacotherapy ($\sim$1 in 1,000 cases). Neutropenia generally occurs within the first 2 months of riluzole pharmacotherapy. Patients should be instructed to report any febrile illness to their prescribing psychologist. Upon report of a febrile illness, white blood cell counts should be obtained. Collaboration with the patient's advanced practice nurse or family physician is indicated.

Prescribe riluzole pharmacotherapy cautiously to patients who

- have kidney or liver dysfunction. Kidney or liver dysfunction may predispose patients to a higher incidence or severity of ADRs, particularly riluzole-induced liver damage, which is manifested by elevated liver enzymes.

Caution patients who are receiving riluzole pharmacotherapy against

- drinking alcohol. The excessive use of alcohol may result in an increased incidence or severity of liver damage. See "Clinically Significant Drug Interactions."
- performing activities that require alertness, judgment, or physical coordination (e.g., driving an automobile, operating dangerous equipment, supervising children) until their response to riluzole pharmacotherapy is known. Riluzole may affect these mental and physical functions adversely.

In addition to these general precautions, caution patients who are receiving riluzole pharmacotherapy to

- inform their prescribing psychologist if they begin or discontinue any other pharmacotherapy while receiving riluzole pharmacotherapy.

CLINICALLY SIGNIFICANT DRUG INTERACTIONS

Concurrent riluzole pharmacotherapy and the following may result in clinically significant drug interactions:

Alcohol Use

Concurrent alcohol use may increase the associated risk of serious hepatotoxicity among patients who are receiving riluzole pharmacotherapy. Advise patients to avoid, or limit, their use of alcohol while receiving riluzole pharmacotherapy.

Pharmacotherapy With Drugs That Are Potentially Hepatotoxic

Concurrent riluzole pharmacotherapy and pharmacotherapy with other drugs that are also known to be potentially hepatotoxic (e.g., allopurinol [Zyloprim®], methyldopa [Aldomet®], sulfasalazine [Azulfidine®]) may increase the incidence and severity of liver damage significantly. Thus, this combination of pharmacotherapy should be avoided.

Tobacco Smoking

Concurrent tobacco smoking may increase the metabolism of riluzole by inducing CYP-1A2. Higher dosages of riluzole may be required for patients who smoke one or more packages of tobacco cigarettes daily.

ADVERSE DRUG REACTIONS

Riluzole pharmacotherapy commonly has been associated with: abdominal pain, asthenia (lack of strength, particularly of cerebellar or muscular origin), circumoral paresthesia, diarrhea, dizziness (vertigo), loss of appetite (anorexia), nausea, pneumonia, reduced lung function, somnolence, and vomiting. Riluzole pharmacotherapy also has been associated with the following ADRs, listed according to body system:

CNS: depression and headache
Cutaneous: eczema, exfoliative dermatitis, peripheral edema, and severe itching (pruritus)
Musculoskeletal: back pain and joint pain (arthralgia)
Respiratory: increased cough and rhinitis (inflammation of the nasal mucosa)

OVERDOSAGE

Clinical data concerning riluzole overdosage are not available. In the absence of such data, riluzole overdosage should be treated as a medical emergency requiring symptomatic medical support of body systems with attention to increasing riluzole elimination. There is no known antidote.

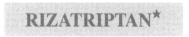
RIZATRIPTAN*

(ri za′ trip tan)

TRADE NAMES

Maxalt®
Maxalt-MLT®

CLASSIFICATION

Antimigraine (vascular serotonin receptor agonist)

APPROVED INDICATIONS FOR NEUROPSYCHOLOGICAL DISORDERS

Pharmacotherapy for the symptomatic management of:

- vascular headaches: migraine headaches, with or without aura. Note: Rizatriptan pharmacotherapy is *not* indicated for the prevention of migraine (i.e., as prophylactic pharmacotherapy), nor is it indicated for the treatment of basilar or hemiplegic migraine.

USUAL DOSAGE AND ADMINISTRATION

Migraine Headaches, With or Without Aura

Adults: Initially, 5 or 10 mg orally. Additional doses, up to the maximum, may be administered at intervals of at least 2 hours.

MAXIMUM: 30 mg orally in any 24-hour period

Women who are, or who may become, pregnant: FDA Pregnancy Category C. Safety and efficacy of rizatriptan pharmacotherapy for women who are pregnant have not been established. Avoid prescribing rizatriptan pharmacotherapy to women who are pregnant. If rizatriptan pharmacotherapy is required, advise patients of potential benefits and possible risk to themselves and the embryo, fetus, or neonate. Collaboration with the patient's obstetrician is indicated.

Women who are breast-feeding: Safety and efficacy of rizatriptan pharmacotherapy for women who are breast-feeding and their neonates and infants have not been established. It is not known whether rizatriptan is excreted in breast milk. Avoid prescribing rizatriptan pharmacotherapy to women who are breast-feeding. If rizatriptan pharmacotherapy is required, breast-feeding probably should be discontinued. If desired, lactation may be maintained and breast-feeding resumed following the discontinuation of short-term rizatriptan pharmacotherapy.

For details and discussion regarding related basic principles of clinical pharmacology, readers are referred to the first text in this series, *The Pharmacologic Basis of Psychotherapeutics: An Introduction for Psychologists.*

Elderly adults: Same as "Adults."

Adults who are receiving concurrent propranolol (Inderal®) pharmacotherapy: Initially, 5 mg orally. The initial dose may be repeated, if required, at intervals of at least 2 hours, according to individual patient response (see "Clinically Significant Drug Interactions").

MAXIMUM: 15 mg orally in any 24-hour period

Children and adolescents younger than 18 years of age: Safety and efficacy of rizatriptan pharmacotherapy for children and adolescents who are younger than 18 years of age have not been established. Rizatriptan pharmacotherapy is *not* recommended for this age group.

Notes, Vascular Headaches: Migraine Headaches, With or Without Aura

Generally, the safety and efficacy of rizatriptan pharmacotherapy for the symptomatic management of more than four migraine headaches in a 30-day period have not been established.

AVAILABLE DOSAGE FORMS, STORAGE, AND COMPATIBILITY

Tablets (Maxalt®), oral: 5, 10 mg
Tablets, orally disintegrating (Maxalt-MLT®): 5, 10 mg (peppermint flavored)

Notes

The orally disintegrating tablets use Zydis® technology that utilizes orally available saliva to dissolve the tablet in seconds without the need for water or other fluids. Each orally disintegrating tablet contains the artificial sweetener aspartame that may pose a theoretical risk to patients who have phenylketonuria (because aspartame is composed of the amino acids, aspartic acid and phenylalanine; each 5 mg orally disintegrating rizatriptan tablet contains ~1 mg of phenylalanine and each 10 mg orally disintegrating rizatriptan tablet contains ~2 mg of phenylalanine). The orally disintegrating tablet is packaged in a blister pack within an outer aluminum pouch.

General instructions for patients: Instruct patients who are receiving rizatriptan pharmacotherapy, as appropriate, to

- administer the rizatriptan orally disintegrating tablet (Maxalt-MLT®) by 1) removing the blister pack, which contains the orally disintegrating tablet, from the outer aluminum pouch; 2) with dry hands, peel open the blister pack; 3) place the orally disintegrating tablet on the tongue; and 4) allow the tablet to dissolve in the mouth and then swallow the saliva (administration with liquid is *not* required).
- ingest each dose of the rizatriptan oral tablets (Maxalt®) whole with adequate liquid chaser (i.e., 60 to 120 ml of water). The rizatriptan oral tablets should *not* be broken, chewed, or crushed.
- safely store rizatriptan dosage forms out of the reach of children in tightly closed, child-resistant containers at controlled room temperature (15° to 30°C; 59° to 86°F).

- obtain an available patient information sheet regarding rizatriptan pharmacotherapy from their pharmacist at the time that their prescription is dispensed. Encourage patients to clarify any questions that they may have regarding rizatriptan pharmacotherapy with their pharmacist or, if needed, to consult their prescribing psychologist.

PROPOSED MECHANISM OF ACTION

Rizatriptan is an agonist for the vascular serotonin receptor subtypes 5-HT_{1B} and 5-HT_{1D}. Activation of these receptors, which are present on cranial arteries, on the basilar artery, and in the vasculature of the dura mater, produces vasoconstriction. The vasoconstriction of these arteries, which are dilated and edematous during a migraine attack, appears to be correlated with migraine relief. In addition, activation of the 5-HT receptors results in inhibition of neuropeptide release and reduces transmission in associated pain pathways.

PHARMACOKINETICS/PHARMACODYNAMICS

Rizatriptan is absorbed rapidly and completely from the GI tract following oral ingestion. However, the bioavailability of rizatriptan is only moderate ($\sim45\%$), primarily due to significant first-pass hepatic metabolism. Peak blood concentrations are obtained within 1 to 2 hours. Food slows the rate, but not the extent, of rizatriptan absorption. Rizatriptan is $\sim15\%$ bound to plasma proteins and has a mean apparent volume of distribution of ~125 liters. Rizatriptan is extensively metabolized. The primary route of metabolism is oxidative deamination by monoamine oxidase-A (MAO-A). Approximately 14% of rizatriptan is excreted in unchanged form in the urine. The half-life of elimination is ~2 to 3 hours.

Significant migraine relief generally is noted within 1 to 2 hours following use. Rizatriptan is efficacious in providing symptomatic relief to $\sim70\%$ of patients who have moderate to severe migraine headaches.

RELATIVE CONTRAINDICATIONS

Angina pectoris
Basilar migraine
Coronary vasospasm (Prinzmetal's angina)
Ergot pharmacotherapy, concurrent or within the previous 24 hours because of possible additive vasoconstriction
Hemiplegic migraine
Hypersensitivity to rizatriptan
Hypertension, uncontrolled
Ischemic heart disease
MAOI pharmacotherapy, concurrent or within the previous 14 days because of the inhibition of rizatriptan metabolism
Myocardial infarction, history of
Myocardial ischemia
Zolmitriptan, or other vascular serotonin receptor agonist, pharmacotherapy, concurrent or within the previous 24 hours because of possible additive vasoconstriction

CAUTIONS AND COMMENTS

Patients who require intermittent, long-term rizatriptan pharmacotherapy and who possess noted risk factors for coronary artery disease (CAD) (e.g., diabetes, hypercholesterolemia, hypertension, obesity, tobacco smoking) are advised to undergo periodic medical evaluation of cardiovascular status in order to reduce the risks associated with rizatriptan pharmacotherapy among patients with unrecognized cardiovascular disease.

Prescribe rizatriptan pharmacotherapy cautiously to patients who

- have liver dysfunction (moderate to severe). The metabolism of rizatriptan may be decreased among these patients and result in significant increases in blood concentrations (i.e., ~30%) and resultant toxicity. Monitor these patients carefully and adjust the dosage, as needed, according to individual patient response.

Caution patients who are receiving rizatriptan pharmacotherapy against

- performing activities that require alertness, judgment, or physical coordination (e.g., driving an automobile, operating dangerous equipment, supervising children) until their response to rizatriptan pharmacotherapy is known. Rizatriptan may cause dizziness and drowsiness and, thus, affect these mental and physical functions adversely.

CLINICALLY SIGNIFICANT DRUG INTERACTIONS

Concurrent rizatriptan pharmacotherapy and the following may result in clinically significant drug interactions:

MAOI Pharmacotherapy

See "Relative Contraindications."

Propranolol Pharmacotherapy

Concurrent propranolol (Inderal®) pharmacotherapy may result in significantly increased rizatriptan blood concentrations (mean increase of ~70%). Rizatriptan dosage adjustment may be required. Monitor these patients carefully and adjust the dosage, as needed, according to individual patient response.

See also "Relative Contraindications."

ADVERSE DRUG REACTIONS

Rizatriptan pharmacotherapy commonly has been associated with chest pain (i.e., feelings of pressure and tightness in the chest), decreased mental acuity, dizziness, feeling of heaviness, neck stiffness, pressure sensation, warm/cold sensations, and weakness (asthenia). Rizatriptan pharmacotherapy also has been associated with the following ADRs, listed according to body system:

Cardiovascular: angina (rare), cardiac dysrhythmias (rare), coronary vasospasm (rare), hypertension (transient), and myocardial infarction (rare)

CNS: cerebral hemorrhage (rare), panic-like symptoms (particularly among patients who have a history of anxiety disorders), drowsiness, seizures (rare), and stroke

Cutaneous: flushing

GI: diarrhea, nausea, and vomiting

Respiratory: shortness of breath (dyspnea)

Miscellaneous: fatigue, hot flashes, tingling sensation, and tremor

OVERDOSAGE

Clinical data concerning rizatriptan overdosage are not available. In the absence of such data, rizatriptan overdosage should be treated as a medical emergency requiring symptomatic support of body systems with attention to increasing rizatriptan elimination. There is no known antidote.

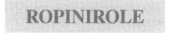

ROPINIROLE

(roe pin′ i role)

TRADE NAME

Requip®

CLASSIFICATION

Antiparkinsonian (benzothiazolamine derivative, non-ergot dopamine D2 receptor agonist)

APPROVED INDICATIONS FOR NEUROPSYCHOLOGICAL DISORDERS

Pharmacotherapy for the symptomatic management of:

- Parkinson's disease: idiopathic

USUAL DOSAGE AND ADMINISTRATION

Parkinson's Disease: Idiopathic

Adults: Initially, 0.75 mg daily orally in three divided doses for seven days. Then increase the daily dosage by 0.75 mg at weekly intervals until a total daily dosage of 3 mg is achieved. If further dosage increase is required, increase the daily dosage by 1.5 mg at weekly intervals until a total daily dosage of 9 mg is achieved. If still further dosage increase is required, increase the daily dosage by 3 mg at weekly intervals until a total daily dosage of 24 mg is achieved.

MAXIMUM: 24 mg daily orally

Women who are, or who may become, pregnant: FDA Pregnancy Category C. Safety and efficacy of ropinirole pharmacotherapy for women who are pregnant have not been established. Avoid prescribing ropinirole pharmacotherapy to women who are pregnant.

Women who are breast-feeding: Safety and efficacy of ropinirole pharmacotherapy for women who are breast-feeding and their neonates and infants have not been established. Avoid prescribing ropinirole pharmacotherapy to women who are breast-feeding.

Elderly adults: Special adjustments to the usual recommended adult dosage are *not* generally required for elderly adult patients. See "Usual Dosage and Administration" for adults.

For details and discussion regarding related basic principles of clinical pharmacology, readers are referred to the first text in this series, *The Pharmacologic Basis of Psychotherapeutics: An Introduction for Psychologists.*

Children and adolescents younger than 18 years of age: Safety and efficacy of ropinirole pharmacotherapy for children and adolescents who are younger than 18 years of age have not been established. Ropinirole pharmacotherapy is *not* recommended for this age group.

Notes, Idiopathic Parkinson's Disease

Ropinirole pharmacotherapy may be prescribed for the symptomatic management of Parkinson's disease alone or in combination with levodopa pharmacotherapy. Generally, combination ropinirole and levodopa pharmacotherapy may effect a reduction in the previous dosage of levodopa. Ropinirole also may elicit a reduced "off" time among a significant minority of patients who have idiopathic Parkinson's disease and who are experiencing a deteriorating response to levodopa pharmacotherapy (i.e., the "on–off" phenomenon).

Discontinuing ropinirole pharmacotherapy: Although not directly associated with the discontinuation of ropinirole pharmacotherapy, confusion and hyperpyrexia (elevated body temperature) have been associated with the abrupt discontinuation of other dopamine agonists. Discontinue ropinirole pharmacotherapy gradually by reducing the dosage over a period of 7 days.

AVAILABLE DOSAGE FORMS, STORAGE, AND COMPATIBILITY

Tablets, oral: 0.25, 0.5, 1, 2, and 5 mg

Notes

General instructions for patients: Instruct patients who are receiving ropinirole pharmacotherapy to

- safely store ropinirole oral tablets out of the reach of children in tightly closed, light- and child-resistant containers at controlled room temperature (15° to 25°C; 59° to 77°F).
- obtain an available patient information sheet regarding ropinirole pharmacotherapy from their pharmacist at the time that their prescription is dispensed. Encourage patients to clarify any questions that they may have regarding ropinirole pharmacotherapy with their pharmacist or, if needed, to consult their prescribing psychologist.

PROPOSED MECHANISM OF ACTION

The exact mechanism of antiparkinsonian action of ropinirole has not yet been fully determined. However, ropinirole is a dopamine receptor agonist with a demonstrated high affinity for D2 receptors and a particularly high affinity for the D3 receptor subtype. Thus, it is thought that ropinirole elicits its action by directly stimulating postsynaptic dopamine receptors within the corpus striatum.

PHARMACOKINETICS/PHARMACODYNAMICS

Ropinirole is well absorbed from the GI tract following oral ingestion with peak blood concentrations occurring within 1 to 2 hours. Food decreases the rate of ropinirole's absorption but does not affect the extent of absorption. The half-life of elimination is ~3 to 4 hours. Additional data are not available.

RELATIVE CONTRAINDICATIONS

Hypersensitivity to ropinirole

CAUTIONS AND COMMENTS

Caution patients who are receiving ropinirole pharmacotherapy against

- performing activities that require alertness, judgment, or physical coordination (e.g., driving an automobile, operating dangerous equipment, supervising children) until their response to ropinirole pharmacotherapy is known. Ropinirole may affect these mental and physical functions adversely.

CLINICALLY SIGNIFICANT DRUG INTERACTIONS

Concurrent ropinirole pharmacotherapy and the following may result in clinically significant drug interactions:

Alcohol Use

Concurrent alcohol use may increase the CNS depressant action of ropinirole. Advise patients to avoid, or limit, their use of alcohol while receiving ropinirole pharmacotherapy.

Ciprofloxacin Pharmacotherapy

Ciprofloxacin (Cipro®), a broad-spectrum antibiotic, inhibits the hepatic microsomal isoenzyme CYP-1A2. This enzyme is the enzyme primarily responsible for the metabolism of ropinirole. Therefore, concurrent ciprofloxacin pharmacotherapy may reduce the metabolism of ropinirole by up to 60%. Collaboration with the prescriber of ciprofloxacin is indicated.

Estrogen Pharmacotherapy

Estrogen pharmacotherapy, primarily ethinyl estradiol, which is found in several combination oral contraceptives (e.g., Brevicon®, Modicon®, Ortho-Novum®, Tri-Norinyl®), may reduce the total body clearance of ropinirole by ~33%. Collaboration with the prescriber of the oral contraceptive is indicated.

Pharmacotherapy With CNS Depressants and Other Drugs That Produce CNS Depression

Concurrent ropinirole pharmacotherapy and pharmacotherapy with opiate analgesics, sedative-hypnotics, or other drugs that produce CNS depression (e.g., antihistamines, phenothiazines, TCAs) may result in additive CNS depression.

ADVERSE DRUG REACTIONS

Ropinirole pharmacotherapy has been commonly associated with the following ADRs: confusion; dizziness; dyspepsia; fatigue; headache; nausea, which may be reduced by ingesting each dose of ropinirole with meals; peripheral edema; somnolence; syncope (fainting); and vomiting. Ropinirole pharmacotherapy also has been associated with the following ADRs, listed according to body system:

Cardiovascular: angina pectoris, heart failure, and postural (orthostatic) hypotension
CNS: agitation, convulsions (rare), depression, hallucinations, and increased sex drive
Cutaneous: cold, clammy skin (rare); dermatitis; and dry skin
GI: dyspepsia, gastritic, gastric ulcer, inflammation of the mouth (stomatitis), and tongue edema
Metabolic/Endocrine: diabetes mellitus, electrolyte abnormalities, glycosuria, gynecomastia, hypothyroidism, and increased blood urea nitrogen
Musculoskeletal: arthrosis, arthropathy, muscle weakness, skeletal pain, and torticollis
Ophthalmic: abnormal accommodation, abnormal sensitivity to light (photophobia), conjunctivitis, and eye pain
Otic: hearing loss
Miscellaneous: neuralgia

OVERDOSAGE

Signs and symptoms of ropinirole overdosage include agitation, chest pain, confusion, dyskinesias, grogginess, nausea, orthostatic hypotension, sedation, and vomiting. Ropinirole overdosage should be treated as a medical emergency requiring symptomatic medical support of body systems with attention to increasing ropinirole elimination. There is no known antidote.

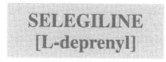

SELEGILINE
[L-deprenyl]

(se le' ji leen)

TRADE NAMES

Atapryl®
Carbex®
Eldepryl®

CLASSIFICATION

Antiparkinsonian (selective type-B MAOI)

APPROVED INDICATIONS FOR NEUROPSYCHOLOGICAL DISORDERS

Adjunctive pharmacotherapy for the symptomatic management of:

* Parkinson's disease. Selegiline pharmacotherapy is prescribed as adjunctive pharmacotherapy. See "Notes, Parkinson's Disease."

USUAL DOSAGE AND ADMINISTRATION

Parkinson's Disease

Adults: 10 mg daily orally in two divided doses. To avoid associated insomnia, these two doses may be prescribed for ingestion with breakfast and lunch.

MAXIMUM: 10 mg daily orally

Women who are, or who may become, pregnant: FDA Pregnancy Category C. Safety and efficacy of selegiline pharmacotherapy for women who are pregnant have not been established. Avoid prescribing selegiline pharmacotherapy to women who are pregnant. If selegiline pharmacotherapy is required, advise patients of potential benefits and possible risks to themselves and the embryo, fetus, or neonate. Collaboration with the patient's obstetrician is indicated.

Women who are breast-feeding: Safety and efficacy of selegiline pharmacotherapy for women who are breast-feeding and their neonates and infants have not been established. Avoid prescribing selegiline pharmacotherapy to women who are breast-feeding. If selegiline pharmacotherapy is required, breast-feeding probably should be discontinued. Collaboration with the patient's pediatrician may be indicated.

For details and discussion regarding related basic principles of clinical pharmacology, readers are referred to the first text in this series, *The Pharmacologic Basis of Psychotherapeutics: An Introduction for Psychologists.*

Elderly: See "Usual Dosage and Administration" for adults.

Children and adolescents younger than 18 years of age: Safety and efficacy of selegiline pharmacotherapy for children and adolescents who are younger than 18 years of age have not been established. Selegiline pharmacotherapy is *not* recommended for this age group.

Notes, Parkinson's Disease

Selegiline pharmacotherapy is approved as an adjunct to levodopa pharmacotherapy for the symptomatic management of Parkinson's disease. When prescribed as an adjunct to levodopa pharmacotherapy, the total daily dosage of levodopa may be reduced by ~10% after 2 or 3 days of selegiline pharmacotherapy. If dyskinesias develop during adjunctive pharmacotherapy, the dosage of levodopa may need to be reduced by an additional 10% to 30%.

MAO-B activity is ~100% inhibited by a selegiline dosage of 10 mg daily. Increasing the dosage of selegiline does *not* increase its therapeutic effect, but does result in 1) the loss of its selectivity for MAO-B and 2) increasing inhibition of MAO-A. Consequently, increasing the dosage of selegiline places patients at an unwarranted risk for the potentially fatal dietary (e.g., tyramine) and drug (e.g., sympathomimetic amines) interactions that are associated with the inhibition of MAO-A.

AVAILABLE DOSAGE FORMS, STORAGE, AND COMPATIBILITY

Capsules, oral: 5 mg
Tablets, oral: 5 mg

Notes

General instructions for patients: Instruct patients who are receiving selegiline pharmacotherapy to

- safely store selegiline oral capsules and tablets out of the reach of children in child-resistant containers at controlled room temperature (15° to 30°C; 59° to 86°F).
- obtain an available patient information sheet regarding selegiline pharmacotherapy from their pharmacist at the time that their prescription is dispensed. Encourage patients to clarify any questions that they may have regarding selegiline pharmacotherapy with their pharmacist or, if needed, to consult their prescribing psychologist.

PROPOSED MECHANISM OF ACTION

Selegiline, particularly at low dosages (i.e., 10 mg daily), is a relatively selective inhibitor of MAO-B, which is found predominantly in the brain. At recommended dosages, selegiline has little effect upon MAO-A, which is found predominantly in the intestines. Selegiline irreversibly inhibits MAO-B within the nigrostriatal pathways in the CNS. This action enhances dopaminergic activity within the substantia nigra by blocking the MAO-B-mediated metabolism of dopamine. Selegiline also prevents the MAO-B-mediated production of the neurotoxin, methyl-4-phenylpyridinium (MPP^+), which selectively destroys neurons within the substantia nigra and contributes to the pathogenesis of Parkinson's disease. Selegiline also may increase dopaminergic activity by interfering with dopamine re-uptake at the synaptic cleft. Active metabolites of selegiline include amphetamine, desmethylselegiline, and methamphetamine. However, the contributions of these metabolites, if any, to selegiline's antiparkinsonian action have not yet been determined.

PHARMACOKINETICS/PHARMACODYNAMICS

The oral availability of selegiline is low (i.e., <10%) because of significant first-pass hepatic metabolism. However, the bioavailability of selegiline may be increased 3- to 4-fold when it is ingested with food. Selegiline is highly bound to plasma proteins (~94%) and has a mean apparent volume of distribution of 2 liters/kg. Selegiline is metabolized rapidly to three active metabolites: L-amphetamine, L-desmethylselegiline, and L-methamphetamine. Mean total body clearance of selegiline is 1500 ml/minute/kg. The mean half-life of elimination for selegiline and its desmethyl metabolite is ~2 hours. The mean half-lives of elimination of its amphetamine and methamphetamine metabolites are 18 hours and 21 hours, respectively. Additional data are not available.

RELATIVE CONTRAINDICATIONS

    Dementia, profound
    Extrapyramidal reactions, such as excessive tremor or tardive dyskinesia
    Hypersensitivity to selegiline
    Fluoxetine and other SSRI pharmacotherapy, concurrent
    Meperidine pharmacotherapy, concurrent
    Nonselective MAOI pharmacotherapy, concurrent
    Peptic ulcer disease, active
    Psychosis, severe
    TCA pharmacotherapy, concurrent

CAUTIONS AND COMMENTS

Caution patients who are receiving selegiline pharmacotherapy against exceeding the recommended dosage. See the "Notes, Parkinson's Disease" subsection of "Usual Dosage and Administration."

CLINICALLY SIGNIFICANT DRUG INTERACTIONS

No clinically significant drug interactions, other than the therapeutic interaction between selegiline and levodopa and those noted in "Relative Contraindications" have been reported in the literature. The drug interactions noted in "Relative Contraindications" (i.e., those involving concurrent selegiline and meperidine, nonselective MAOI, SSRI, or TCA pharmacotherapy) generally involve risk for the development of hyperpyrexia and death as a result of nonselective inhibition of MAO. The relative risk for these interactions increases significantly when the maximal recommended dosage of selegiline is exceeded.

ADVERSE DRUG REACTIONS

Selegiline pharmacotherapy commonly has been associated with insomnia and nausea. Selegiline pharmacotherapy also has been associated with the following ADRs, listed according to body system:

Cardiovascular: angina pectoris, palpitations, postural (orthostatic) hypotension, syncope, and tachycardia

CNS: anxiety, behavioral disturbances, confusion, delusions, depression, dizziness, euphoria, hallucinations, headache, hypersexuality, lightheadedness, mania, and vivid dreams (nightmares)

Genitourinary: anorgasmia, prostatic hypertrophy, and urinary retention

GI: abdominal pain and dry mouth

Musculoskeletal: back pain and leg pain

Ophthalmic: double vision (diplopia) and sensitivity to light (photosensitivity)

OVERDOSAGE

Clinical data concerning selegiline overdosage are limited. Signs and symptoms of selegiline overdosage may include psychomotor agitation, seizures, and severe hypotension. Selegiline overdosage should be treated as a medical emergency requiring symptomatic medical support of body systems with attention to increasing selegiline elimination. There is no known antidote.

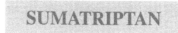

SUMATRIPTAN

(soo ma trip′ tan)

TRADE NAME

Imitrex®

CLASSIFICATION

Antimigraine (vascular serotonin receptor agonist)

APPROVED INDICATIONS FOR NEUROPSYCHOLOGICAL DISORDERS

Pharmacotherapy for the symptomatic management of:

- vascular headaches: migraine headaches, with or without aura. Note: Sumatriptan pharmacotherapy is *not* indicated for the prevention of migraine (i.e., as prophylactic pharmacotherapy) *nor* is it indicated for the treatment of basilar migraine.

USUAL DOSAGE AND ADMINISTRATION

Migraine Headaches, With or Without Aura

Adults: Sumatriptan pharmacotherapy may be prescribed as injectable, intranasal, or oral pharmacotherapy according to the following recommendations:

INJECTABLE PHARMACOTHERAPY: A single 6-mg subcutaneous injection per migraine attack. Subsequent migraine attacks may be treated with similar dosage provided that a *minimum* of one hour has elapsed since the previous dose.
Maximum   12 mg subcutaneously (i.e., two 6-mg subcutaneous injections) in any 24-hour period

INTRANASAL PHARMACOTHERAPY: 5 to 20 mg intranasally (i.e., one to four sumatriptan 5-mg intranasal sprays [or a single sumatriptan 20 mg intranasal spray] into a single nostril) per migraine attack. Subsequent migraine attacks may be treated with similar dosages provided that a *minimum* of two hours has elapsed since the previous dose.
Maximum   40 mg intranasally (i.e., eight sumatriptan 5-mg intranasal sprays) in any 24-hour period

ORAL PHARMACOTHERAPY: 25, 50, or 100 mg orally per migraine attack. Subsequent migraine attacks can be treated with a dosage up to 100 mg provided that a *minimum* of two hours has elapsed since the previous dose.

For details and discussion regarding related basic principles of clinical pharmacology, readers are referred to the first text in this series, *The Pharmacologic Basis of Psychotherapeutics: An Introduction for Psychologists.*

Maximum   200 mg orally (i.e., two sumatriptan 100-mg oral tablets) in any 24-hour period

Women who are, or who may become, pregnant: FDA Pregnancy Category C. Safety and efficacy of sumatriptan pharmacotherapy for women who are pregnant have not been established. Avoid prescribing sumatriptan pharmacotherapy to women who are pregnant. If sumatriptan pharmacotherapy is required, advise patients of potential benefits and possible risks to themselves and the embryo, fetus, or neonate. Collaboration with the patient's obstetrician is indicated.

Women who are breast-feeding: Safety and efficacy of sumatriptan pharmacotherapy for women who are breast-feeding and their neonates and infants have not been established. However, sumatriptan is excreted in breast milk. Avoid prescribing sumatriptan pharmacotherapy to women who are breast-feeding. If sumatriptan pharmacotherapy is required, breast-feeding probably should be discontinued. If desired, lactation may be maintained and breast-feeding resumed following the discontinuation of short-term sumatriptan pharmacotherapy.

Elderly adults: Safety and efficacy of sumatriptan pharmacotherapy for elderly adults who are 65 years of age and older have not been established. Sumatriptan pharmacotherapy is *not* recommended for this age group.

Adults who have mild to moderate liver dysfunction: 50 mg orally per migraine attack. Subsequent migraine attacks may be treated with a similar dosage provided that a *minimum* of four hours has elapsed since the previous dose.

MAXIMUM: 100 mg orally (i.e., two sumatriptan 50-mg oral tablets) in any 24-hour period

Children and adolescents younger than 18 years of age: Safety and efficacy of sumatriptan pharmacotherapy for children and adolescents who are younger than 18 years of age have not been established. Sumatriptan pharmacotherapy is *not* recommended for this age group.

Notes, Vascular Headaches: Migraine Headaches, With or Without Aura

The sumatriptan injectable is for subcutaneous use only. *Never* inject sumatriptan intravenously. A burning sensation commonly is experienced at the subcutaneous injection site of sumatriptan. Other ADRs (e.g., dizziness, fatigue, tightness in the chest) also frequently have been associated with the subcutaneous injection of sumatriptan.

AVAILABLE DOSAGE FORMS, STORAGE, AND COMPATIBILITY

Injectable, subcutaneous: 6 mg/0.5 ml in pre-filled syringes
Intranasal spray: 5, 20 mg in unit-dose spray devices
Tablets, oral: 25, 50, 100 mg

Notes

The 100 mg tablets are generally only available in Canada and Europe.

General instructions for patients: Instruct patients who are receiving sumatriptan pharmacotherapy, as appropriate, to

- administer each dose of the sumatriptan injectable subcutaneously on the outside thigh using the autoinjector supplied by the manufacturer.
- administer each dose of the sumatriptan intranasal spray into one nostril *only* using the single-dose unit supplied by the manufacturer. The nasal spray unit is ready to use and should *not* be primed.
- ingest each dose of the sumatriptan oral tablets whole with adequate liquid chaser (i.e., 60 to 120 ml of water). The sumatriptan oral tablets should *not* be broken, chewed, or crushed.
- safely store sumatriptan dosage forms out of the reach of children in tightly closed, light- and child-resistant containers at controlled room temperature (2° to 30°C; 36° to 86°F).
- obtain an available patient information sheet regarding sumatriptan pharmacotherapy from their pharmacist at the time that their prescription is dispensed. Encourage patients to clarify any questions that they may have regarding sumatriptan pharmacotherapy with their pharmacist or, if needed, to consult their prescribing psychologist.

PROPOSED MECHANISM OF ACTION

Sumatriptan is an agonist for the vascular serotonin receptor subtype 5-HT$_{1D}$. Activation of this receptor, which is present on cranial arteries, on the basilar artery, and in the vasculature of the dura mater, produces vasoconstriction. The vasoconstriction of these arteries, which are dilated and edematous during a migraine attack, appears to be correlated with migraine relief.

PHARMACOKINETICS/PHARMACODYNAMICS

The bioavailability of sumatriptan following oral ingestion or intranasal insufflation is low (~15%), primarily due to significant first-pass hepatic metabolism. However, following subcutaneous injection, sumatriptan's bioavailability is ~100%. It is ~15% bound to plasma proteins and has a mean apparent volume of distribution of 0.7 liters/kg. Sumatriptan is extensively metabolized in the liver. Approximately 25% of sumatriptan is excreted in unchanged form in the urine. The mean half-life of elimination is ~2 hours and the mean total body clearance is ~1 liter/kg/hour.

Significant migraine relief generally is noted within 15 minutes following either subcutaneous injection or intranasal insufflation. Significant migraine relief generally is noted within 1 hour following oral ingestion. Sumatriptan is efficacious in providing symptomatic relief to ~75% of patients with moderate to severe migraine headaches.

RELATIVE CONTRAINDICATIONS

Angina pectoris
Basilar migraine
Cardiac dysrhythmias, particularly tachycardias
Cerebrovascular accident, recent history of
Coronary vasospasm (Prinzmetal's angina)
Ergot pharmacotherapy, concurrent or within the previous 24 hours because of possible additive vasoconstriction

Hemiplegic migraine
Hypersensitivity to sumatriptan
Hypertension, uncontrolled
Ischemic heart disease
Lithium pharmacotherapy
MAOI pharmacotherapy, concurrent or within the previous 14 days
Myocardial infarction, history of
SSRI pharmacotherapy because of possible "serotonin syndrome"
Zolmitriptan, or other vascular serotonin receptor agonist, pharmacotherapy, concurrent or within the previous 24 hours because of possible additive vasoconstriction

CAUTIONS AND COMMENTS

Caution patients who are receiving sumatriptan pharmacotherapy against

- performing activities that require alertness, judgment, or physical coordination (e.g., driving an automobile, operating dangerous equipment, supervising children) until their response to sumatriptan pharmacotherapy is known. Sumatriptan may affect these mental and physical functions adversely.

CLINICALLY SIGNIFICANT DRUG INTERACTIONS

No clinically significant drug interactions involving sumatriptan pharmacotherapy have been reported to date other than those noted under "Relative Contraindications" (i.e., ergot, lithium, MAOI, SSRI, and zolmitriptan pharmacotherapy).

ADVERSE DRUG REACTIONS

Sumatriptan pharmacotherapy has been commonly associated with chest pain (i.e., feelings of tightness and pressure in the chest); dizziness; fatigue; feeling of heaviness; neck stiffness; pressure sensation; taste disturbances after intranasal administration; transient local burning sensation, erythema, or pain at the injection site after subcutaneous injection; and weakness. Sumatriptan pharmacotherapy also has been associated with the following ADRs, listed according to body system:

Cardiovascular: angina (rare), cardiac dysrhythmias (rare), coronary vasospasm (rare), and hypertension (transient)
CNS: drowsiness, panic-like symptoms (particularly in patients with a history of anxiety disorder), and seizures (rare)
Cutaneous: flushing
GI: nausea and vomiting
Miscellaneous: tingling sensation

OVERDOSAGE

Clinical data concerning sumatriptan overdosage are not available. In the absence of such data, sumatriptan overdosage should be treated as a medical emergency requiring symptomatic medical support of body systems with attention to increasing sumatriptan elimination. There is no known antidote.

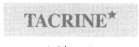

TACRINE*

(tak′ reen)

TRADE NAME

Cognex®

CLASSIFICATION

Nootropic (centrally acting reversible anticholinesterase)

APPROVED INDICATIONS FOR NEUROPSYCHOLOGICAL DISORDERS

Adjunctive pharmacotherapy for the symptomatic management of:

- dementia of the Alzheimer's type: mild to moderate

USUAL DOSAGE AND ADMINISTRATION

Adults: Initially, 40 mg daily orally in four divided doses. After a minimum of six weeks with bi-monthly monitoring of aminotransferase (ALT/SGPT) serum concentrations, the dosage may be increased to 80 mg daily orally in four divided doses. For adult patients who have elevations in ALT/SGPT serum concentrations, see the table "Tacrine Dosage Adjustments for Adult Patients With Elevations in Aminotransferase (ALT/SGPT) Serum Concentrations."

MAXIMUM: 160 mg daily orally

Women who are, or who may become, pregnant: FDA Pregnancy Category C. Safety and efficacy of tacrine pharmacotherapy for women who are pregnant have not been established. Avoid prescribing tacrine pharmacotherapy to women who are pregnant. If tacrine pharmacotherapy is required, advise patients of potential benefits and possible risks to themselves and the embryo, fetus, or neonate. Collaboration with the patient's obstetrician is indicated.

Women who are breast-feeding: Safety and efficacy of tacrine pharmacotherapy for women who are breast-feeding and their neonates and infants have not been established. Avoid prescribing tacrine pharmacotherapy to women who are breast-feeding. If tacrine pharmacotherapy is required, breast-feeding probably should be discontinued. Collaboration with the patient's pediatrician may be indicated.

Elderly adults: See "Usual Dosage and Administration" for adults.

For details and discussion regarding related basic principles of clinical pharmacology, readers are referred to the first text in this series, *The Pharmacologic Basis of Psychotherapeutics: An Introduction for Psychologists.*

Tacrine dosage adjustments for adult patients with elevations in aminotransferase (ALT/SGPT) serum concentrations.

ALT/SGPT serum concentrations	Tacrine dosage adjustment
Up to 3 times the upper limit of normal	No dosage adjustment is necessary. If the ALT serum concentration is >2 times the upper limit of normal, monitor ALT weekly until the concentration returns to normal.
3 to 5 times the upper limit of normal	Reduce the dosage by 40 mg daily and monitor serum ALT concentrations weekly. Dosage may be resumed at the usual initial dose after ALT concentrations have returned to normal levels.
>5 times, but <10 times, the upper limit of normal	Withhold tacrine pharmacotherapy and closely monitor the patient for signs and symptoms of tacrine-induced hepatitis. A rechallenge with the usual initial dosage of tacrine can be considered after ALT serum concentrations have returned to normal levels.
≥10 times the upper limit of normal	Clinical experience is limited. These patients may be subjected to risk for serious or fatal liver damage. Therefore, tacrine pharmacotherapy is *not* recommended. See "Relative Contraindications."

Children and adolescents younger than 18 years of age: Safety and efficacy of tacrine pharmacotherapy for children and adolescents who are younger than 18 years of age have not been established. Tacrine pharmacotherapy is *not* recommended for this age group.

Notes, Mild to Moderate Dementia of the Alzheimer's Type

Each dose of tacrine oral capsules should be ingested on an empty stomach 1 hour before, or 2 hours after, the ingestion of food or beverages to assure maximal absorption and related therapeutic benefit.

AVAILABLE DOSAGE FORMS, STORAGE, AND COMPATIBILITY

Capsules, oral: 10, 20, 30, 40 mg

Notes

General instructions for patients: Instruct patients who are receiving tacrine pharmacotherapy, or those assisting them with their pharmacotherapy, to do the following, as appropriate:

- ingest each dose of the tacrine oral capsules on an empty stomach 1 hour before, or 2 hours after, ingesting foods or beverages.
- safely store tacrine oral capsules out of the reach of children in tightly closed, child-resistant containers at controlled room temperature (15° to 30°C; 59° to 86°F).
- obtain an available patient information sheet regarding tacrine pharmacotherapy from their pharmacist at the time that their prescription is dispensed. Encourage patients to

clarify any questions that they may have regarding tacrine pharmacotherapy with their pharmacist or, if needed, to consult their prescribing psychologist.

PROPOSED MECHANISM OF ACTION

One of the early pathophysiologic changes associated with Alzheimer's disease is the selective loss of cholinergic neurons in the cerebral cortex, hippocampus, and nucleus basalis. This pathophysiologic change results in a relative deficiency of acetylcholine and, thus, memory loss and cognitive deficits. The exact mechanism of tacrine's action in regard to the treatment of Alzheimer's disease has not been fully determined. However, it appears to be related to the following mechanisms: 1) inactivation of cholinesterases, including acetylcholinesterase, which, in turn, inhibits the hydrolysis of the acetylcholine that is released from functioning neurons; and 2) blockade of axonal potassium channels, which, in turn, stimulates the release of acetylcholine.

PHARMACOKINETICS/PHARMACODYNAMICS

Tacrine is rapidly but poorly absorbed (<20%) following oral ingestion. Ingestion with food further reduces the oral availability of tacrine by an additional ~30% to 40%. Peak tacrine blood concentrations are achieved within 1 hour. Tacrine is ~50% bound to plasma proteins and has a mean apparent volume of distribution of 10 liters/kg. Tacrine is extensively metabolized in the liver, primarily by cytochrome P450 isoenzyme CYP1A2. Less than 1% of tacrine is excreted in unchanged form in the urine. The mean half-life of elimination is ~3 hours and the mean total body clearance is ~2 liters/kg/hour.

RELATIVE CONTRAINDICATIONS

Aminotransferase serum concentrations that exceed 10 times the upper limit of normal
Hypersensitivity to tacrine
Jaundice, associated with the elevation of the total serum bilirubin concentration above 3 mg/100 ml (i.e., 3 mg %)

CAUTIONS AND COMMENTS

Caution patients who are receiving tacrine pharmacotherapy, or those assisting them with their pharmacotherapy against

- abrupt discontinuation of tacrine pharmacotherapy. The abrupt discontinuation of tacrine pharmacotherapy may result in a significant decline in cognitive performance.

CLINICALLY SIGNIFICANT DRUG INTERACTIONS

Concurrent tacrine pharmacotherapy and the following may result in clinically significant drug interactions:

Anticholinergic Pharmacotherapy

Concurrent tacrine and anticholinergic (e.g., atropine) pharmacotherapy may result in the antagonism of the anticholinergic by tacrine. Tacrine increases the synaptic concentration of acetylcholine.

Cimetidine Pharmacotherapy

Concurrent tacrine and cimetidine (Tagamet®) pharmacotherapy may result in an increase in the bioavailability of tacrine by ~50%. Dosage adjustment of tacrine generally is not required unless troublesome ADRs are noted.

Fluvoxamine Pharmacotherapy

Tacrine is extensively metabolized in the liver by the hepatic microsomal enzymes, particularly cytochrome P450 isoenzyme CYP1A2. Fluvoxamine (Luvox®), a potent inhibitor of CYP1A2, significantly inhibits the metabolism of tacrine. Concurrent pharmacotherapy may significantly increase tacrine's blood concentrations and exacerbate related ADRs.

Parasympathomimetic Pharmacotherapy

Parasympathomimetics (e.g., bethanechol [Urecholine®]) stimulate the parasympathetic nervous system to release acetylcholine at nerve endings. Tacrine stimulates the release of acetylcholine and inhibits its metabolism by acetylcholinersterase. Thus, concurrent pharmacotherapy is expected to produce additive or synergistic effects.

Pharmacotherapy With Succinylcholine and Related Depolarizing Skeletal Muscle Relaxants

Concurrent tacrine pharmacotherapy may decrease the metabolism of succinylcholine (Anectine®) and related drugs by means of inactivation of cholinesterases. Prolonged neuromuscular blockade and apnea may result from this interaction. Patients must be monitored closely.

Theophylline Pharmacotherapy

Concurrent tacrine and theophylline pharmacotherapy may result in a 2-fold increase in the average blood concentration and half-life of elimination of theophylline. When concurrent pharmacotherapy is required, the blood concentrations of theophylline should be monitored and the theophylline dosage adjusted accordingly. Collaboration with the prescriber of the theophylline pharmacotherapy is indicated.

Tobacco Smoking

Concurrent tobacco smoking of one or more packages of tobacco cigarettes daily may increase the metabolism of tacrine by means of induction of the hepatic microsomal isoenzyme

CYP-1A2. Tacrine blood concentrations among smokers are, on average, approximately one-third the blood concentrations seen in non-smokers. Close patient monitoring and higher tacrine dosages generally are required for patients who smoke one or more packages of tobacco cigarettes daily.

ADVERSE DRUG REACTIONS

Tacrine pharmacotherapy commonly has been associated with dizziness, elevated serum transaminase concentrations, and headache. Tacrine pharmacotherapy also has been associated with the following ADRs, listed according to body system:

CNS: agitation, confusion, convulsions, incoordination (ataxia), and nervousness
Cutaneous: rash and sweating (increased)
GI: abdominal pain, dyspepsia, loss of appetite (anorexia), nausea, and vomiting
Musculoskeletal: joint pain (arthralgia) and muscle pain (myalgia)
Respiratory: runny nose (rhinitis)

OVERDOSAGE

Signs and symptoms of tacrine overdosage may result in cholinergic crisis and bradycardia, cardiovascular collapse, convulsions, hypotension, muscle weakness, nausea, salivation (excessive), sweating, and vomiting. Tacrine overdosage should be treated as a medical emergency requiring symptomatic medical support of body systems with attention to increasing tacrine elimination. Tertiary anticholinergics, such as atropine, may be used as antidotes for tacrine overdosage.

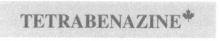

TETRABENAZINE*

(tet′ ra ben a zeen)

TRADE NAME

Nitoman®

CLASSIFICATION

Centrally acting monoamine depletor

APPROVED INDICATIONS FOR NEUROPSYCHOLOGICAL DISORDERS

Pharmacotherapy for the symptomatic management of:

- hyperkinetic movement disorders: hemiballismus; Huntington's chorea; senile chorea; tardive dyskinesia; tic disorders (e.g., Tourette's disorder [Gilles de la Tourette syndrome]) and other hyperkinetic movement disorders

USUAL DOSAGE AND ADMINISTRATION

Hyperkinetic Movement Disorders

Adults: Initially, 25 to 37.5 mg daily orally in two or three divided doses. Increase the daily dosage by 12.5 mg at intervals of three to five days according to individual patient response.

MAXIMUM: 200 mg daily orally in divided doses. Most patients tolerate a maximal daily dosage of 75 mg.

Women who are, or who may become, pregnant: FDA Pregnancy Category "not established." Safety and efficacy of tetrabenazine pharmacotherapy for women who are pregnant have not been established. However, tetrabenazine has been used for many years and no cases of congenital malformations (i.e., birth defects) have been reported. Avoid prescribing tetrabenazine pharmacotherapy to women who are pregnant. If tetrabenazine pharmacotherapy is required, advise patients of potential benefits and possible risks to themselves and the embryo, fetus, or neonate. Collaboration with the patient's obstetrician is indicated.

Women who are breast-feeding: Safety and efficacy of tetrabenazine pharmacotherapy for women who are breast-feeding and their neonates and infants have not been established. Tetrabenazine is excreted in breast milk. Avoid prescribing tetrabenazine pharmacotherapy to women who are breast-feeding. If tetrabenazine pharmacotherapy is required, breast-feeding probably should be discontinued.

For details and discussion regarding related basic principles of clinical pharmacology, readers are referred to the first text in this series, *The Pharmacologic Basis of Psychotherapeutics: An Introduction for Psychologists.*

Elderly, frail, or debilitated patients: Generally prescribe lower dosages for elderly, frail, or debilitated patients. These patients may be more sensitive to the pharmacologic actions of tetrabenazine (e.g., dose-related Parkinsonian-like ADRs) than are younger or healthier adult patients.

Children and adolescents younger than 18 years of age: Initially, 12.5 mg daily orally in two divided doses. Gradually increase the dosage, if needed, according to individual patient response.

Notes, Hyperkinetic Movement Disorders

- Do *not* prescribe tetrabenazine for the treatment of levodopa-induced dyskinetic/choreiform movements.
- Patients who fail to respond to tetrabenazine pharmacotherapy within 7 days are not likely to benefit from either an increase in dosage or combined pharmacotherapy.

AVAILABLE DOSAGE FORMS, STORAGE, AND COMPATIBILITY

Tablets, oral: 25 mg

Notes

General instructions for patients: Instruct patients who are receiving tetrabenazine pharmacotherapy to

- safely store tetrabenazine oral tablets out of the reach of children in tightly closed, child-resistant containers at controlled room temperature (15° to 30°C; 59° to 86°F).
- obtain an available patient information sheet regarding tetrabenazine pharmacotherapy from their pharmacist at the time that their prescription is dispensed. Encourage patients to clarify any questions that they may have regarding tetrabenazine pharmacotherapy with their pharmacist or, if needed, to consult their prescribing psychologist.

PROPOSED MECHANISM OF ACTION

Tetrabenazine interferes with the vesicular storage of biogenic amines, including dopamine, norepinephrine, and serotonin. In this regard, its pharmacologic activity resembles that of the antihypertensive, reserpine (Serpasil®). However, it differs in having much less peripheral activity and in having a much shorter duration of action (i.e., ~24 hours). Hydroxytetrabenazine appears to be the principal active metabolite of tetrabenazine that elicits its effects primarily within the brain. Tetrabenazine also displays antidopaminergic activity within the corpus striatum.

PHARMACOKINETICS/PHARMACODYNAMICS

Tetrabenazine is absorbed erratically from the GI tract following oral ingestion and is subject to extensive first-pass hepatic metabolism. Virtually all of the oral dose that is absorbed is metabolized to the principal active metabolite, hydroxytetrabenazine. Additional data are not available.

RELATIVE CONTRAINDICATIONS

Depression
Hypersensitivity to tetrabenazine
Levodopa-induced dyskinetic/choreiform movements
MAOI pharmacotherapy, concurrent or within 14 days
Parkinson's disease

CAUTIONS AND COMMENTS

Caution patients who are receiving tetrabenazine pharmacotherapy against

- performing activities that require alertness, judgment, or physical coordination (e.g., driving an automobile, operating dangerous equipment, supervising children). Tetrabenazine can cause drowsiness and postural (orthostatic) hypotension. Thus, it may affect these mental and physical functions adversely.

CLINICALLY SIGNIFICANT DRUG INTERACTIONS

Tetrabenazine pharmacotherapy and the following may result in clinically significant drug interactions:

Alcohol Use

Concurrent alcohol use may increase the drowsiness, postural (orthostatic) hypotension, and other related actions of tetrabenazine (see "Adverse Drug Reactions"). Advise patients to avoid, or limit, their use of alcohol while receiving tetrabenazine pharmacotherapy.

Antidepressant Pharmacotherapy

Concurrent tetrabenazine pharmacotherapy and antidepressant pharmacotherapy may result in excessive CNS stimulation and hypertension. If concurrent pharmacotherapy is required, monitor patients closely for related signs and symptoms.

Levodopa Pharmacotherapy

Tetrabenazine pharmacotherapy exacerbates the signs and symptoms of Parkinson's disease and, therefore, significantly reduces the therapeutic action of levodopa.

Pharmacotherapy With CNS Depressants and Other Drugs That Produce CNS Depression

Concurrent tetrabenazine pharmacotherapy with opiate analgesics, sedative-hypnotics, or other drugs that produce CNS depression (e.g., antihistamines, phenothiazines, TCAs) may result in additive CNS depression.

ADVERSE DRUG REACTIONS

Tetrabenazine pharmacotherapy commonly has been associated with depression, drowsiness, fatigue, parkinsonian signs and symptoms, and weakness. Tetrabenazine pharmacotherapy also has been associated with the following ADRs, listed according to body system:

Cardiovascular: hypotension
CNS: agitation, akathisia, anxiety, confusion, disorientation, dizziness, insomnia, irritability, nervousness, and restlessness
GI: drooling, epigastric pain, nausea, and vomiting

OVERDOSAGE

Signs and symptoms of tetrabenazine overdosage include drowsiness, hypotension, hypothermia, and sweating (excessive). Tetrabenazine overdosage requires emergency symptomatic medical support of body systems with attention to increasing tetrabenazine elimination. There is no known antidote.

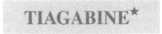
TIAGABINE*

(tye ag′ a been)

TRADE NAME

Gabitril®

CLASSIFICATION

Anticonvulsant (selective GABA uptake inhibitor)

APPROVED INDICATIONS FOR NEUROPSYCHOLOGICAL DISORDERS

Pharmacotherapy for the adjunctive symptomatic management of:

- seizure disorders: partial onset seizures that are refractory to conventional pharmacotherapy

USUAL DOSAGE AND ADMINISTRATION

Seizure Disorders: Partial Seizures

Adults: Initially, 4 mg daily orally in a single dose. Increase the daily dosage at weekly intervals by 4 to 8 mg as indicated by individual patient response. Most patients benefit from 32 to 56 mg daily orally in two to four divided doses.

MAXIMUM: 56 mg daily orally

Women who are, or who may become, pregnant: FDA Pregnancy Category C. Safety and efficacy of tiagabine pharmacotherapy for women who are pregnant have not been established. Avoid prescribing tiagabine pharmacotherapy to women who are pregnant. If tiagabine pharmacotherapy is required, advise patients of potential benefits and possible risks to themselves and the embryo, fetus, or neonate. Collaboration with the patient's obstetrician is indicated.

Women who are breast-feeding: Safety and efficacy of tiagabine pharmacotherapy for women who are breast-feeding and their neonates and infants have not been established. Avoid prescribing tiagabine pharmacotherapy to women who are breast-feeding. If tiagabine pharmacotherapy is required, breast-feeding probably should be discontinued.

For details and discussion regarding related basic principles of clinical pharmacology, readers are referred to the first text in this series, *The Pharmacologic Basis of Psychotherapeutics: An Introduction for Psychologists.*

Elderly, frail, or debilitated patients: Generally prescribe lower dosages of tiagabine for elderly, frail, or debilitated patients. These patients may be more sensitive to the pharmacologic actions of tiagabine than are younger or healthier adult patients.

Adult patients who have liver dysfunction: Prescribe lower dosages of tiagabine for adult patients who have liver dysfunction. The total body clearance of tiagabine is decreased among these patients.

Children younger than 12 years of age: Safety and efficacy of tiagabine pharmacotherapy for children who are younger than 12 years of age have not been established. Tiagabine pharmacotherapy is *not* recommended for this age group.

Adolescents: Initially, 4 mg daily orally in a single dose. Increase the daily dosage at weekly intervals by 4 mg according to individual patient response.

MAXIMUM: 32 mg daily orally

Notes, Seizure Disorders: Partial Seizures

Discontinuing tiagabine pharmacotherapy: Gradually reduce the dosage of tiagabine, if possible, over a period of several days. The abrupt discontinuation of tiagabine pharmacotherapy may result in "withdrawal seizures."

AVAILABLE DOSAGE FORMS, STORAGE, AND COMPATIBILITY

Tablets, oral: 4, 12, 16, 20 mg

Notes

General instructions for patients: Instruct patients who are receiving tiagabine pharmacotherapy to

- ingest each dose of the tiagabine oral tablets with food in order to decrease associated ADRs.
- safely store tiagabine oral tablets out of the reach of children in tightly closed, light- and child-resistant containers at controlled room temperature (15° to 25°C; 59° to 77°F).
- obtain an available patient information sheet regarding tiagabine pharmacotherapy from their pharmacist at the time that their prescription is dispensed. Encourage patients to clarify any questions that they may have regarding tiagabine pharmacotherapy with their pharmacist or, if needed, to consult their prescribing psychologist.

PROPOSED MECHANISM OF ACTION

GABA is the major inhibitory neurotransmitter within the CNS. Tiagabine selectively and reversibly inhibits the re-uptake of GABA into presynaptic neurons and glial cells following synaptic release. Thus, synaptic concentrations of GABA are increased, GABAergic transmission is enhanced, and seizure activity is reduced.

PHARMACOKINETICS/PHARMACODYNAMICS

Tiagabine is rapidly and well absorbed following oral ingestion ($F = 0.9$). Peak blood concentrations are achieved within 1 hour. The ingestion of tiagabine with food decreases the rate but not the extent of tiagabine absorption. Tiagabine is highly bound to plasma proteins ($\sim$96%) and is widely distributed throughout the body with an apparent volume of distribution of $\sim$1 liter/kg. Tiagabine is extensively metabolized by the process of oxidation and glucuronidation in the liver by the hepatic cytochrome P450 isoenzyme CYP-3A. Less than 3% is excreted in unchanged form in the urine. The total body clearance of tiagabine is $\sim$13 liters/hour. The mean half-life of elimination is $\sim$7 hours.

RELATIVE CONTRAINDICATIONS

Hypersensitivity to tiagabine

CAUTIONS AND COMMENTS

Caution patients who are receiving tiagabine pharmacotherapy against

- performing activities that require alertness, judgment, or physical coordination (e.g., driving an automobile, operating dangerous equipment, supervising children) until their response to tiagabine pharmacotherapy is known. Tiagabine may affect these mental and physical functions adversely.

In addition to this general precaution, caution patients who are receiving tiagabine pharmacotherapy to

- inform their prescribing psychologist if they begin or discontinue any other pharmacotherapy while receiving tiagabine pharmacotherapy.

CLINICALLY SIGNIFICANT DRUG INTERACTIONS

Concurrent tiagabine pharmacotherapy and the following may result in clinically significant drug interactions:

Alcohol Use

Concurrent alcohol use may increase the CNS depressant action of tiagabine. Advise patients to avoid, or limit, their use of alcohol while receiving tiagabine pharmacotherapy.

Carbamazepine Pharmacotherapy

Concurrent tiagabine and carbamazepine (Tegretol®) pharmacotherapy may result in an increased total body clearance of tiagabine by up to 70%. An increase in the dosage of tiagabine may be required.

Pharmacotherapy With CNS Depressants and Other Drugs That Produce CNS Depression

Concurrent tiagabine pharmacotherapy and pharmacotherapy with opiate analgesics, sedative-hypnotics, or other drugs that produce CNS depression (e.g., antihistamines, phenothiazines, TCAs) may result in additive CNS depression.

Phenobarbital or Primidone Pharmacotherapy

Concurrent tiagabine and phenobarbital (Luminal®) or primidone (Mysoline®) pharmacotherapy may result in an increased total body clearance of tiagabine by up to 70%. An increase in the dosage of tiagabine may be required.

Phenytoin Pharmacotherapy

Concurrent tiagabine and phenytoin (Dilantin®) pharmacotherapy may result in an increased total body clearance of tiagabine by up to 70%. Monitor patient response closely and adjust the dosage accordingly. An increase in the dosage of tiagabine may be required.

ADVERSE DRUG REACTIONS

Tiagabine pharmacotherapy commonly has been associated with abnormal thinking (difficulty with attention and concentration), asthenia (weakness, particularly of cerebellar or muscular origin), dizziness, nervousness, somnolence, and tremor. Tiagabine pharmacotherapy also has been associated with the following ADRs, listed according to body system:

Cardiovascular: hypertension, palpitation, syncope, and tachycardia
CNS: confusion, depression, emotional lability, euphoria, and migraine
GI: diarrhea, gingivitis, and nausea
Musculoskeletal: arthralgia

OVERDOSAGE

Signs and symptoms of tiagabine overdosage include agitation, confusion, hostility, impaired consciousness, myoclonus, somnolence, speech impairment, and weakness. Tiagabine overdosage requires emergency symptomatic medical support of body systems with attention to increasing tiagabine elimination. There is no known antidote.

TOLCAPONE
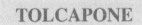

(tole′ ka pone)

TRADE NAME

Tasmar®

CLASSIFICATION

Antiparkinsonian (reversible catechol-O-methyltransferase [COMT] inhibitor)

APPROVED INDICATIONS FOR NEUROPSYCHOLOGICAL DISORDERS

Adjunctive pharmacotherapy for the symptomatic management of:

- Parkinson's disease: idiopathic. Tolcapone pharmacotherapy should be prescribed *only* as adjunctive pharmacotherapy with levodopa pharmacotherapy. See "Notes, Idiopathic Parkinson's Disease." See also "Cautions and Comments."

USUAL DOSAGE AND ADMINISTRATION

Parkinson's Disease: Idiopathic

Adults: 300 to 600 mg daily orally in three divided doses. See "Notes, Idiopathic Parkinson's Disease."

MAXIMUM: 600 mg daily orally

Women who are, or who may become, pregnant: FDA Pregnancy Category C. Safety and efficacy of tolcapone pharmacotherapy for women who are pregnant have not been established. Avoid prescribing tolcapone pharmacotherapy to women who are pregnant.

Women who are breast-feeding: Safety and efficacy of tolcapone pharmacotherapy for women who are breast-feeding and their neonates and infants have not been established. Avoid prescribing tolcapone pharmacotherapy to women who are breast-feeding.

Elderly patients and those who have kidney dysfunction: Generally, no special adjustments to the usual recommended adult dosage are required for elderly patients or those who have kidney dysfunction. Kidney dysfunction does not appear to significantly affect tolcapone pharmacokinetics. See "Notes, Idiopathic Parkinson's Disease."

For details and discussion regarding related basic principles of clinical pharmacology, readers are referred to the first text in this series, *The Pharmacologic Basis of Psychotherapeutics: An Introduction for Psychologists.*

Children and adolescents younger than 18 years of age: Safety and efficacy of tolcapone pharmacotherapy for children and adolescents who are younger than 18 years of age have not been established. Tolcapone pharmacotherapy is *not* recommended for this age group.

Notes, Idiopathic Parkinson's Disease

Tolcapone pharmacotherapy generally allows, and in many cases requires, a reduction in the total dosage of levodopa by ~30%, on average, in order to decrease associated ADRs.

Initiating tolcapone pharmacotherapy: Because of the potential for severe life-threatening ADRs (see "Adverse Drug Reactions"), the potential risks and benefits of tolcapone pharmacotherapy should be fully discussed with the patient and/or responsible family members prior to the initiation of pharmacotherapy. Informed consent should be obtained from the patient.

Tolcapone pharmacotherapy is prescribed *only* as an adjunct to the symptomatic management of Parkinson's disease among patients who are receiving levodopa pharmacotherapy (see "Proposed Mechanism of Action"). It is recommended that the first daily dose of tolcapone be ingested together with the first daily dose of levodopa. The subsequent two doses of tolcapone should be ingested 6 and 12 hours later, respectively.

Discontinuing tolcapone pharmacotherapy: In order to avoid the occurrence of a relatively rare, but potentially fatal, syndrome that resembles the neuroleptic malignant syndrome, the levodopa dosage should be correspondingly increased when tolcapone adjunctive pharmacotherapy is discontinued. The signs and symptoms of this syndrome include altered consciousness, elevated serum creatinine phosphokinase levels, elevated temperature (hyperpyrexia), and muscular rigidity.

AVAILABLE DOSAGE FORMS, STORAGE, AND COMPATIBILITY

Tablets, oral: 100, 200 mg

Notes

General instructions for patients: Instruct patients who are receiving adjunctive tolcapone pharmacotherapy to

- safely store tolcapone oral tablets out of the reach of children in child-resistant containers at controlled room temperature (15° to 30 °C; 59° to 86 °F).
- immediately report to their prescribing psychologist any signs and symptoms of liver toxicity: anorexia (loss of appetite), clay-colored stools, dark-colored urine, fatigue, jaundice, lethargy, pruritus, and right upper quadrant tenderness.
- obtain an available patient information sheet regarding tolcapone pharmacotherapy from their pharmacist at the time that their prescription is dispensed. Encourage patients to clarify any questions that they may have regarding tolcapone pharmacotherapy with their pharmacist or, if needed, to consult their prescribing psychologist.

PROPOSED MECHANISM OF ACTION

Levodopa, a synthetic dopamine precursor, is metabolized by both aromatic L-amino acid decarboxylase and COMT to an inactive metabolite (3-0-methyldopa). Tolcapone, a reversible COMT inhibitor, prolongs the half-life of elimination of levodopa and increases dopamine levels in the corpus striatum. Thus, tolcapone decreases the "off" time among patients who have idiopathic Parkinson's disease and are experiencing a deteriorating response to levodopa pharmacotherapy (i.e., are experiencing the "on–off" phenomenon).

PHARMACOKINETICS/PHARMACODYNAMICS

Tolcapone is rapidly absorbed from the GI tract following oral ingestion. Peak blood concentrations are achieved in ~2 hours. Oral bioavailability is good ($F = 0.7$). Food may decrease the bioavailability of tolcapone by 10% to 20%. Tolcapone is highly bound to plasma proteins (i.e., >99%) and has a relatively small apparent volume of distribution (~9 liters). Tolcapone is metabolized extensively to several inactive metabolites. Less than 1% is excreted in unchanged form in the urine. The total body clearance is ~7 liters/hour. The half-life of elimination is 2 to 3 hours.

RELATIVE CONTRAINDICATIONS

Hypersensitivity to tolcapone
Liver dysfunction (see "Adverse Drug Reactions")
Nonselective MAOI (e.g., phenelzine [Nardil®], tranylcypromine [Parnate®]) pharmacotherapy, concurrent

CAUTIONS AND COMMENTS

Because of the risk of potentially fatal, acute fulminant liver failure, tolcapone pharmacotherapy generally should be reserved for patients who meet all of the following criteria: 1) have Parkinson's disease, 2) are receiving fixed-ratio combination levodopa and carbidopa pharmacotherapy, 3) are experiencing fluctuations in therapeutic response (i.e., "on–off" phenomenon), and either 4a) are not responding satisfactorily to other adjunctive pharmacotherapy, or 4b) are not appropriate candidates for other adjunctive pharmacotherapy.

Prescribe adjunctive tolcapone pharmacotherapy cautiously to patients who

- have postural (orthostatic) hypotension. A higher incidence of postural hypotension and related syncope (fainting) have been noted among patients receiving adjunctive tolcapone pharmacotherapy. Patients who have a history of postural hypotension prior to the initiation of tolcapone pharmacotherapy appear to be at particular risk.

Caution patients who are receiving adjunctive tolcapone pharmacotherapy against

- performing activities that require alertness, judgment, or physical coordination (e.g., driving an automobile, operating dangerous equipment, supervising children) until their response to tolcapone pharmacotherapy is known. Tolcapone may affect these mental and physical functions adversely.

In addition to this general precaution, caution patients who are receiving adjunctive tolcapone pharmacotherapy to

- inform their prescribing psychologist if they begin or discontinue any other pharmacotherapy while receiving tolcapone pharmacotherapy.

CLINICALLY SIGNIFICANT DRUG INTERACTIONS

Concurrent adjunctive tolcapone pharmacotherapy and the following may result in clinically significant drug interactions:

Pharmacotherapy With Drugs Metabolized by COMT

Tolcapone is an inhibitor of COMT. Therefore, the metabolism of any drugs metabolized by COMT (e.g., methyldopa [Aldomet®], apomorphine, dobutamine [Dobutrex®], epinephrine [Adrenalin®], and isoproterenol [Isuprel®]) is expected to be reduced with a concomitant increase in the blood concentrations of these drugs. In the absence of reported clinical experience, a reduction in the dosage of these drugs should be considered together with careful clinical monitoring for possible ADRs. Collaboration with other prescribers is indicated in order to provide optimal pharmacotherapy.

ADVERSE DRUG REACTIONS

Adjunctive tolcapone pharmacotherapy commonly has been associated with diarrhea, dyskinesia, dystonia, and loss of appetite (anorexia). Tolcapone pharmacotherapy also has been associated with the following ADRs, listed according to body system:

CNS: confusion, dizziness, and headache
Hepatic: *Acute fulminant liver failure resulting in death.* Although relatively rare (i.e., 3 reported deaths in ~40,000 patient-years of worldwide use), the reported incidence of this ADR is 10- to 100-fold higher than the background incidence in the general population. In order to prevent or minimize the occurrence of this potentially fatal ADR, the following are recommended: 1) do *not* initiate tolcapone pharmacotherapy for patients who have significant liver dysfunction; 2) regularly monitor liver function tests (i.e., SGPT/ALT, SGOT/AST) every 2 weeks for the first year, ever 4 weeks for the next 6 months, and every 8 weeks thereafter; 3) discontinue tolcapone pharmacotherapy immediately when signs and symptoms of possible liver dysfunction are noted; and 4) do *not* reinitiate tolcapone pharmacotherapy for patients who have previously discontinued tolcapone pharmacotherapy because of associated liver dysfunction.
Renal: intensified yellow discoloration of the urine (a harmless ADR, but one necessitating appropriate patient education)
Miscellaneous: *Note*: Because adjunctive tolcapone pharmacotherapy inhibits the metabolism of levodopa, also monitor patients for ADRs associated with levodopa pharmacotherapy (*see the* levodopa monograph).

OVERDOSAGE

In the absence of reported clinical experience with tolcapone overdosage, it is expected that tolcapone overdosage would require symptomatic medical support of body systems with attention to increasing tolcapone elimination. There is no known antidote. (See also the levodopa monograph, "Overdosage.")

TOPIRAMATE

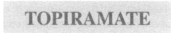

(toe pyre′ a mate)

TRADE NAME

Topamax®

CLASSIFICATION

Anticonvulsant (sulfamate-substituted monosaccharide)

APPROVED INDICATIONS FOR NEUROPSYCHOLOGICAL DISORDERS

Pharmacotherapy for the symptomatic management of:

- seizure disorders: partial onset seizures among patients who are refractory to more conventional anticonvulsant pharmacotherapy

USUAL DOSAGE AND ADMINISTRATION

Seizure Disorders: Partial Onset Seizures Among Patients Who Are Refractory to More Conventional Anticonvulsant Pharmacotherapy

Adults: Initially, 50 mg daily orally in two divided doses. Increase the daily dosage at weekly intervals by 50 mg according to individual patient response.

MAINTENANCE: The usual maintenance dosage is 400 mg daily orally in two divided doses.

MAXIMUM: 800 mg daily orally. Note that dosages in excess of 400 mg daily generally have not resulted in increased therapeutic benefit, but have increased the incidence and severity of ADRs.

Women who are, or who may become, pregnant: FDA Pregnancy Category C. Safety and efficacy of topiramate pharmacotherapy for women who are pregnant have not been established. Avoid prescribing topiramate pharmacotherapy to women who are pregnant. If topiramate pharmacotherapy is required, advise patients of potential benefits and possible risks to themselves and the embryo, fetus, or neonate. Collaboration with the patient's obstetrician is indicated.

For details and discussion regarding related basic principles of clinical pharmacology, readers are referred to the first text in this series, *The Pharmacologic Basis of Psychotherapeutics: An Introduction for Psychologists.*

Women who are breast-feeding: Safety and efficacy of topiramate pharmacotherapy for women who are breast-feeding and their neonates and infants have not been established. Avoid prescribing topiramate pharmacotherapy to women who are breast-feeding. If topiramate pharmacotherapy is required, breast-feeding probably should be discontinued.

Elderly, frail, or debilitated patients: Age alone does not appear to have a significant effect on the clearance of topiramate. However, generally prescribe lower dosages for elderly, frail, or debilitated patients. These patients may be more sensitive to the pharmacologic actions of topiramate than are younger or healthier adult patients.

Adult patients who have kidney dysfunction: Initially, 50 mg daily orally in two divided doses. Adjust the dosage according to individual patient response.

MAXIMUM: 200 mg daily orally

Children and adolescents younger than 18 years of age: Safety and efficacy of topiramate pharmacotherapy for children and adolescents who are younger than 18 years of age have not been established. Topiramate pharmacotherapy is *not* recommended for this age group.

Notes, Seizure Disorders: Partial Onset Seizures Among Patients Who Are Refractory to More Conventional Anticonvulsant Pharmacotherapy

Topiramate oral tablets may be ingested without regard to meals.

Discontinuing topiramate pharmacotherapy: Avoid discontinuing topiramate pharmacotherapy abruptly. Whenever possible, gradually discontinue topiramate pharmacotherapy by reducing the daily dosage by 100 mg at weekly intervals until it is discontinued completely. The abrupt discontinuation of topiramate pharmacotherapy has been associated with "withdrawal seizures."

AVAILABLE DOSAGE FORMS, STORAGE, AND COMPATIBILITY

Tablets, oral: 25, 100, 200 mg

Notes

General instructions for patients: Instruct patients who are receiving topiramate pharmacotherapy to

- safely store topiramate oral tablets out of the reach of children in tightly closed, child-resistant containers at controlled room temperature (15° to 30°C; 59° to 86°F).
- swallow each dose of the topiramate oral tablets whole with adequate liquid chaser (e.g., 60 to 120 ml of water) without breaking, chewing, or crushing the tablets.
- obtain an available patient information sheet regarding topiramate pharmacotherapy from their pharmacist at the time that their prescription is dispensed. Encourage patients to clarify any questions that they may have regarding topiramate pharmacotherapy with their pharmacist or, if needed, to consult their prescribing psychologist.

PROPOSED MECHANISM OF ACTION

The exact mechanism of topiramate's anticonvulsant action has not been fully determined. However, it appears to be related to the following mechanisms: 1) inhibition of voltage-dependent sodium ion channels, which, in turn, reduce the frequency at which action potentials are generated when neurons are subjected to a sustained depolarization; 2) potentiation of the activity of GABA at some subtypes of $GABA_A$ receptors; and 3) antagonism of the ability of kainate to activate the glutamate receptor. Topiramate also is a weak inhibitor of some isoenzymes of carbonic anhydrase. This action accounts for several of topiramate's ADRs.

PHARMACOKINETICS/PHARMACODYNAMICS

Topiramate is rapidly and well absorbed following oral ingestion ($F = 0.8$). Peak blood concentrations are achieved within 2 to 3 hours. The ingestion of food does not significantly affect the bioavailability of topiramate. Topiramate is only slightly bound to plasma proteins ($\sim$15%). It has an apparent volume of distribution of $\sim$0.7 liters/kg. Approximately 70% of topiramate is excreted in unchanged form in the urine. The total body clearance is $\sim$25 ml/minute. The half-life of elimination is $\sim$21 hours.

RELATIVE CONTRAINDICATIONS

Hypersensitivity to topiramate

CAUTIONS AND COMMENTS

Prescribe topiramate pharmacotherapy cautiously to patients who

- are at risk for the development of kidney stones (nephrolithiasis). Risk factors for kidney stone formation include the following: 20 to 50 years of age; hypercalciuria (elevated calcium levels in the urine); male gender; positive family history of kidney stones; and prior kidney stone formation.

Caution patients who are receiving topiramate pharmacotherapy against

- performing activities that require alertness, judgment, or physical coordination (e.g., driving an automobile, operating dangerous equipment, supervising children) until their response to topiramate pharmacotherapy is known. Topiramate may affect these mental and physical functions adversely.

In addition to this general precaution, caution patients who are receiving topiramate pharmacotherapy to

- drink an appropriate amount of water daily so that adequate hydration is maintained. Adequate hydration reduces the risk for kidney stone formation.
- inform their prescribing psychologist if they begin or discontinue any other pharmacotherapy while receiving topiramate pharmacotherapy.

CLINICALLY SIGNIFICANT DRUG INTERACTIONS

Concurrent topiramate pharmacotherapy and the following may result in clinically significant drug interactions:

Alcohol Use

Concurrent alcohol use may increase the CNS depressant action of topiramate. Advise patients to avoid, or limit, their use of alcohol while receiving topiramate pharmacotherapy.

Carbamazepine Pharmacotherapy

Concurrent topiramate and carbamazepine (Tegretol®) pharmacotherapy can reduce the blood concentrations of topiramate by ~40%. Although blood concentrations of topiramate are not correlated directly with therapeutic efficacy, monitor patients closely and adjust the dosage, if needed, according to individual patient response.

Estrogen Pharmacotherapy

Concurrent topiramate pharmacotherapy may reduce the efficacy of estrogen, particularly low-dose (e.g., 20 μg) estrogen oral contraceptives. Advise women who are receiving estrogen pharmacotherapy of this potential interaction. Alternative methods of contraception may be required. Collaboration with the prescriber of the estrogen pharmacotherapy is indicated.

Pharmacotherapy With Acetazolamide and Other Carbonic Anhydrase Inhibitors

Concurrent topiramate and acetazolamide (Diamox®) or other carbonic anhydrase inhibitor pharmacotherapy may promote kidney stone formation by reducing urinary citrate excretion and increasing urinary pH. Avoid concurrent topiramate pharmacotherapy and pharmacotherapy with acetazolamide or other carbonic anhydrase inhibitors. Particularly avoid concurrent pharmacotherapy among patients who are at risk for kidney stone formation (see "Cautions and Comments").

Pharmacotherapy With CNS Depressants and Other Drugs That Produce CNS Depression

Concurrent topiramate pharmacotherapy and pharmacotherapy with opiate analgesics, sedative-hypnotics, or other drugs that produce CNS depression (e.g., antihistamines, phenothiazines, TCAs) may result in additive CNS depression.

Pharmacotherapy With Drugs That Are Metabolized by the Cytochrome P450 Isoenzyme CYP2C19

Topiramate inhibits the enzyme activity of CYP2C19. Thus, concurrent pharmacotherapy may result in increased blood concentrations of drugs metabolized by CYP2C19 (e.g., diazepam

[Valium®], mephenytoin [Mesantoin®], omeprazole [Prilosec®]) with resultant increased ADRs and toxicity.

Phenytoin Pharmacotherapy

Concurrent topiramate and phenytoin (Dilantin®) pharmacotherapy can reduce the blood concentrations of topiramate by ~60%. Although blood concentrations of topiramate are not correlated directly with therapeutic efficacy, monitor patients closely and adjust the topiramate dosage, if needed, according to individual patient response.

ADVERSE DRUG REACTIONS

Topiramate pharmacotherapy commonly has been associated with the following ADRs: confusion, difficulty concentrating, dizziness, fatigue, incoordination (ataxia), loss of appetite (anorexia), nervousness, nystagmus, paresthesia (sensation of numbness, prickling, or tingling), psychomotor slowing, somnolence (prolonged drowsiness), speech and language impairment, and weight loss. Topiramate pharmacotherapy also has been associated with the following ADRs, listed according to body system:

CNS: aggression, agitation, anxiety, apathy, and depression
GI: abdominal pain and nausea
Ophthalmic: double vision (diplopia)
Renal: kidney stones (nephrolithiasis) (see "Cautions and Comments")

OVERDOSAGE

Clinical data concerning topiramate overdosage are not available. In the absence of such data, topiramate overdosage should be treated as a medical emergency requiring symptomatic medical support of body systems with attention to increasing topiramate elimination. There is no known antidote.

TRAMADOL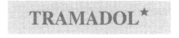*

(tra′ ma dole)

TRADE NAME

Ultram®

CLASSIFICATION

Opiate analgesic congener (mixed agonist/antagonist). *Note*: Although acting at the opiate receptor (see "Proposed Mechanism of Action"), tramadol is *not* a natural or synthetic derivative of opium. Therefore, it is *not* a true or classical opiate analgesic. Consequently, tramadol is *not* subject to control under the U.S. Federal Controlled Substances Act.

See also "Opiate Analgesics, General Monograph."

APPROVED INDICATIONS FOR NEUROPSYCHOLOGICAL DISORDERS

Adjunctive pharmacotherapy for the symptomatic management of:

- pain disorders: acute and chronic pain, moderate to severe

USUAL DOSAGE AND ADMINISTRATION

Acute and Chronic Pain, Moderate to Severe

Adults: 50 to 100 mg orally every four to six hours as required for the relief of moderate to severe pain

MAXIMUM: 400 mg daily orally is the generally recommended maximal daily dosage, particularly for patients who require long-term tramadol pharmacotherapy.

Women who are, or who may become, pregnant: FDA Pregnancy Category C. Safety and efficacy of tramadol pharmacotherapy for women who are pregnant have not been established. Avoid prescribing tramadol pharmacotherapy to women who are pregnant. If tramadol pharmacotherapy is required, advise patients of potential benefits and possible risks to themselves and the embryo, fetus, or neonate. Collaboration with the patient's obstetrician and pediatrician is indicated.

For details and discussion regarding related basic principles of clinical pharmacology, readers are referred to the first text in this series, *The Pharmacologic Basis of Psychotherapeutics: An Introduction for Psychologists.*

Women who are breast-feeding: Safety and efficacy of tramadol pharmacotherapy for women who are breast-feeding and their neonates and infants have not been established. Although only a small amount (i.e., ~0.1%) of the maternal dose is excreted in breast milk, avoid prescribing tramadol pharmacotherapy to women who are breast-feeding. If tramadol pharmacotherapy is required, breast-feeding probably should be discontinued. If desired, lactation may be maintained and breast-feeding resumed following the discontinuation of short-term tramadol pharmacotherapy.

Elderly, frail, or debilitated patients: Initially, 200 mg daily orally in four divided doses. Gradually increase the dosage, if needed, according to individual patient response. Generally prescribe lower dosages for elderly, frail, or debilitated patients. These patients may be more sensitive to the pharmacologic actions of tramadol than are younger or healthier adult patients.

MAXIMUM: 300 mg daily orally is the general maximal dosage for patients who are 75 years of age or older.

Patients who have kidney or liver dysfunction: 100 to 200 mg daily orally in two divided doses, at 12-hour intervals.

Children and adolescents younger than 16 years of age: Safety and efficacy of tramadol pharmacotherapy for children and adolescents who are younger than 16 years of age have not been established. Tramadol pharmacotherapy is *not* recommended for this age group.

Notes, Acute or Chronic Pain, Moderate to Severe

Discontinuing tramadol pharmacotherapy: Gradually discontinue tramadol pharmacotherapy. The abrupt discontinuation of tramadol pharmacotherapy, particularly high-dosage or long-term pharmacotherapy, may result in an acute withdrawal reaction. The signs and symptoms of this reaction include anxiety, diarrhea, hallucinations (rare), insomnia, nausea, pain, piloerection, rigors, sweating, tremors, and upper respiratory tract symptoms.

AVAILABLE DOSAGE FORMS, STORAGE, AND COMPATIBILITY

Tablets, oral: 50 mg

Notes

General instructions for patients: Instruct patients who are receiving tramadol pharmacotherapy to

- safely store tramadol oral tablets out of the reach of children in tightly closed, child-resistant containers at controlled room temperature (15° to 25°C; 59° to 77°F).
- obtain an available patient information sheet regarding tramadol pharmacotherapy from their pharmacist at the time that their prescription is dispensed. Encourage patients to clarify any questions that they may have regarding tramadol pharmacotherapy with their pharmacist or, if needed, to consult their prescribing psychologist.

PROPOSED MECHANISM OF ACTION

The exact mechanism of the analgesic action of tramadol has not yet been fully determined. However, both tramadol and its active metabolite, M1, selectively bind to the mu-opiate receptors. This binding is thought to account primarily for their observed analgesic action. In addition, tramadol inhibits the re-uptake of selective monoamines (i.e., norepinephrine, serotonin). This action may contribute to the analgesic action of tramadol and to potential drug interactions (see "Clinically Significant Drug Interactions").

PHARMACOKINETICS/PHARMACODYNAMICS

Tramadol is well absorbed from the GI tract following oral ingestion ($F = 0.75$). The ingestion of food does not affect the rate or extent of tramadol absorption. Peak blood concentrations are achieved by $\sim$2 hours. Tramadol is only partially bound to plasma proteins ($\sim$20%) and has an apparent volume of distribution of $\sim$3 liters/kg. Tramadol is metabolized extensively to several metabolites including an active metabolite, M1. Approximately 30% of tramadol is excreted in unchanged form in the urine. The mean half-life of elimination is $\sim$6 hours. Analgesia generally occurs within 1 hour following oral ingestion, peaks within 2 to 3 hours, and lasts for 3 to 6 hours. Tramadol-induced analgesia is only partially antagonized by naloxone (Narcan®).

RELATIVE CONTRAINDICATIONS

CNS depressant intoxication, acute
Hypersensitivity to tramadol or opiate analgesics
Opiate addiction and habituation, history of

CAUTIONS AND COMMENTS

Tramadol is addicting and habituating. It has a high abuse potential. Prescribe tramadol pharmacotherapy cautiously to patients who have histories of problematic patterns of alcohol or other abusable psychotropic use. See also "Relative Contraindications."

Tramadol pharmacotherapy reportedly is associated with a risk of seizures. This risk is increased with dosages exceeding the recommended maximal dosage. Tramadol pharmacotherapy also has been associated with an increased risk for seizures among patients who concurrently are receiving MAOIs, opiate analgesics, SSRIs, TCAs, or other pharmacotherapy that may decrease the seizure threshold.

Cautiously prescribe tramadol pharmacotherapy for patients who

- have histories of seizure disorders. Seizures have been associated with tramadol pharmacotherapy. An increased risk is noted for patients who have a history of seizure disorders, particularly those who are receiving concurrent antidepressant or antipsychotic pharmacotherapy.

Caution patients who are receiving tramadol pharmacotherapy against

- performing activities that require alertness, judgment, or physical coordination (e.g., driving an automobile, operating dangerous equipment, supervising children) until their response to tramadol pharmacotherapy is known. Tramadol may affect these mental and physical functions adversely.

In addition to this general precaution, caution patients who are receiving tramadol pharmacotherapy to

- inform their prescribing psychologist if they begin or discontinue any other pharmacotherapy while receiving tramadol pharmacotherapy.

CLINICALLY SIGNIFICANT DRUG INTERACTIONS

Concurrent tramadol pharmacotherapy and the following may result in clinically significant drug interactions:

Alcohol Use

Concurrent alcohol use may increase the CNS depressant action of tramadol. Advise patients to avoid, or limit, their use of alcohol while receiving tramadol pharmacotherapy.

Carbamazepine Pharmacotherapy

Carbamazepine (Tegretol®) induces the hepatic microsomal enzymes (e.g., the CYP2D6 isoenzyme of cytochrome P450) that are primarily responsible for the metabolism of tramadol. Patients who are receiving long-term carbamazepine pharmacotherapy of up to 800 mg daily may require twice the usual recommended dosage of tramadol.

Pharmacotherapy With CNS Depressants and Other Drugs That Produce CNS Depression

Concurrent tramadol pharmacotherapy and pharmacotherapy with opiate analgesics, sedative-hypnotics, or other drugs that produce CNS depression (e.g., antihistamines, phenothiazines, TCAs) may result in additive CNS depression.

See also "Cautions and Comments."

ADVERSE DRUG REACTIONS

Tramadol pharmacotherapy commonly has been associated with asthenia, constipation, dizziness, headache, nausea, severe itching (pruritus), somnolence, and vomiting. Tramadol pharmacotherapy also has been associated with the following ADRs, listed according to body system:

Cardiovascular: vasodilation
CNS: anxiety, confusion, euphoria, hallucinations, nervousness, and seizures
Cutaneous: rash
Genitourinary: urinary frequency and urinary retention
GI: abdominal pain, diarrhea, dry mouth, dyspepsia, flatulence, and loss of appetite (anorexia)
Musculoskeletal: hypertonia
Miscellaneous: malaise and sweating

OVERDOSAGE

Signs and symptoms of tramadol overdosage include respiratory depression and seizures. Tramadol overdosage can be potentially fatal. Thus, tramadol overdosage should be treated as a medical emergency requiring symptomatic medical support of body systems with attention to increasing tramadol elimination. There is no known antidote. Naloxone (Narcan®) pharmacotherapy for the management of tramadol overdosage does *not* consistently counteract the associated lethality of tramadol overdosage. Naloxone reverses only some of the signs and symptoms associated with tramadol overdosage and may actually *increase* the risk for seizures.

TRIHEXYPHENIDYL
[Benzhexol]

(trye hex ee fen′ i dil)

TRADE NAMES

Aparkane®
Artane®
Trihexane®
Trihexyphen®

CLASSIFICATION

Antiparkinsonian (tertiary amine antimuscarinic)

APPROVED INDICATIONS FOR NEUROPSYCHOLOGICAL DISORDERS

Adjunctive pharmacotherapy for the symptomatic management of:

- Parkinson's disease. Trihexyphenidyl is indicated for all forms of Parkinson's disease including idiopathic and drug-induced. Trihexyphenidyl is prescribed as adjunctive pharmacotherapy with other antiparkinsonian drugs.

USUAL DOSAGE AND ADMINISTRATION

Parkinson's Disease

Adults: Initially, 1 mg daily orally in a single dose. Increase the dosage by 2-mg increments at three to five day intervals, according to individual patient response.

MAXIMUM: 15 mg daily orally

Women who are, or who may become, pregnant: FDA Pregnancy Category "not established." Safety and efficacy of trihexyphenidyl pharmacotherapy for women who are pregnant have not been established. Avoid prescribing trihexyphenidyl pharmacotherapy to women who are pregnant. If trihexyphenidyl pharmacotherapy is required, advise patients of potential benefits and possible risks to themselves and the embryo, fetus, or neonate. Collaboration with the patient's obstetrician is indicated.

For details and discussion regarding related basic principles of clinical pharmacology, readers are referred to the first text in this series, *The Pharmacologic Basis of Psychotherapeutics: An Introduction for Psychologists.*

Women who are breast-feeding: Safety and efficacy of trihexyphenidyl pharmacotherapy for women who are breast-feeding and their neonates and infants have not been established. Avoid prescribing trihexyphenidyl pharmacotherapy to women who are breast-feeding. If trihexyphenidyl pharmacotherapy is required, breast-feeding probably should be discontinued. Collaboration with the patient's pediatrician may be indicated.

Elderly, frail, or debilitated patients: Generally prescribe lower dosages for elderly, frail, or debilitated patients. These patients may be more sensitive to the pharmacologic actions of trihexyphenidyl than are younger or healthier adult patients.

Children and adolescents younger than 18 years of age: Safety and efficacy of trihexyphenidyl pharmacotherapy for children and adolescents who are younger than 18 years of age have not been established. Trihexyphenidyl pharmacotherapy is *not* recommended for this age group.

Notes, Parkinson's Disease

Maximal therapeutic benefit from trihexyphenidyl pharmacotherapy is in the range of 20% to 30% improvement among 50% to 75% of patients. Trihexyphenidyl usually is prescribed as adjunctive pharmacotherapy with other antiparkinsonian drugs. When adjunctive trihexyphenidyl pharmacotherapy is prescribed with levodopa pharmacotherapy, it may be necessary to reduce the dosage of each drug according to individual patient response.

For many patients, trihexyphenidyl pharmacotherapy is best tolerated when the total daily dosage is divided into three doses and ingested with meals.

AVAILABLE DOSAGE FORMS, STORAGE, AND COMPATIBILITY

Elixir, oral: 2 mg/5 ml (contains 5% alcohol)
Tablets, oral: 2, 5 mg

Notes

Patients who are receiving adjunctive trihexyphenidyl pharmacotherapy require a gonioscope evaluation and close monitoring of intraocular pressure at regular intervals. Collaboration with the patient's ophthalmologist is indicated.

General instructions for patients: Instruct patients who are receiving adjunctive trihexyphenidyl pharmacotherapy to

- safely store the trihexyphenidyl oral elixir and oral tablets out of the reach of children in tightly closed, child-resistant containers at controlled room temperature (15° to 30°C; 59° to 86°F).
- obtain an available patient information sheet regarding adjunctive trihexyphenidyl pharmacotherapy from their pharmacist at the time that their prescription is dispensed. Encourage patients to clarify any questions that they may have regarding adjunctive trihexyphenidyl pharmacotherapy with their pharmacist or, if needed, to consult their prescribing psychologist.

PROPOSED MECHANISM OF ACTION

The exact mechanism of trihexyphenidyl's antiparkinsonian action has not yet been fully determined. It appears to act by the following mechanisms: 1) the blockade of cholinergic receptors in the basal ganglia, which, in turn, blocks efferent nerve impulses; and 2) the central inhibition of cerebral motor centers.

PHARMACOKINETICS/PHARMACODYNAMICS

Trihexyphenidyl is absorbed rapidly from the GI tract following oral ingestion. The onset of action occurs within 1 hour. Peak effects occur within 2 to 3 hours. The duration of action is 6 to 12 hours. Additional data are not available.

RELATIVE CONTRAINDICATIONS

Children who are younger than 3 years of age
Hypersensitivity to trihexyphenidyl
Narrow-angle glaucoma
Tardive dyskinesia

CAUTIONS AND COMMENTS

Caution patients who are receiving trihexyphenidyl pharmacotherapy against

- performing activities that require alertness, judgment, or physical coordination (e.g., driving an automobile, operating dangerous equipment, supervising children) until their response to adjunctive trihexyphenidyl pharmacotherapy is known. Trihexyphenidyl may affect these mental and physical functions adversely.

Prescribe trihexyphenidyl pharmacotherapy cautiously to patients who

- have glaucoma; obstructive disease of the genitourinary or GI tracts; or prostatic hypertrophy. The anticholinergic actions of trihexyphenidyl may affect these medical conditions adversely. Monitor these patients closely for anticholinergic effects. Collaboration with the patient's advanced practice nurse, family physician, or ophthalmologist is recommended.

CLINICALLY SIGNIFICANT DRUG INTERACTIONS

Concurrent trihexyphenidyl pharmacotherapy and the following may result in clinically significant drug interactions:

Alcohol Use

Concurrent alcohol use may increase the CNS depressant action of trihexyphenidyl. Advise patients to avoid, or limit, their use of alcohol while receiving trihexyphenidyl pharmacotherapy.

Anticholinergic Pharmacotherapy and Pharmacotherapy With Other Drugs That Produce Significant Anticholinergic Actions

Concurrent trihexyphenidyl pharmacotherapy and pharmacotherapy with anticholinergics (e.g., atropine) or other drugs that produce significant anticholinergic actions (e.g., phenothiazines, tricyclic antidepressants) may result in additive or synergistic anticholinergic effects. These effects include heat stroke and paralytic ileus. Instruct patients to promptly report the occurrence of fever, heat intolerance, or constipation. Collaboration with the patient's ophthalmologist is required for periodic gonioscope evaluation and monitoring of intraocular pressure.

Pharmacotherapy With CNS Depressants and Other Drugs That Produce CNS Depression

Concurrent trihexyphenidyl pharmacotherapy and pharmacotherapy with opiate analgesics, sedative-hypnotics, or other drugs that produce CNS depression (e.g., antihistamines, phenothiazines, TCAs) may result in additive CNS depression.

ADVERSE DRUG REACTIONS

Adjunctive trihexyphenidyl pharmacotherapy commonly has been associated with ADRs related to its anticholinergic action. These ADRs include blurred vision, dizziness, dryness of the mouth, nausea, and nervousness. Adjunctive trihexyphenidyl pharmacotherapy also has been associated with the following ADRs, listed according to body system:

Cardiovascular: postural (orthostatic) hypotension and tachycardia
CNS: confusion, drowsiness, and headache
Cutaneous: rash
Genitourinary: urinary hesitancy and urinary retention
GI: constipation and vomiting
Ophthalmic: abnormal dilation of the pupils (mydriasis) and increased intraocular pressure
Miscellaneous: weakness

OVERDOSAGE

Signs and symptoms of trihexyphenidyl overdosage are primarily related to its anticholinergic actions and include clumsiness, CNS depression, confusion, drowsiness, dryness and flushing of the skin, shortness of breath, severe dryness of the mouth and throat, tachycardia, and warmth. Trihexyphenidyl overdosage requires emergency symptomatic medical support of body systems with attention to increasing trihexyphenidyl elimination. Physostigmine (Antilirium®) is a specific antidote. However, physostigmine generally is *not* recommended for the treatment of anticholinergic toxicity because of 1) the ADRs associated with its use (e.g., asystole, seizures); and 2) its relative contraindication for use among patients who have asthma, cardiovascular disease, gangrene, and mechanical obstruction of the GI or genitourinary tracts.

VALPROIC ACID
[Divalproex sodium; Sodium valproate; Valproate sodium]

(val proe' ik)

TRADE NAMES

Depacon® (valproate sodium)
Depakene® (valproic acid)
Depakote® (divalproex sodium)
Epival® (divalproex sodium)

CLASSIFICATION

Anticonvulsant (valproic acid derivative)

APPROVED INDICATIONS FOR NEUROPSYCHOLOGICAL DISORDERS

Pharmacotherapy for the management of:

- seizure disorders. Valproic acid pharmacotherapy is indicated for the prophylactic and symptomatic management of simple or complex absence seizures, including petit mal seizures.
- vascular headaches: migraine headache. Valproic acid pharmacotherapy is indicated for the prophylactic management of migraine headache.

USUAL DOSAGE AND ADMINISTRATION

Seizures Disorders: Simple or Complex Absence Seizures

Adults: Initially, 15 mg/kg daily intravenously or orally. Gradually increase the dosage by 5 to 10 mg/kg/day every seven days according to individual patient response (i.e., until seizures are controlled or ADRs preclude further increases in dosage).

MAXIMUM: 60 mg/kg daily intravenously or orally

Women who are, or who may become, pregnant: FDA Pregnancy Category D. Valproic acid crosses the placenta and achieves higher blood concentrations in the embryo, fetus, or neonate than in the mother. Valproic acid pharmacotherapy during pregnancy has been associated with congenital malformations (i.e., birth defects). These congenital malformations include

For details and discussion regarding related basic principles of clinical pharmacology, readers are referred to the first text in this series, *The Pharmacologic Basis of Psychotherapeutics: An Introduction for Psychologists.*

cardiovascular malformations and anomalies involving various other body systems, cranial defects, and spina bifida. The incidence of neural tube defects among neonates born to women who received valproic acid pharmacotherapy during the first trimester of pregnancy is significantly increased (e.g., risk of spinal bifida is ~1% to 2%). Liver failure resulting in the deaths of a neonate and an infant have been reported following the maternal use of valproic acid during pregnancy. Do *not* prescribe valproic acid pharmacotherapy to women who are pregnant. Caution women to avoid pregnancy while receiving valproic acid pharmacotherapy.

Women who are breast-feeding: Safety and efficacy of valproic acid pharmacotherapy for women who are breast-feeding and their neonates and infants have not been established. Valproic acid in the form of valproate is excreted in breast milk in concentrations reportedly up to 10% of maternal blood concentrations. Although this concentration of valproic acid generally poses little significant risk to neonates and infants who are breast-feeding, rare, apparently idiosyncratic, cases of hepatic failure have been reported. Avoid prescribing valproic acid pharmacotherapy to women who are breast-feeding. If valproic acid pharmacotherapy is required, breast-feeding should be discontinued. Collaboration with the patient's pediatrician may be indicated.

Elderly, frail, or debilitated patients: Generally prescribe lower dosages of valproic acid for elderly, frail, or debilitated patients. Gradually increase the dosage, if needed, according to individual patient response. These patients may be more sensitive to the pharmacologic actions of valproic acid than are younger or healthier adult patients.

Children 2 years of age and older: Initially, 15 mg/kg daily intravenously or orally. Gradually increase the dosage by 5 to 10 mg/kg/day every seven days according to individual patient response (i.e., until seizures are controlled or ADRs preclude further increases in dosage). Note: Dosage is the same as for adults.

Notes, Seizure Disorders: Simple or Complex Absence Seizures

Initiating and maintaining valproic acid pharmacotherapy: Evaluate liver function (e.g., obtain liver function tests) prior to initiating valproic acid pharmacotherapy and at regular intervals, especially during the first 6 months of pharmacotherapy. Collaboration with the patient's family physician or a specialist (e.g., internist) may be required. Discontinue valproic acid pharmacotherapy immediately if liver dysfunction is suspected or medically confirmed. Unfortunately, in rare cases, liver dysfunction has progressed among some patients following the discontinuation of valproic acid pharmacotherapy. The frequency of ADRs, particularly elevated liver enzymes, may be dose related. The benefit of higher dosages must be weighed against the potential for the increased frequency or severity of ADRs, including possible liver toxicity. See also "Cautions and Comments."

For patients who require a total daily dosage of valproic acid that exceeds 250 mg, divide the total daily dosage according to the table "Recommended Divided Doses for Valproic Acid for Seizure Disorder Dosages Exceeding 250 mg Daily."

Injectable pharmacotherapy: Prior to use, dilute the injectable with at least 50 ml of sterile dextrose (5%) for injection, lactated Ringer's solution, or sodium chloride (0.9%) for injection. Infuse at a rate ≤20 mg/minute. A minimal infusion time of 60 minutes will help to minimize associated ADRs.

Recommended divided doses for valproic acid for seizure disorder dosages exceeding 250 mg daily (based upon patient body weight and an initial dosage of 15 mg/kg/day).

Body weight	Total daily dosage	Divided dose (mg) (equivalent to valproic acid)		
		Dose 1	Dose 2	Dose 3
10 to 24.9 kg	250 mg	0	0	250 mg
25 to 39.9 kg	500 mg	250 mg	0	250 mg
40 to 59.9 kg	750 mg	250 mg	250 mg	250 mg
60 to 74.9 kg	1000 mg	250 mg	250 mg	500 mg
75 to 89.9 kg	1250 mg	500 mg	250 mg	500 mg
etc.	etc.	etc.		

Safely and appropriately discard any unused portion of the vial of injectable valproate sodium (Depacon®), as well as any unused diluted injectable solution, within 24 hours. Replace intravenous valproic acid pharmacotherapy with oral valproic acid pharmacotherapy as soon as it is clinically feasible.

Vascular Headaches: Migraine Headache Prophylaxis

Adults: 500 mg daily orally in two divided doses

MAXIMUM: 1000 mg daily orally

Women who are, or who may become, pregnant: FDA Pregnancy Category D. Valproic acid crosses the placenta and achieves higher blood concentrations in the embryo, fetus, or neonate than in the mother. Valproic acid pharmacotherapy during pregnancy has been associated with congenital malformations (i.e., birth defects). These congenital malformations include cardiovascular malformations and anomalies involving various other body systems, cranial defects, and spina bifida. The incidence of neural tube defects among neonates born to women who received valproic acid pharmacotherapy during the first trimester of pregnancy is increased significantly (e.g., risk of spinal bifida is ~1% to 2%). Liver failure resulting in the death of a neonate and an infant have been reported following the maternal use of valproic acid during pregnancy. Do *not* prescribe valproic acid pharmacotherapy to women who are pregnant. Caution women to avoid pregnancy while receiving valproic acid pharmacotherapy.

Women who are breast-feeding: Safety and efficacy of valproic acid pharmacotherapy for women who are breast-feeding and their neonates and infants have not been established. Valproic acid in the form of valproate is excreted in breast milk in concentrations reportedly up to 10% of maternal blood concentrations. Although this concentration of valproic acid generally poses little significant risk to neonates and infants who are breast-feeding, rare, apparently idiosyncratic, cases of hepatic failure have been reported. Avoid prescribing valproic acid pharmacotherapy to women who are breast-feeding. If valproic acid pharmacotherapy is required, breast-feeding should be discontinued. Collaboration with the patient's pediatrician may be indicated.

Elderly, frail, or debilitated patients: Generally prescribe lower dosages of valproic acid for *elderly, frail, or debilitated patients.* Gradually increase the dosage, if needed, according to individual patient response. These patients may be more sensitive to the pharmacologic actions of valproic acid than are younger or healthier adult patients.

Children and adolescents younger than 18 years of age: Safety and efficacy of valproic acid pharmacotherapy for the prophylactic management of migraine headaches among children and adolescents have not been established. Valproic acid pharmacotherapy for this indication is *not* recommended for this age group.

Notes, Vascular Headaches: Migraine Headache Prophylaxis

Initiating and maintaining valproic acid pharmacotherapy: Evaluate liver function (e.g., obtain liver function tests) prior to initiating valproic acid pharmacotherapy and at regular intervals, especially during the first 6 months of pharmacotherapy. Collaboration with the patient's family physician or a specialist (e.g., internist) may be required. Discontinue valproic acid pharmacotherapy immediately if liver dysfunction is suspected or medically confirmed. Unfortunately, in rare cases, liver dysfunction has progressed among some patients following the discontinuation of valproic acid pharmacotherapy. The frequency of ADRs, particularly elevated liver enzymes, may be dose related. The benefit of higher dosages must be weighed against the potential for the increased frequency or severity of ADRs, including possible liver toxicity. See also "Cautions and Comments."

AVAILABLE DOSAGE FORMS, STORAGE, AND COMPATIBILITY

Capsules, oral (soft): 250, 500 mg (Depakene®)
Capsules, oral sprinkle: 125 mg (Depakote® Sprinkle)
Injectable, intravenous: 100 mg/ml (Depacon®)
Syrup, oral: 250 mg/5 ml (Depakene®)
Tablets, oral enteric-coated: 125, 250, 500 mg (Epival®)
Tablets, oral enteric-coated extended-release: 125, 250, 500 mg (Depakote®)

Notes

All oral dosage formulations are listed in terms of valproic acid equivalents, even though some (e.g., Depakote®, Epival®) contain the valproic acid prodrug, divalproex sodium.

Depakote® Sprinkle oral capsules contain coated particles. The entire contents of each capsule may be sprinkled on a small amount (5 ml) of cold soft food (e.g., applesauce, pudding) immediately prior to ingestion. Caution patients against chewing the coated particles.

Depakene® 500 mg oral capsules contain tartrazine (FD & C Yellow No. 5). Tartrazine has been associated with hypersensitivity reactions (e.g., bronchial asthma) among susceptible patients, particularly those who have a hypersensitivity to aspirin.

Safety store valproate sodium injectable vials at controlled room temperature (15° to 30°C; 59° to 86°F). Each ml of the injectable form (Depacon®) contains valproate sodium equivalent to 100 mg of valproic acid.

General instructions for patients: Instruct patients who are receiving valproic acid pharmacotherapy to

- ingest each dose of the valproic acid oral capsules, syrup, or tablets with food to decrease associated GI irritation.
- swallow each dose of the valproic acid soft oral capsules whole without breaking or chewing to avoid associated local irritation of the mouth and throat.
- avoid ingesting valproic acid oral enteric-coated tablets within 1 hour of ingesting antacids or milk. Concurrent ingestion may, theoretically, destroy the enteric coating of the tablets and result in gastric irritation and loss of efficacy. Also instruct them to swallow each dose of the valproic acid oral enteric-coated tablets whole without breaking, chewing, or crushing with adequate liquid chaser (e.g., 60 to 120 ml of water). Breaking, chewing, or crushing the enteric tablets may result in gastric irritation and loss of efficacy.
- safely store valproic acid oral dosage forms out of the reach of children in tightly closed, child-resistant containers at controlled room temperature (15° to 30°C; 59° to 86°F). Divalproex sodium capsules containing coated particles should be stored at 15° to 25°C (59° to 77°F).
- obtain an available patient information sheet regarding valproic acid pharmacotherapy from their pharmacist at the time that their prescription is dispensed. Encourage patients to clarify any questions that they may have regarding valproic acid pharmacotherapy with their pharmacist or, if needed, to consult their prescribing psychologist.

PROPOSED MECHANISM OF ACTION

Valproic acid appears to elicit its anticonvulsant action by means of increasing the availability of GABA, an inhibitory neurotransmitter, within the CNS. However, the exact mechanisms of its anticonvulsant and antimigraine actions have not been determined.

PHARMACOKINETICS/PHARMACODYNAMICS

Divalproex sodium dissociates in the GI tract into valproic acid, which, in turn, becomes valproate ion. Valproic acid is rapidly and virtually completely absorbed ($\sim$100%) following oral ingestion ($F \simeq 1$). Absorption may be delayed slightly if divalproex sodium is ingested with meals. However, ingesting divalproex sodium with meals does not affect total absorption. Thus, the ingestion of the various oral formulations of divalproex sodium with food, or their substitution with each other, should not be clinically problematic. However, any change in dosage or formulation, or any change in concurrent pharmacotherapy, should be accompanied with close monitoring of valproate blood concentrations and individual patient response. Peak blood concentrations are achieved within 1 to 5 hours. Valproate ion is moderately to highly plasma protein bound (80% to 95%, concentration dependent) and has an apparent volume of distribution of $\sim$0.2 liters/kg. Valproic acid is metabolized extensively by the liver with less than 4% excreted in unchanged form in the urine. The mean total body clearance is $\sim$0.5 liters/hour. The mean half-life of elimination is $\sim$12 hours.

Therapeutic Drug Monitoring

Blood concentrations of 50 to 125 μg/ml (350 to 875 μmol/liter) were achieved and generally well tolerated by 80% of patients receiving valproic acid pharmacotherapy. These blood concentrations may be used as a *general* guide. However, a direct relationship between the valproic acid blood concentration and clinical response has not been clearly established. Therefore, the dosage must be ultimately determined by individual patient response. It generally is recommended that blood samples be obtained from trough concentrations just prior to the next dose. However, in cases of suspected overdosage, samples may be obtained at any time.

RELATIVE CONTRAINDICATIONS

Children, younger than 2 years of age (see "Cautions and Comments")
Hypersensitivity to divalproex sodium or valproic acid
Liver disease, active
Liver dysfunction, severe
Pregnancy

CAUTIONS AND COMMENTS

Prescribe valproic acid pharmacotherapy cautiously to patients who

- are receiving pharmacotherapy with several different drugs for the prophylactic and symptomatic management of seizure disorders (or the prophylactic management of migraine headaches). See "Clinically Significant Drug Interactions."
- have histories of liver dysfunction. Fatal liver failure has been reported during the first 6 months of valproic acid pharmacotherapy. These deaths generally have occurred among infants and children younger than 2 years of age. In addition to valproic acid pharmacotherapy, these infants and children were receiving anticonvulsant pharmacotherapy with several different drugs, and also had congenital metabolic disorders, severe seizure disorders and mental retardation, or other organic brain disease. Thus, valproic acid pharmacotherapy was not implicated conclusively. Although the incidence of fatal hepatotoxicity decreases significantly among progressively older patient groups, monitor liver function carefully and observe all patients for non-specific signs and symptoms of liver dysfunction. These signs and symptoms include facial edema, lethargy, loss of appetite (anorexia), malaise, and vomiting. See "Relative Contraindications."

Caution patients who are receiving valproic acid pharmacotherapy against

- performing activities that require alertness, judgment, and physical coordination (e.g., driving an automobile, operating dangerous equipment, supervising children) until their response to valproic acid is known. Valproic acid may affect these mental and physical functions adversely.

In addition to this general precaution, caution patients who are receiving valproic acid pharmacotherapy to

- inform their prescribing psychologist if they begin or discontinue any other pharmacotherapy while receiving valproic acid pharmacotherapy.

In addition to these general precautions for patients, caution women to

- inform their prescribing psychologist if they become, or intend to become, pregnant while receiving valproic acid pharmacotherapy so that their pharmacotherapy can be safely discontinued and appropriately replaced, if needed.

CLINICALLY SIGNIFICANT DRUG INTERACTIONS

Concurrent valproic acid pharmacotherapy and the following may result in clinically significant drug interactions:

Alcohol Use

Concurrent alcohol use may increase the CNS depressant action of valproic acid. Advise patients to avoid, or limit, their use of alcohol while receiving valproic acid pharmacotherapy.

Amitriptyline Pharmacotherapy

Valproic acid may decrease the first-pass hepatic metabolism of amitriptyline and inhibit its systemic metabolism. This interaction may result in a significant increase in amitriptyline's bioavailability. Amitriptyline blood concentrations may be increased by approximately one-third.

Anticonvulsant Pharmacotherapy

Concurrent valproic acid pharmacotherapy may displace diazepam (Valium®) or phenytoin (Dilantin®) from plasma protein binding sites. Thus, this interaction may result in an increase in diazepam's or phenytoin's anticonvulsant and other actions. (See also "Phenobarbital Pharmacotherapy," below.)

Pharmacotherapy With CNS Depressants and Other Drugs That Produce CNS Depression

Concurrent valproic acid pharmacotherapy and pharmacotherapy with opiate analgesics, sedative-hypnotics, or other drugs that produce CNS depression (e.g., antihistamines, phenothiazines) may result in additive CNS depression.

Pharmacotherapy With Drugs That Induce Hepatic Enzyme Metabolism

Hepatic enzyme inducers (e.g., carbamazepine, phenobarbital, phenytoin, primidone) may decrease valproic acid blood concentrations. This interaction may result in a lowered therapeutic response to valproic acid pharmacotherapy. (See also "Phenobarbital Pharmacotherapy," below.)

Phenobarbital Pharmacotherapy

Concurrent valproic acid pharmacotherapy may increase phenobarbital blood concentrations by decreasing its hepatic metabolism. This interaction may result in phenobarbital toxicity. (See also "Pharmacotherapy With Drugs That Induce Hepatic Enzyme Metabolism" and "Pharmacotherapy With CNS Depressants and Other Drugs That Produce CNS Depression.")

ADVERSE DRUG REACTIONS

Valproic acid pharmacotherapy traditionally has been indicated for the prophylactic and symptomatic management of seizure disorders. Thus, the following ADRs, listed according to body system, have been ascribed in the available literature to valproic acid alone, or in combination with other anticonvulsants that are indicated for the management of seizure disorders. More data are needed. Several ADRs (e.g., anemia, hepatotoxicity, irregular menses) may require appropriate collaboration with the patient's advanced practice nurse, family physician, or a specialist (e.g., gynecologist) for appropriate evaluation and management.

Cardiovascular: edema of the extremities

CNS: sedation, particularly with concurrent CNS depressant pharmacotherapy. This ADR usually may be managed with a reduction in dosage. Other ADRs affecting the CNS include aggression, behavioral deterioration, depression, dizziness, emotional upset, hyperactivity, incoordination (ataxia), and psychosis, which may be dose related. In rare cases, coma has been associated with valproic acid alone or in combination with phenobarbital pharmacotherapy. Also, in rare cases, encephalopathy with fever has occurred following the initiation of valproic acid pharmacotherapy. This ADR may occur among patients who have no evidence of liver dysfunction or inappropriate valproic acid blood concentrations. Recovery usually occurs upon discontinuation of valproic acid pharmacotherapy.

Cutaneous: erythema multiforme, generalized itching (pruritus), hair loss (transient), lupus erythematosus, sensitivity to light (photosensitivity), and Stevens–Johnson syndrome. Fatal epidermal necrolysis has been reported involving a 6-month-old infant who was receiving multiple combination pharmacotherapy, including valproic acid.

Genitourinary: involuntary urination (enuresis). Also see information on the metabolic/endocrine system, below.

GI: indigestion, nausea, and vomiting commonly have been associated with the initiation of valproic acid pharmacotherapy. These ADRs usually are transient and generally do not require the discontinuation of valproic acid pharmacotherapy. Other ADRs affecting the GI system include abdominal cramps, constipation, and diarrhea. An increased appetite with some associated weight gain, or a loss of appetite with some associated weight loss (anorexia), also has been observed with valproic acid pharmacotherapy. Replacing valproic acid pharmacotherapy with divalproex sodium pharmacotherapy may be of benefit for patients who experience troublesome ADRs affecting the GI system.

Hematologic: anemia, including macrocytic anemia with or without folate deficiency; bone marrow depression; eosinophilia; hypofibrinogenemia; inhibition of the secondary phase of platelet aggregation with an altered bleeding time, bruising, hemorrhage, hematoma, and petechiae; leukopenia; lymphocytosis; macrocytosis; and thrombocytopenia

Hepatic: minor elevations of liver enzyme tests, which may be dose related, and abnormal changes in other liver function tests, including increases in serum bilirubin. These changes in liver function tests occasionally may indicate potentially serious hepatotoxicity.

Metabolic/Endocrine: abnormal absence of menses (amenorrhea), abnormal breast enlargement, abnormal lactation (galactorrhea), abnormal thyroid function tests, acute intermittent porphyria, hyperammonemia, hyponatremia, inappropriate antidiuretic hormone (ADH) secretion, irregular menses, and parotid gland swelling. Fatal hyperglycemia has been reported among patients who had pre-existing nonketotic hyperglycemia. Valproic acid pharmacotherapy also has been associated with fatal pancreatitis.

Musculoskeletal: abnormal muscle tremor, which may be dose related, or involuntary jerking movements of the hands, feet, or tongue (asterixis); difficulty speaking due to tongue and other muscular dysfunction (dysarthria); and weakness

Ocular: double vision (diplopia) and "spots before the eyes"

Otic: hearing loss, which may be irreversible
Miscellaneous: fever

OVERDOSAGE

Signs and symptoms of valproic acid overdosage include somnolence, heart block, and deep coma. Deaths have been associated with valproic acid overdosage. Valproic acid overdosage requires emergency symptomatic medical support of body systems with attention to increasing valproic acid elimination. The opiate analgesic antagonist, naloxone (Narcan®), reportedly reverses the CNS depression associated with valproic acid overdosage. Caution is required when naloxone pharmacotherapy is used for patients who have histories of seizure disorders because it may also reverse, theoretically, valproic acid's anticonvulsant actions. There is no known antidote.

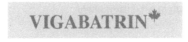

VIGABATRIN

(vye ga′ ba trin)

TRADE NAME

Sabril®

CLASSIFICATION

Anticonvulsant (irreversible inhibitor of gamma-aminobutyric acid transaminase [GABA-T])

APPROVED INDICATIONS FOR NEUROPSYCHOLOGICAL DISORDERS

Adjunctive pharmacotherapy for the prophylactic and symptomatic management of:

- seizure disorders. Vigabatrin pharmacotherapy is prescribed as adjunctive pharmacotherapy for patients whose seizure disorders have not been satisfactorily controlled by less toxic, conventional anticonvulsant pharmacotherapy alone; vigabatrin pharmacotherapy also is indicated as initial monotherapy for the symptomatic management of infantile spasms (West syndrome).

USUAL DOSAGE AND ADMINISTRATION

Seizure Disorders

Adults: Initially, 1 to 2 grams daily orally in a single dose or two divided doses. Increase the dosage by 0.5 grams daily, if required, according to individual patient response.

MAXIMUM: 4 grams daily orally

Women who are, or who may become, pregnant: FDA Pregnancy Category "not established." Safety and efficacy of vigabatrin pharmacotherapy for women who are pregnant have not been established. Do *not* prescribe vigabatrin pharmacotherapy to women who are pregnant. (See "Relative Contraindications.")

Women who are breast-feeding: Safety and efficacy of vigabatrin pharmacotherapy for women who are breast-feeding and their neonates and infants have not been established. Do *not* prescribe vigabatrin pharmacotherapy to women who are breast-feeding. (See "Relative Contraindications.")

For details and discussion regarding related basic principles of clinical pharmacology, readers are referred to the first text in this series, *The Pharmacologic Basis of Psychotherapeutics: An Introduction for Psychologists.*

Elderly, frail, or debilitated patients, and those who have kidney dysfunction: Generally prescribe lower dosages of vigabatrin for elderly, frail, or debilitated patients and those who have kidney dysfunction. These patients may be more sensitive to the pharmacologic actions of vigabatrin than are younger or healthier adult patients.

Children and adolescents younger than 18 years of age: Initially, 40 mg/kg/day orally in a single dose or two divided doses. *Alternatively*, vigabatrin pharmacotherapy may be initiated at a dosage of 500 mg daily orally and increased by 500-mg increments at weekly intervals according to individual patient response. See the table "Recommended Vigabatrin Dosages for Children."

Recommended vigabatrin dosages for children.

Body weight	Usual daily vigabatrin dosage
10 to 15 kg	0.5 to 1 gram
16 to 30 kg	1 to 1.5 grams
31 to 50 kg	1.5 to 3 grams
>50 kg	2 to 4 grams

Infants (for the symptomatic management of infantile spasms): 50 to 100 mg/kg/day orally in two divided doses. Adjust the dosage according to individual patient response.

MAXIMUM: 150 mg/kg/day orally

Notes, Seizure Disorders

Initiating and maintaining adjunctive vigabatrin pharmacotherapy: As adjunctive pharmacotherapy, vigabatrin is *added* to the patient's existing anticonvulsant pharmacotherapy in order to improve the prophylactic and symptomatic management of the seizure disorder.

Vigabatrin pharmacotherapy reportedly has been associated with a number of ADRs affecting the ophthalmic system (see "Adverse Drug Reactions"). Therefore, ophthalmological examinations, including expert mydriatic peripheral fundus examinations and visual field perimetry, are recommended prior to the initiation of vigabatrin pharmacotherapy and every three months during the entire course of pharmacotherapy. Patients should be regularly evaluated in regard to changes in visual field or acuity and encouraged to immediately report any such changes to their prescribing psychologist. Collaboration with the patient's ophthalmologist is required.

Discontinuing adjunctive vigabatrin pharmacotherapy: In order to minimize the risk of the occurrence of rebound seizures associated with the abrupt discontinuation of vigabatrin pharmacotherapy, gradually reduce the vigabatrin dosage, if possible, by 0.5 grams every 1 to 2 weeks before completely discontinuing vigabatrin pharmacotherapy.

AVAILABLE DOSAGE FORMS, STORAGE, AND COMPATIBILITY

Powder, oral: 500 mg (in individual sachets)
Tablets, oral: 500 mg

Notes

For *children and adults,* dissolve the entire contents of the sachet(s) in 240 ml (one glassful) of cold or room temperature water, juice, or milk immediately before oral ingestion. For *infants,* dissolve the entire contents of the sachet(s) in 10 ml of fruit juice or water and administer the appropriate amount using an oral dosing syringe. Note that the manufacturer suggests that the dosage can also be administered in milk or the infant's formula; however, this practice is not recommended because of the potential of having the infant "go off" of their milk or formula (i.e., essential source of fluid and nutrition).

General instructions for patients: Instruct patients who are receiving vigabatrin pharmacotherapy to

- safely store vigabatrin oral dosage forms out of the reach of children in tightly closed, light- and child-resistant containers at controlled room temperature (15° to 30°C; 59° to 86°F).
- obtain an available patient information sheet regarding vigabatrin pharmacotherapy from their pharmacist at the time that their prescription is dispensed. Encourage patients to clarify any questions that they may have regarding vigabatrin pharmacotherapy with their pharmacist or, if needed, to consult their prescribing psychologist.

PROPOSED MECHANISM OF ACTION

Vigabatrin's anticonvulsant action is due to its irreversible inhibition of GABA-T and the resultant increased levels of the inhibitory neurotransmitter, GABA in the brain.

PHARMACOKINETICS/PHARMACODYNAMICS

Vigabatrin is absorbed rapidly and well following oral ingestion ($F = 0.8$). Peak blood concentrations are achieved within 2 hours. The ingestion of vigabatrin with food has no significant effect on either the rate or extent of absorption. Vigabatrin only is slightly plasma protein bound (i.e., ~5%), but is widely distributed throughout the body. Its mean apparent volume of distribution is 0.8 liters/kg. Approximately 80% is excreted in unchanged form in the urine. The half-life of elimination is ~8 hours and the total body clearance is ~2 ml/kg/minute.

Note that because the time it takes the target enzyme (i.e., GABA-T) to biologically replenish itself is significantly longer than the half-life of elimination of vigabatrin, the duration of pharmacologic activity of vigabatrin is predicated on this factor rather than its half-life of elimination. Thus, even though vigabatrin's half-life of elimination is ~8 hours, it can be dosed effectively once or twice daily.

RELATIVE CONTRAINDICATIONS

Breast-feeding
Hypersensitivity to vigabatrin
Pregnancy

CAUTIONS AND COMMENTS

Prescribe vigabatrin pharmacotherapy cautiously to patients who

- have histories of psychosis. These patients may be predisposed to the occurrence of vigabatrin-related behavioral disturbances, which include aggression and psychotic episodes.
- have myoclonic seizures. Patients who have myoclonic seizures may be particularly likely to experience an *increase* in seizure frequency in response to vigabatrin pharmacotherapy.

Caution patients who are receiving vigabatrin pharmacotherapy against

- performing activities that require alertness, judgment, or physical coordination (e.g., driving an automobile, operating dangerous equipment, supervising children) until their response to vigabatrin pharmacotherapy is known. Vigabatrin may affect these mental and physical functions adversely.

CLINICALLY SIGNIFICANT DRUG INTERACTIONS

Concurrent vigabatrin pharmacotherapy and the following may result in clinically significant drug interactions:

Alcohol Use

Concurrent alcohol use may increase the CNS depressant action of vigabatrin. Advise patients to avoid, or limit, their use of alcohol while receiving vigabatrin pharmacotherapy.

Pharmacotherapy With CNS Depressants and Other Drugs That Produce CNS Depression

Concurrent vigabatrin pharmacotherapy and pharmacotherapy with opiate analgesics, sedative-hypnotics, or other drugs that produce CNS depression (e.g., antihistamines, phenothiazines, TCAs) may result in additive CNS depression.

Phenytoin Pharmacotherapy

Vigabatrin pharmacotherapy has been associated in several published studies and reports with a decrease ($\sim$20%) in phenytoin (Dilantin®) blood concentrations. This decrease in phenytoin blood concentrations may be delayed for a few weeks following the initiation of concurrent pharmacotherapy with vigabatrin. The mechanism of this drug interaction has not yet been determined and several other published controlled studies have failed to support this interaction. Concurrent phenytoin and vigabatrin pharmacotherapy requires careful monitoring of phenytoin blood concentrations and patient response. Carefully adjust the dosage of phenytoin accordingly.

ADVERSE DRUG REACTIONS

Vigabatrin pharmacotherapy commonly has been associated with drowsiness, fatigue, hyperactivity among children, somnolence, and weight gain. Vigabatrin pharmacotherapy also has been associated with the following ADRs, listed according to body system:

CNS: aggression, agitation, confusion, depression, dizziness, headache, incoordination (ataxia), insomnia, irritability, memory impairment, nervousness, paradoxical exacerbation of seizures (particularly in children), psychosis, and slurred speech
GI: abdominal pain, constipation, nausea, and vomiting
Ophthalmic: double vision (diplopia), optic atrophy, optic disk pallor (bilateral), optic neuritis, peripheral retinal atrophy (subtle), and visual field constriction (see "Notes, Seizure Disorders, Initiating and Maintaining Vigabatrin Pharmacotherapy")
Miscellaneous: loss or lack of strength (asthenia)

OVERDOSAGE

Clinical data concerning vigabatrin overdosage are limited. Signs and symptoms of vigabatrin overdosage include coma, delirium (loss of orientation to time and place), dizziness, drowsiness, impaired concentration, labile affect, loss of consciousness, and tremor. Vigabatrin overdosage should be treated as a medical emergency requiring symptomatic medical support of body systems with attention to increasing vigabatrin elimination. There is no known antidote.

ZOLMITRIPTAN

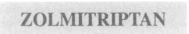

(zole mi trip′ tan)

TRADE NAME

Zomig®

CLASSIFICATION

Antimigraine (vascular serotonin receptor agonist)

APPROVED INDICATIONS FOR NEUROPSYCHOLOGICAL DISORDERS

Pharmacotherapy for the *symptomatic management* of:

- vascular headaches: migraine headaches, with or without aura. Note: zolmitriptan pharmacotherapy is *not* indicated for the *prevention* of migraine (i.e., as prophylactic pharmacotherapy) nor is it indicated for the treatment of basilar or hemiplegic migraine.

USUAL DOSAGE AND ADMINISTRATION

Migraine Headaches With or Without Aura

Adults: 2.5 mg orally per migraine attack. Subsequent migraine attacks may be treated with 2.5 to 5 mg orally provided that a *minimum* of two hours has elapsed since the previous dose.

MAXIMUM: 10 mg orally in any 24-hour period

Women who are, or who may become, pregnant: FDA Pregnancy Category C. Safety and efficacy of zolmitriptan pharmacotherapy for women who are pregnant have not been established. Avoid prescribing zolmitriptan pharmacotherapy to women who are pregnant. If zolmitriptan pharmacotherapy is required, advise patients of potential benefits and possible risks to themselves and the embryo, fetus, or neonate. Collaboration with the patient's obstetrician is indicated.

Women who are breast-feeding: Safety and efficacy of zolmitriptan pharmacotherapy for women who are breast-feeding and their neonates and infants have not been established. Avoid prescribing zolmitriptan pharmacotherapy to women who are breast-feeding. If zolmitriptan pharmacotherapy is required, breast-feeding probably should be discontinued. If desired, lactation may be maintained and breast-feeding resumed following the discontinuation of short-term zolmitriptan pharmacotherapy.

For details and discussion regarding related basic principles of clinical pharmacology, readers are referred to the first text in this series, *The Pharmacologic Basis of Psychotherapeutics: An Introduction for Psychologists.*

Elderly, frail, or debilitated patients: Generally prescribe lower dosages of zolmitriptan for elderly, frail, or debilitated patients. These patients may be more sensitive to the pharmacologic actions of zolmitriptan than are younger or healthier adult patients.

Adults who have mild to moderate liver dysfunction: 1 to 2.5 mg orally per migraine attack. Subsequent migraine attacks may be treated with a similar dosage provided that a *minimum* of 2 hours has elapsed since the previous dose.

MAXIMUM: 5 mg orally in any 24-hour period

Children and adolescents younger than 18 years of age: Safety and efficacy of zolmitriptan pharmacotherapy for children and adolescents who are younger than 18 years of age have not been established. Zolmitriptan pharmacotherapy is *not* recommended for this age group.

AVAILABLE DOSAGE FORMS, STORAGE, AND COMPATIBILITY

Tablets, oral: 2.5, 5 mg

Notes

General instructions for patients: Instruct patients who are receiving zolmitriptan pharmacotherapy to

- safely store zolmitriptan oral tablets out of the reach of children in tightly closed, light- and child-resistant containers at controlled room temperature (2° to 30°C; 36° to 86°F).
- obtain an available patient information sheet regarding zolmitriptan pharmacotherapy from their pharmacist at the time that their prescription is dispensed. Encourage patients to clarify any questions that they may have regarding zolmitriptan pharmacotherapy with their pharmacist or, if needed, to consult their prescribing psychologist.

PROPOSED MECHANISM OF ACTION

Zolmitriptan is an agonist for the vascular serotonin receptor subtypes 5-HT_{1B} and 5-HT_{1D}. Activation of these receptors within the trigeminal system treats migraine headache attacks by means of the following mechanisms: 1) acting at central serotonin receptor sites; 2) blocking the release of neuropeptides that cause inflammation; 3) depolarizing neurons at peripheral sites in the cranium; and 4) constricting associated blood vessels.

PHARMACOKINETICS/PHARMACODYNAMICS

Zolmitriptan is absorbed rapidly following oral ingestion, but has limited bioavailability ($F = 0.5$). Peak blood concentrations are achieved within 2 hours. The ingestion of food does not affect the bioavailability of zolmitriptan. Zolmitriptan is metabolized in the liver and has an active metabolite, N-desmethylzolmitriptan. Zolmitriptan and its active metabolite are only minimally bound to plasma proteins (~25%). Approximately 10% of zolmitriptan is excreted in unchanged form in the urine. The half-life of elimination of both zolmitriptan and its active metabolite is ~3 hours. The mean total body clearance of zolmitriptan is 9 ml/kg/minute.

RELATIVE CONTRAINDICATIONS

Angina pectoris
Basilar migraine
Cardiac dysrhythmias, particularly tachycardia
Cerebrovascular accident, recent history of
Coronary vasospasm (Prinzmetal's angina)
Ergot pharmacotherapy, concurrent or within the previous 24 hours
Hemiplegic migraine
Hypersensitivity to zolmitriptan
Hypertension, uncontrolled
Ischemic heart disease
MAOI pharmacotherapy, concurrent or within the previous 14 days
Myocardial infarction, history of
SSRI pharmacotherapy, concurrent
Sumatriptan, or other vascular serotonin receptor agonist pharmacotherapy, concurrent or within the previous 24 hours

CAUTIONS AND COMMENTS

Caution patients who are receiving zolmitriptan pharmacotherapy against

- performing activities that require alertness, judgment, and physical coordination (e.g., driving an automobile, operating dangerous equipment, supervising children) until their response to zolmitriptan is known. Zolmitriptan may affect these mental and physical functions adversely.

In addition to this general precaution, caution patients who are receiving zolmitriptan pharmacotherapy to

- inform their prescribing psychologist if they begin or discontinue any other pharmacotherapy while receiving zolmitriptan pharmacotherapy.

CLINICALLY SIGNIFICANT DRUG INTERACTIONS

Concurrent zolmitriptan pharmacotherapy and the following may result in clinically significant drug interactions:

Alcohol Use

Concurrent alcohol use may increase the CNS depressant action of zolmitriptan. Advise patients to avoid, or limit, their use of alcohol while receiving zolmitriptan pharmacotherapy.

Cimetidine Pharmacotherapy

Concurrent cimetidine (Tagamet®) pharmacotherapy may significantly inhibit the hepatic metabolism of zolmitriptan. This interaction may result in a 100% increase (i.e., doubling) of zolmitriptan blood concentrations and its half-life of elimination.

Ergot Pharmacotherapy

Concurrent zolmitriptan and ergot (e.g., dihydroergotamine [Migranal®], ergotamine [Ergomar®]) pharmacotherapy may result in prolonged vasospastic reactions (see "Relative Contraindications").

MAOI Pharmacotherapy

Concurrent zolmitriptan and MAOI (e.g., phenelzine [Nardil®], tranylcypromine [Parnate®]) pharmacotherapy may result in an increased incidence and severity of ADRs associated with zolmitriptan (see "Relative Contraindications").

Pharmacotherapy With CNS Depressants and Other Drugs That Produce CNS Depression

Concurrent zolmitriptan pharmacotherapy and pharmacotherapy with opiate analgesics, sedative-hypnotics, or other drugs that produce CNS depression (e.g., antihistamines, phenothiazines) may result in additive CNS depression.

Propranolol Pharmacotherapy

Concurrent propranolol (Inderal®) pharmacotherapy may significantly inhibit the metabolism of zolmitriptan. This interaction may result in increased zolmitriptan blood concentrations and a longer half-life of elimination of zolmitriptan, but lower blood concentrations of its active metabolite (i.e., N-desmethylzolmitriptan). These pharmacokinetic changes appear to largely counterbalance each other and negate the need for dosage adjustment. However, patients should be carefully monitored and the dosage of zolmitriptan adjusted accordingly.

SSRI Pharmacotherapy

Concurrent zolmitriptan pharmacotherapy and SSRI (e.g., fluoxetine [Prozac®], paroxetine [Paxil®]) pharmacotherapy may increase the risk for the serotonin syndrome, including signs and symptoms of hyperreflexia, incoordination, and weakness (see "Relative Contraindications").

Sumatriptan and Other 5-HT$_1$ Agonist Pharmacotherapy

Concurrent pharmacotherapy with zolmitriptan and other 5-HT$_1$ agonists, such as sumatriptan (Imitrex®), may result in prolonged vasospastic reactions and increased risk for the serotonin syndrome (see "Relative Contraindications").

ADVERSE DRUG REACTIONS

Zolmitriptan pharmacotherapy commonly has been associated with dizziness, loss or lack of strength (asthenia), nausea, paresthesia, and somnolence. Zolmitriptan pharmacotherapy also has been associated with the following ADRs, listed according to body system:

Cardiovascular: chest pain, hypertension, and palpitations
CNS: anxiety, depression, and insomnia
Cutaneous: rash
GI: dry mouth, dyspepsia, and vomiting
Musculoskeletal: back pain, leg cramps, muscular pain (myalgia), and muscular weakness and abnormal fatigue (myasthenia)
Miscellaneous: diminished sense of touch (hypesthesia), pain and pressure sensations, sweating, and warm and cold sensations

OVERDOSAGE

Clinical data concerning zolmitriptan overdosage are not available. In the absence of such data, zolmitriptan overdosage should be treated as a medical emergency requiring symptomatic medical support of body systems with attention to increasing sumatriptan elimination. There is no known antidote.

References[1,2]

Adkins, J.C., & Noble, S. (1998). Tiagabine: A review of its pharmacodynamic and pharmacokinetic properties and therapeutic potential in the management of epilepsy. *Drugs, 55,* 437–460.

Airaudo, C.B., Gayte-Sorbier, A., Bianchi, C., & Verdier, M. (1993). Interactions between six psychotherapeutic drugs and plastic containers. *International Journal of Clinical Pharmacology, Therapy and Toxicology, 31,* 261–266.

Alcohol-medication interactions. (1995, January). *Alcohol Alert, 27,* 1–3.

Alcohol-medication interactions. (1995, January). *National Institute on Alcohol Abuse and Alcoholism, 237,* 1–4.

Anand, R., Gharabawi, G., & Enz, A. (1996). Efficacy and safety results of the early phase studies with Exelon® (ENA-713) in Alzheimer's Disease: An overview. *Journal of Drug Development and Clinical Practice, 8,* 1–8.

Andringa, G., Vermeulen, R.J., Drukarch, B., Stoof, J.C., & Cools, A.R. (1998). Dopamine receptor subtypes as targets for the pharmacotherapy of Parkinson's disease. *Advances in Pharmacology, 42,* 792–795.

Antiepileptic drugs. (1998). *Prescriber's Letter, 4,* 9–10.

Ashton, H. (1994). Guidelines for the rational use of benzodiazepines. When and what to use. *Drugs, 48,* 25–40.

Ashton, H. (1994). The treatment of benzodiazepine dependence. *Addiction, 89,* 1535–1541.

Bailey, R.T., Jr., Bonavina, L., Nwakama, P.E., DeMeester, T.R., & Cheng, S.C. (1990). Influence of dissolution rate and pH of oral medications on drug-induced esophageal injury. *DICP. The Annals of Pharmacotherapy, 24,* 571–573.

Bapna, J.S. (1989). Education on the concept of essential drugs and rationalized drug use. *Clinical Pharmacology & Therapeutics, 45,* 217–219.

---

[1]The references cited were used in the writing of this text. They were integrated with over 30 years of clinical experience and academic knowledge of each of the coauthors. As noted in the "Preface to *The Pharmacologic Basis of Psychotherapeutics: An Introduction for Psychologists,*" this text and the others in this series were based on the "Hierarchical Series of Graduate and Postgraduate Courses in Pharmacopsychology" that were developed by the coauthors in 1989 and continue to be taught at the University of Alberta by them. Thus, the references are not meant to provide an exhaustive review of the related literature, but may be better interpreted as a starting point. Additional comprehensive referencing, particularly to earlier classical and initial foundational works in the field, can be found in previous textbooks by the coauthors.

[2]The references are meant to provide readers with examples that document clinical neuropharmacopsychologic data, including ADRs and drug interactions, which are presented in the individual neuropsychotropic drug monographs of this text. They are not meant to provide an exhaustive review of the related literature, but may be better interpreted as a starting point. For this reason, secondary reviews have been cited where possible. Readers are encouraged to perform current CD-ROM searches of relevant computerized databases (e.g., Medline, PsychLIT) to obtain additional references. Although the Internet provides databases reporting ADRs and drug interactions, these reports generally have *not* been reviewed externally and should be interpreted with caution.

Baranki, J.V., & Pigeau, R.A. (1997). Self-monitoring cognitive performance during sleep deprivation: Effects of modafinil, d-amphetamine and placebo. *Journal of Sleep Research, 6,* 84–91.

Bazil, M.K., & Bazil, C.W. (1997). Recent advances in the pharmacotherapy of epilepsy. *Clinical Therapeutics, 19,* 369–382.

Becker, R.E., Colliver, J.A., Markwell, S.J., Moriearty, P.L., Unni, L.K., & Vieari, S. (1996). Double-blind, placebo-controlled study of metrifonate, an acetylcholinesterase inhibitor, for Alzheimer disease. *Alzheimer Disease and Associated Disorders, 10,* 124–131.

Becquemont, L., Ragueneau, I., Le Bot, M.A., Riche, C., Funck-Brentano, C., & Jaillon, P. (1997). Influence of the CYP1A2 inhibitor fluvoxamine on tacrine pharmacokinetics in humans. *Clinical Pharmacology and Therapeutics, 61,* 619–627.

Ben-Menachem, E. (1995). Vigabatrin. *Epilepsia, 36*(Suppl. 2), S95-S104.

Benet, L.Z., & Pagliaro, L.A. (1986). Pharmacokinetic considerations in drug response. In A.M. Pagliaro & L.A. Pagliaro (Eds.), *Pharmacologic aspects of nursing* (pp. 118–129). St. Louis, MO: Mosby.

Bernus, I., Dickinson, R.G., Hooper, W.D., & Eadie, M.J. (1997). Anticonvulsant therapy in aged patients: Clinical pharmacokinetic considerations. *Drugs & Aging, 10,* 278–289.

Besset, A., Chetrit, M., Carlander, B., & Billiard, M. (1996). Use of modafinil in the treatment of narcolepsy: A long term follow-up study. *Neurophysiologie Clinique, 26,* 60–66.

Bhatara, V.S., & Bandettini, F. (1993). Serotonin syndrome and drug interactions [Letter]. *Clinical Pharmacology & Therapeutics, 53,* 230.

Biegon, A., & Volkow, N.D. (Eds.). (1995). *Sites of drug action in the human brain.* Boca Raton, FL: CRC.

Blaisdell, G.D. (1994). Akathisia: A comprehensive review and treatment summary. *Pharmacopsychiatry, 27,* 139–146.

Block, L.H. (1983). Drug interactions in the geriatric client. In L.A. Pagliaro & A.M. Pagliaro (Eds.), *Pharmacologic aspects of aging* (pp. 140–191). St. Louis, MO: Mosby.

Bloomer, J.C., Clarkie, S.E., & Chenery, R.J. (1997). In vitro identification of the P450 enzymes responsible for the metabolism of ropinirole. *Drug Metabolism and Disposition, 25,* 840–844.

Bloomfield, S.S., Cissell, G.B., Mitchell, J., Barden, T.P., Kaiko, R.F., Fitzmartin, R.D., Grandy, R.P., Komorowski, J., & Goldenheim, P.D. (1993). Analgesic efficacy and potency of two oral controlled-release morphine preparations. *Clinical Pharmacology and Therapeutics, 53,* 469–478.

Bomhof, M.A., Heywood, J., Pradalier, A., Enahoro, H., Winter, P., & Hassani, H. (1998). Tolerability and efficacy of naratriptan tablets with long-term treatment (6 months). *Cephalalgia, 18,* 33–37.

Bostrom-Ezrati, J., Dibble, S., & Rizzuto, C. (1990). Intravenous therapy management: Who will develop insertion site symptoms? *Applied Nursing Research, 3,* 146–152.

Brefel, C., Thalamas, C., Rayet, S., Lopez-Gil, A., Fitzpatrick, K., Bullman, S., Citerone, D.R., Taylor, A.C., Montastruc, J.L., & Rascol, O. (1998). Effect of food on the pharmacokinetics of ropinirole in parkinsonian patients. *British Journal of Clinical Pharmacology, 45,* 412–415.

Bristow, M.R. (1993). Changes in myocardial and vascular receptors in heart failure. *Journal of the American College of Cardiology, 22*(4, Suppl. A), 61A–71A.

Brodde, O.E. (1993). Beta-adrenoceptors in cardiac disease. *Pharmacology & Therapeutics, 60,* 405–430.

Brooks, D.J., Torjanski, N., & Burn, D.J. (1995). Ropinirole in the symptomatic treatment of Parkinson's disease. *Journal of Neural Transmission, 45*(Suppl.), 231–238.

Brosen, K. (1995). Drug interactions and the cytochrome P450 system. The role of cytochrome P450 1A2. *Clinical Pharmacokinetics, 29*(Suppl. 1), 20–25.

Broughton, R.J., Fleming, J.A., George, C.F., Hill, J.D., Kryger, M.H., Moldofsky, H., Montplaisir, J.Y., Morehouse, R.L., Moscovitch, A., & Murphy, W.F. (1997). Randomized, double-blind, placebo-controlled crossover trial of modafinil in the treatment of excessive daytime sleepiness in narcolepsy. *Neurology, 49,* 444–451.

Bruera, E., Legris, M.A., & Kuehn, N. (1990). Hypodermoclysis for the administration of fluids and narcotic analgesics in patients with advanced cancer. *Journal of Pain and Symptom Management, 5,* 218–220.

Butler, S.H. (1986). Analgesics and narcotic antagonists. In A.M. Pagliaro & L.A. Pagliaro (Eds.), *Pharmacologic aspects of nursing* (pp. 299–324). St. Louis, MO: Mosby.

Caccia, S., & Garattini, S. (1990). Formation of active metabolites of psychotropic drugs: An updated review of their significance. *Clinical Pharmacokinetics, 18,* 434–459.

Cardella, J.F., Fox, P.S., & Lawler, J.B. (1993). Interventional radiologic placement of peripherally inserted central catheters. *Journal of Vascular & Interventional Radiology, 4,* 653–660.

Cohen, M.R., & Davis, N.M. (1992). Free flow associated with electronic infusion devices: An underestimated danger. *Hospital Pharmacy, 27,* 384–390.

Combination therapy with lamotrigine and topiramate. (1998). *Facts and Comparisons Drug Link, 2,* 46–47.

Connolly, M.J. (1993). Ageing, late-onset asthma and the beta-adrenoceptor. *Pharmacology & Therapeutics, 60,* 389–404.

Cooper, J.R., Bloom, F.E., & Roth, R.H. (1996). *The biochemical basis of neuropharmacology* (7th ed.). New York: Oxford University Press.

Corso, D.M., Pucino, F., DeLeo, J.M., Calis, K.A., & Gallelli, J.F. (1992). Development of a questionnaire for detecting potential adverse drug reactions. *The Annals of Pharmacotherapy, 26,* 890–892.

Costa, E., & Guidotti, A. (1996). Benzodiazepines on trial: A research strategy for their rehabilitation. *Trends in Pharmacological Sciences, 17,* 192–200.

Dalen, P., Alvan, G., Wakelkamp, M., & Olsen, H. (1996). Formation of meprobamate from carisoprodol is catalysed by CYP2C19. *Pharmacogenetics, 6,* 387–394.

Davie, M.B., Cook, M.J., & Ng, C. (1996). Vigabatrin overdose (letter). *Medical Journal of Australia, 165,* 403.

Diagnostic and statistical manual of mental disorders (4th ed.) (DSM-IV). (1994). Washington, DC: American Psychiatric Association.

Dichter, M.A., & Brodie, M.J. (1996). New antiepileptic drugs. *New England Journal of Medicine, 334,* 1583–1590.

DiPadova, C., Roine, R., Frezza, M., Gentry, R.T., Baraona, E., & Lieber, C.S. (1992). Effects of ranitidine on blood alcohol levels after ethanol ingestion. *Journal of the American Medical Association, 267,* 83–86.

Dixon, R.M., Meire, H.B., Evans, D.H., Watt, H., On, N., Posner, J., & Rolan, P.E. (1997). Peripheral vascular effects and pharmacokinetics of the antimigraine compound, zolmitriptan, in combination with oral ergotamine in healthy volunteers. *Cephalalgia, 17,* 639–646.

Dixon, R., & Warrander, A. (1997). The clinical pharmacokinetics of zolmitriptan. *Cephalalgia, 17* (Suppl. 18), 15–20.

Dowson, A.J. (1997). 311C90: Patient profiles and typical case histories of migraine management. *Neurology, 48*(Suppl. 3), S20–S23.

Drug/drug interaction: Fluoxetine/Phenytoin. (1994). *Drug Evaluations Monitor, 2,* 7.

Drugs that cause psychiatric symptoms. (1993). *Medical Letter on Drugs and Therapeutics, 35,* 65–70.

Drugs for pain. (1998). *The Medical Letter, 40,* 79–84.

Dunham, D. (1998). Naratriptan hydrochloride (Amerge). *Prescriber's Letter, 5,* 16.

Elwes, R.D., & Binnie, C.D. (1996). Clinical pharmacokinetics of newer antiepileptic drugs: Lamotrigine, vigabatrin, gabapentin and oxcarbazepine. *Clinical Pharmacokinetics, 30,* 403–415.

Evans, R.J., Miranda, R.N., Jordan, J., & Krolikowski, F.J. (1995). Fatal acute pancreatitis caused by valproic acid. *American Journal of Forensic Medicine & Pathology, 16,* 62–65.

Fernstrom, M.H. (1995). Drugs that cause weight gain. *Obesity Research, 3*(Suppl. 4), 435S–439S.

Ferrari, M.D. (1997). 311C90: Increasing the options for therapy with effective acute antimigraine 5HT$_{1B/1D}$ receptor agonists. *Neurology, 448*(Suppl. 3), S21–S24.

Ferraro, L., Antonelli, T., O'Connor, W.T., Tanganelli, S., Rambert, F., & Fuxe, K. (1997). The antinarcoleptic drug modafinil increases glutamate release in thalamic areas and hippocampus. *Neuroreport, 8,* 2882–2887.

Friesen, A.J.D. (1983). Adverse drug reactions in the geriatric client. In L.A. Pagliaro & A.M. Pagliaro (Eds.), *Pharmacologic aspects of aging* (pp. 257–293). St. Louis, MO: Mosby.

Fromm, M.F. (1997). Loss of analgesic effect of morphine due to coadministration of rifampin. *Pain, 72,* 261–267.

Fry, J.M. (1998). Treatment modalities for narcolepsy. *Neurology, 50*(Suppl. 2), S43–S48.

Fugati, Y., Otani, K., & Abe, J. (1996). Growth suppression in children receiving acetazolamide with antiepileptic drugs. *Pediatric Neurology, 15,* 323–326.

Garcia, B., Zaborras, E., Areas, V., Obeso, G., Jimenez, I., de Juana, P., & Bermejo, T. (1992). Interaction between isoniazid and carbamazepine potentiated by cimetidine [Letter]. *The Annals of Pharmacotherapy, 26,* 841.

Geller, J.L., Gaulin, B.D., & Barreira, P.J. (1992). A practitioner's guide to use of psychotropic medication in liquid form. *Hospital and Community Psychiatry, 43,* 969–971.

Generali, J.A. (1996). Drug-nutrient interactions: New drug update. *Drug Newsletter, 15*(6), 42–44.

Generali, J.A. (1996). Serotonin syndrome. *Drug Newsletter, 15*(10), 76–77.

Generali, J.A. (1998). Unlabelled use of medications. *Drug Link, 2*(1), 2–4.

Gibaldi, M. (1992). Drug interactions: Part I. *The Annals of Pharmacotherapy, 26,* 709–713.

Gibaldi, M. (1992). Drug interactions: Part II. *The Annals of Pharmacotherapy, 26,* 829–834.

Gidal, B.E., Crismon, M.L., Wagner, M.L., Fagan, S.C., Privitera, M.D., Dalmady-Israel, C., & Graves, N.M. (1996). Current developments in neurology, Part II: Advances in the pharmacotherapy of Alzheimer's disease, Parkinson's disease, and stroke. *Annals of Pharmacotherapy, 30,* 1446–1451.

Gidal, B.E., DeCerce, J., Bockbrader, H.N., Gonzalez, J., Kruger, S., Pitterle, M.E., Rutecki, P., & Ransay, R.E. (1998). Gabapentin bioavailability: Effect of dose and frequency of administration in adult patients with epilepsy. *Epilepsy Research, 31,* 91–99.

Gidal, B.E., Maly, M.M., Kowalski, J.W., Rutecki, P.A., Pitterle, M.E., & Cook, D.E. (1998). Gabapentin absorption: Effect of mixing with foods of varying macronutrient composition. *Annals of Pharmacotherapy, 32,* 405–409.

Gidal, B.E., Wagner, M.L., Privitera, M.D., Dalmady-Israel, C., Crismon, M.L., Fagan, S.C., & Graves, N.M. (1996). Current developments in neurology, Part I: Advances in the pharmacotherapy of headache, epilepsy, and multiple sclerosis. *Annals of Pharmacotherapy, 30,* 1272–1276.

Gijsman, H., Kramer, M.S., Sargent, J., Tuchman, M., Matzura-Wolfe, D., Polis, A., Teall, J., Block, G., & Ferrari, M.D. (1997). Double-blind, placebo-controlled, dose-finding study of rizatriptan (MK-462) in the acute treatment of migraine. *Cephalalgia, 17,* 647–651.

Gillotin, C., Bagnis, C., Mamet, J.P., Peck, R.W., & Deray, G. (1997). No need to adjust the dose of 311C90 (zolmitriptan), a novel anti-migraine treatment, in patients with renal failure not requiring dialysis. *International Journal of Clinical Pharmacology and Therapeutics, 35,* 522–526.

Ginkgo biloba for dementia. (1998). *The Medical Letter, 40,* 63–64.

Gitlin, M.J. (1994). Psychotropic medications and their effects on sexual function: Diagnosis, biology, and treatment approaches. *Journal of Clinical Psychiatry, 55,* 406–413.

Glue, P., Banfield, C.R., Perhach, J.L., Mather, G.G., Racha, J.K., & Levy, R.H. (1997). Pharmacokinetic interactions with felbamate: In vitro-in vivo correlation. *Clinical Pharmacokinetics, 33,* 214–224.

Gold, L.H., & Balster, R.L. (1996). Evaluation of the cocaine-like discriminative stimulus effects and reinforcing effects of modafinil. *Psychopharmacology, 126,* 286–292.

Goshman, L. (1997). New drug: Tolcapone (Tasmar). *Prescriber's Letter, 4,* 47.

Gottwald, M.D., Bainbridge, J.L., Dowling, G.A., Aminoff, M.J., & Alldredge, B.K. (1997). New pharmacotherapy for Parkinson's disease. *Annals of Pharmacotherapy, 31,* 1205–1217.

Graham, D.R., Keldermans, M.M., Klemm, L.W., Semenza, N.J., & Shafer, M.L. (1991). Infectious complications among patients receiving home intravenous therapy with peripheral, central, or peripherally placed central venous catheters. *American Journal of Medicine, 91*(3B), 95S–100S.

Gram, L. (1996). Pharmacokinetics of new antiepileptic drugs. *Epilepsia, 37*(Suppl. 6), S12–S16.

Grozinger, M., Hartter, S., Hiemke, C., Griese, E.U., & Roschke, J. (1998). Interaction of modafinil and clomipramine as comedication in a narcoleptic patient. *Clinical Neuropharmacology, 21,* 127–129.

Guerrini, R., Belmonte, A., & Genton, P. (1998). Antiepileptic drug-induced worsening of seizures in children. *Epilepsia, 39*(Suppl. 3), S2–S10.

Hansten, P.D. (1986). Drug interactions. In A.M. Pagliaro & L.A. Pagliaro (Eds.), *Pharmacologic aspects of nursing* (pp. 170–179). St. Louis, MO: Mosby.

Hansten, P.D. (1995). Pediatric drug interactions. In L.A. Pagliaro & A.M. Pagliaro (Eds.), *Problems in pediatric drug therapy* (3rd ed.) (pp. 463–504). Hamilton, IL: Drug Intelligence.

Heckmann, J.G., Niedermeier, W., & Neundorfer, B. (1998). Indications for acetazolamide in neurology. *Internist, 39,* 221.

Hensley, J.R. (1991). Continuous SC morphine for cancer pain. *American Journal of Nursing,* 98–101.

Hoener, B. (1986). Drug availability and distribution. In A.M. Pagliaro & L.A. Pagliaro (Eds.), *Pharmacologic aspects of nursing* (pp. 78–94). St. Louis, MO: Mosby.

Holsboer, F., Grasser, A., Friess, E., & Wiedemann, K. (1994). Steroid effects on central neurons and implications for psychiatric and neurological disorders. *Annals of the New York Academy of Sciences, 746,* 345–359.

Human, S.E., & Nestler, E.J. (1996). Initiation and adaptation: A paradigm for understanding psychotropic drug action. *American Journal of Psychiatry, 153,* 151–162.

Janai, H. (1990). Adverse drug reactions: United States experience. Part I. *Pediatric Infectious Disease Journal, 9,* S115–S116.

Janicak, P.G. (1993). The relevance of clinical pharmacokinetics and therapeutic drug monitoring. Anticonvulsant mood stabilizers and antipsychotics. *Journal of Clinical Psychiatry, 54*(Suppl.), 35–41.

Joyce, T.H. (1993). Topical anesthesia and pain management before venipuncture. *The Journal of Pediatrics, 22*(5, part 2), S24–S29.

Kalow, W. (1993). Pharmacogenetics: Its biologic roots and the medical challenge. *Clinical Pharmacology & Therapeutics, 54,* 235–241.

Kane, J.M., Jeste, D.V., & Barnes, T.R.E. (1992). *Tardive dyskinesia: A task force report of the American Psychiatric Association.* Washington, DC: American Psychiatric Association.

Kane, J.M., & Lieberman, J.A. (Eds.). (1992). *Adverse effects of psychotropic drugs.* New York: Guilford.

Keck, P.E., Caroff, S.N., & McElroy, S.L. (1995). Neuroleptic malignant syndrome and malignant hyperthermia: End of a controversy? *Journal of Neuropsychiatry & Clinical Neurosciences, 7,* 135–144.

Kehoe, W.A. (1998). Gabapentin for psychiatric disorders. *Prescriber's Letter, 5,* 64.

Kehoe, W.A. (1998). Using anticonvulsants in women of childbearing age. *Prescriber's Letter, 5,* 68–69.

Ketter, T.A., Flockhart, D.A., Post, R.M., Denicoff, K., Pazzaglia, P.J., Marangell, L.B., George, M.S., & Callahan, A.M. (1995). The emerging role of cytochrome P450 3A in psychopharmacology. *Journal of Clinical Psychopharmacology, 15,* 387–398.

Kirvela, M., Lindgren, L., Seppala, T., & Olkkola, K.T. (1996). The pharmacokinetics of oxycodone in uremic patients undergoing renal transplantation. *Journal of Clinical Anesthesia, 8,* 13–18.

Klassen, A., Elkind, A., Asgharnejad, M., Webster, C., & Laurenza, A. (1997). Naratriptan is effective and well tolerated in the acute treatment of migraine: Results of a double-blind, placebo-controlled, parallel-group study. *Headache, 37,* 640–645.

Koch, K.E. (1990). Use of standardized screening procedures to identify adverse drug reactions. *American Journal of Hospital Pharmacy, 47,* 1314–1320.

Kopala, L.C. (1996). Risperidone for child and adolescent schizophrenia. *Child & Adolescent Psychopharmacology News, 1*(2), 1–4.

Kostowski, W. (1995). Recent advances in the GABA-A-benzodiazepine receptor pharmacology. *Polish Journal of Pharmacology, 47,* 237–246.

Kornhuber, J., & Weller, M. (1997). Psychotogenicity and N-methyl-D-aspartame receptor antagonism: Implications for neuroprotective pharmacotherapy. *Biological Psychiatry, 41,* 135–144.

Kramer, K.S., Matzura-Wolfe, D., Polis, A., Getson, A., Amaranen, P.G., Solbach, M.P., McHugh, W., Feighner, J., Silberstein, S., & Reines, S.A. (1998). A placebo-controlled crossover study of rizatriptan in the treatment of multiple migraine attacks. *Neurology, 51,* 773–781.

Kuhlman, J.J., Lalani, S., Magluilo, J., Levine, B., Darwin, W.D., Johnson, R.E., & Cone, E.J. (1996). Human pharmacokinetics of intravenous, sublingual, and buccal buprenorphine. *Journal of Analytical Toxicology, 20,* 369–378.

Lamotrigine. (1998). *Facts and Comparisons Drug Link, 2* (10), 1.

Latimer, P.R. (1995). Tardive dyskinesia: A review. *Canadian Journal of Psychiatry, 40*(Suppl. 2), S49–S54.

Lieberman, A., Ranhosky, A., & Korts, D. (1997). Clinical evaluation of pramipexole in advanced Parkinson's disease. *Neurology, 49,* 162–168.

Longmore, J., Hargreaves, R.J., Boulanger, C.M., Brown, M.J., Desta, B., Ferro, A., Schofield, W.N., Taylor, A.A., & Hill, R.G. (1997). Comparison of the vasoconstrictor properties of the 5-HT1D-receptor agonists rizatriptan (MK-462) and sumatriptan in human isolated coronary artery: Outcome of two independent studies using different experimental protocols. *Functional Neurology, 12,* 3–9.

Lou, G., Montgomery, P.R., & Sitar, D.S. (1996). Bioavailability and pharmacokinetic disposition of tacrine in elderly patients with Alzheimer's Disease. *Journal of Psychiatry and Neuroscience, 21,* 334–339.

MacMorran, W.S., & Krahn, L.E. (1997). Adverse cutaneous reactions to psychotropic drugs. *Psychosomatics, 38,* 413–422.

Marti-Masso, J.F., Lopez de Munain, A., & Lopez de Dicastillo, G. (1992). Ataxia following gastric bleeding due to omeprazole-benzodiazepine interaction. *Annals of Pharmacotherapy, 26,* 429–430.

Martin, G. (1997). Receptor specificity and trigemino-vascular inhibitory actions of a novel 5HT 1B/1D receptor partial agonist, 311C90 (zolmitriptan). *British Journal of Pharmacology, 121,* 157–164.

Mathew, N.T., Asgharnejad, M., Peykamian, M., & Laurenza, A. (1997). Naratriptan is effective and well tolerated in the acute treatment of migraine: Results of a double-blind, placebo-controlled, crossover study. *Neurology, 49,* 1485–1490.

McDuffee, A.T., & Tobias, J.D. (1995). Seizure after flumazenil administration in a pediatric patient. *Pediatric Emergency Care, 11,* 186–187.

McLean, D.R. (1986). Antiparkinsonian medications and stimulants. In A.M. Pagliaro & L.A. Pagliaro (Eds.), *Pharmacologic aspects of nursing* (pp. 382–404). St. Louis MO: Mosby.

McLean, D.R. (1986). Drugs used to treat epilepsy. In A.M. Pagliaro & L.A. Pagliaro (Eds.), *Pharmacologic aspects of nursing* (pp. 405–432). St. Louis, MO: Mosby.

Medication errors. (1996). *Prescriber's Letter, 3*(12), 72.

Meyer, F.P., Tröger, U., & Röhl, F.-W. (1996). Pharmacoepidemiology and drug utilization. *Clinical Pharmacology & Therapeutics, 60,* 347–352.

Mitchell, J.F., & Pawlicki, K.S. (1994). Oral dosage forms that should not be crushed: 1994 revision. *Hospital Pharmacy, 29,* 666–668, 670–675.

Moulin, D.E., Kreeft, J.H., Murray-Parsons, N., & Bouquillon, A.I. (1991). Comparison of continuous subcutaneous and intravenous hydromorphone infusions for management of cancer pain. *The Lancet, 337,* 465–468.

Murray, M. (1992). P450 enzymes: Inhibition mechanisms, genetic regulation and effects of liver disease. *Clinical Pharmacokinetics, 23,* 132–146.

Naganuma, H., & Fujii, I. (1994). Incidence and risk factors in neuroleptic malignant syndrome. *Acta Psychiatrica Scandinavica, 90,* 424–426.

Nagel, T.R., & Schunk, J.E. (1995). Felbamate overdose: A case report and discussion of a new antiepileptic drug. *Pediatric Emergency Care, 11,* 369–371.

Naranjo, C.A., Shear, N.H., & Lanctot, K.L. (1992). Advances in the diagnosis of adverse drug reactions. *Journal of Clinical Pharmacology, 32,* 897–904.

Natsch, S., Hekster, Y.A., Keyser, A., Deckers, C.L., Meinardi, H., Renier, W.O. (1997). Newer anticonvulsant drugs: Role of pharmacology, drug interactions and adverse drug reactions in drug choice. *Drug Safety, 17,* 228–240.

Nestler, E.J. (1992). Molecular mechanisms of drug addiction. *Journal of Neuroscience, 12,* 2439–2450.

New drugs. (1998). *Facts and Comparisons Drug Link, 2,* 17.

Newest anticonvulsant, tiagabine, not yet in trials. (1998). *Psychopharmacology Update, 9* (9), 7.

New "triptans" and other drugs for migraine. (1998). *The Medical Letter, 40,* 97–100.

Nilsson, A., Boman, I., Wallin, B., & Rotstein, A. (1994). The EMLA patch – a new type of local anaesthetic application for dermal analgesia in children. *Anaesthesia, 49,* 70–72.

Ogbru, O. (1997). Drug interactions with grapefruit juice. *Drug Link, 1* (8), 59–61.

Olkkola, K.T., Backman, J.T., & Neuvonen, P.J. (1994). Midazolam should be avoided in patients receiving the systemic antimycotics ketoconazole or itraconazole. *Clinical Pharmacology and Therapeutics, 55,* 481–485.

O'Mara, N.B., & Nahata, M.C. (1995). Drugs excreted in human breast milk. In L.A. Pagliaro & A.M. Pagliaro (Eds.), *Problems in pediatric drug therapy* (3rd ed.) (pp. 245–335). Hamilton, IL: Drug Intelligence.

Oshika, T. (1995). Ocular adverse effects of neuropsychiatric agents. *Drug Safety, 12,* 256–263.

Palmer, K.J., & Spencer, C. (1997). Zolmitriptan. *CNS Drugs, 7* (6), 468–478.

Pagliaro, A.M. (1985, October). Diet, vitamins, and nutrient interactions with drugs in the elderly. *Proceedings of the International Holistic Gerontology Symposium.* Ponoka, Alberta, Canada.

Pagliaro, A.M. (1995). Administering drugs to infants, children, and adolescents. In L.A. Pagliaro & A.M. Pagliaro (Eds.), *Problems in pediatric drug therapy* (3rd ed., pp. 1–101). Hamilton, IL: Drug Intelligence.

Pagliaro, A.M., & Pagliaro, L.A. (Eds.). (1986). *Pharmacologic aspects of nursing.* St. Louis, MO: Mosby.

Pagliaro, A.M., & Pagliaro, L.A. (1996). *Substance use among children and adolescents: Its nature, extent, and effects from conception to adulthood.* New York: Wiley.

Pagliaro, A.M., & Pagliaro, L.A. (1997). Teratogenic effects of in utero exposure to alcohol and other abusable psychotropics. In P. Budetti & M. Haack (Eds.), *Drug-dependent mothers and their children: Issues in public policy and public health* (pp. 31–63). New York: Springer-Verlag.

Pagliaro, L.A. (1985, October). Drug interactions in the elderly: Overview and basic principles. *Proceedings of the International Holistic Gerontology Symposium.* Ponoka, Canada.

Pagliaro, L.A. (1986). Mechanisms of drug action. In A.M. Pagliaro & L.A. Pagliaro (Eds.), *Pharmacologic aspects of nursing* (pp. 71–77). St. Louis, MO: Mosby.

Pagliaro, L.A. (1994). Pharmacopsychology updates: Attention-deficit/hyperactivity disorder. *Psymposium, 4*(3), 14–15.

Pagliaro, L.A. (1995). Pharmacopsychology updates: Drugs and sexual (dys)function. *Psymposium, 4*(6), 20–21.

Pagliaro, L.A. (1995). Pharmacopsychology updates: Psychotropic teratogens. *Psymposium, 5*(1), 18–19.

Pagliaro, L.A. (1995). The straight dope: A consideration of substance-induced disorders. *Psynopsis, 17*(Spring), 14.

Pagliaro, L.A. (1996). The effects of psychotropics on learning and memory: An overview. *Alberta Correctional Education Journal* [Special issue: *Proceedings of the ACEA Conference '96*], 8–15.

Pagliaro, L.A. (1995). Pharmacopsychology updates: Drug prescription privileges for psychologists. *Psymposium, 5*(4), 11–12.

Pagliaro, L.A. (1996). Should Canadian psychologists follow the APA trend and seek prescription privileges?: Of course they should! – An invited critical commentary of Dozois and Dobson. *Canadian Psychology, 36*(4), 305–312.

Pagliaro, L.A. (1997, Fall). Face to face: First nurses, now psychologists. *Innovation, 12.*

Pagliaro, L.A., & Benet, L.Z. (1975). Critical compilation of terminal half-lives, percent excreted unchanged, and changes of half-life in renal and hepatic dysfunction for studies in humans with references. *Journal of Pharmacokinetics and Biopharmaceutics, 3,* 333–383.

Pagliaro, L.A., & Locock, R.A. (1992). Nutritional products. In *Self-medication: Reference for health professionals* (4th ed.). Ottawa, ON, Canada: Canadian Pharmaceutical Association.

Pagliaro, L.A., Maguire, T., & Pagliaro, A.M. (1997). Significant interaction between Librium® and Antabuse®. *The American Journal of Pharmacopsychology, 1*(2), 4–5.

Pagliaro, L.A., & Pagliaro, A.M. (Eds.). (1983). *Pharmacologic aspects of aging.* St Louis, MO: Mosby.

Pagliaro, L.A., & Pagliaro, A.M. (1986). Adverse drug reaction index. In A. M. Pagliaro & L.A. Pagliaro (Eds.), *Pharmacologic aspects of nursing* (pp. 1727–1745). St. Louis, MO: Mosby.

Pagliaro, L.A., & Pagliaro, A.M. (1986). Age-dependent drug selection and response. In A.M. Pagliaro & L.A. Pagliaro (Eds.), *Pharmacologic aspects of nursing* (pp. 130–139). St. Louis, MO: Mosby.

Pagliaro, L.A., & Pagliaro, A.M. (1991). Drug induced automatism: Psychological aspects [Abstract]. *Canadian Psychology, 32,* 204.

Pagliaro, L.A., & Pagliaro, A.M. (1992). Drug induced aggression. *The Medical Psychotherapist, 8*(2–3), 9.

Pagliaro, L.A., & Pagliaro, A.M. (1992). Pharmacopsychology as distinct from psychopharmacology: The initial results of a historical and philosophical inquiry [Abstract]. *Canadian Psychology, 33,* 437.

Pagliaro, L.A., & Pagliaro, A.M. (1993). Carbamazepine-induced Stevens–Johnson syndrome. *Hospital and Community Psychiatry, 44,* 999–1000.

Pagliaro, L.A., & Pagliaro, A.M. (1995). Alcoholic cognitive impairment and reliability of eyewitness testimony: A forensic case report. *The Medical Psychotherapist, 11*(1), 9–10.

Pagliaro, L.A., & Pagliaro, A.M. (1995). Drug prescription privileges for Canadian psychologists: Attainable and necessary. *Canadian Clinical Psychologist, 5*(3), 2–5.

Pagliaro, L.A., & Pagliaro, A.M. (Eds.). (1995). *Problems in pediatric drug therapy* (3rd ed.). Hamilton, IL: Drug Intelligence.

Pagliaro, L.A., & Pagliaro, A.M. (1996). Alcohol and other substance use among the disabled. In K. Anchor (Ed.), *The disability analysis handbook* (pp. 107–137). Nashville, TN: American Board of Disability Analysts.

Pagliaro, L.A., & Pagliaro, A.M. (1997). Teaching clinical pharmacology to prescribing psychologists [Abstract]. *Clinical Pharmacology & Therapeutics, 61*(2), 219.

Pagliaro, L.A., & Pagliaro, A.M. (1998). *The pharmacologic basis of psychotherapeutics: An introduction for psychologists.* Washington, DC: Brunner/Mazel.

Pagliaro, L.A., & Pagliaro, A.M. (1999). *Psychologists' psychotropic drug reference.* Philadelphia, PA: Brunner/Mazel.

Pagliaro, L.A., & Pagliaro, A.M. (in preparation). *Clinical pharmacopsychotherapeutics for psychologists.* Philadelphia, PA: Brunner/Mazel.

Pagliaro, L.A., Pagliaro, A.M., Henderson, D., Kirchen, M., & Uibel, B. (1997). The effects of drugs upon cognition, learning, and memory [Abstract]. *Canadian Psychology, 38*(2a), 4.

Parkinson Study Group (1997). Safety and efficacy of pramipexole in early Parkinson's Disease. *Journal of the American Medical Association, 278,* 125–130.

Patel, S.V. (1995). Pharmacotherapy of cognitive impairment in Alzheimer's disease: A review. *Journal of Geriatric Psychiatry and Neurology, 8*(2), 81–95.

Peck, R.W., Seaber, E.J., Dixon, R., Gillotin, C.G., Weatherley, B.C., Layton, G., & Posner, J. (1997). The interaction between propranolol and the novel antimigraine agent zolmitriptan (311C90). *British Journal of Clinical Pharmacology, 44,* 595–599.

Perucca, E. (1996). Pharmacokinetic profile of topiramate in comparison with other antiepileptic drugs. *Epilepsia, 37*(Suppl. 2), S8–S13.

Perucca, E. (1996). The new generation of antiepileptic drugs: Advantages and disadvantages. *British Journal of Clinical Pharmacology, 42,* 531–543.

Perucca, E., & Bialer, M. (1996). The clinical pharmacokinetics of the newer antiepileptic drugs: Focus on topiramate, zonisamide and tiagabine. *Clinical Pharmacokinetics, 31,* 29–46.

Petursson, H. (1994). The benzodiazepine withdrawal syndrome. *Addiction, 89,* 1455–1459.

Popli, A.P., Kando, J.C., Pillay, S.S., Tohen, M., & Cole, J.O. (1995). Occurrence of seizures related to psychotropic medication among psychiatric inpatients. *Psychiatric Services, 46*(5), 486.

Potentially life-threatening rash may occur with lamotrigine. (1998). *Psychopharmacology Update, 9*(9), 8.

Pranzatelli, M.R., & Nadi, N.S. (1995). Mechanisms of action of antiepileptic and antimyoclonic drugs. *Advances in Neurology, 67,* 329–360.

Prosser, T.R., & Kamysz, P.L. (1990). Multidisciplinary adverse drug reaction surveillance program. *American Journal of Hospital Pharmacy, 47,* 1334–1339.

Rambeck, B., Specht, U., & Wolf, P. (1996). Pharmacokinetic interactions of the new antiepileptic drugs. *Clinical Pharmacokinetics, 31,* 309–324.

Randomized trial of modafinil for the treatment of pathological somnolence in narcolepsy. *Annals of Neurology, 43,* 88–97.

Reiss, W.G., & Oles, K.S. (1996). Acetazolamide in the treatment of seizures. *Annals of Pharmacotherapy, 30,* 514–519.

Ritschel, W.A. (1983). Pharmacokinetics in the aged. In L.A. Pagliaro & A.M. Pagliaro (Eds.), *Pharmacologic aspects of aging.* St. Louis, MO: Mosby.

Roberts, J.W., Cora-Locatelli, G., Bravi, D. (1993). Catechol-O-methyltransferase inhibitor tolcapone prolongs levodopa/carbidopa action in parkinsonian patients. *Neurology, 43,* 2685–2688.

Sachdeo, R.C., Leroy, R.F., Krauss, G.L., Drake, M.E., Green, P.M., Leppik, I.E., Shu, V.S., Ringham, G.L., & Sommerville, K.W. (1997). Tiagabine therapy for complex partial seizures: A dose frequency study. *Archives of Neurology, 54,* 595–601.

Sachdev, P. (1995). The epidemiology of drug-induced akathisia: Part I. Acute akathisia. *Schizophrenia Bulletin, 21,* 431–449.

Sachdev, P. (1995). The epidemiology of drug-induced akathisia: Part II. Chronic, tardive, and withdrawal akathisias. *Schizophrenia Bulletin, 21,* 451–461.

Santanello, N.C., Polis, A.B., Hartmaier, S.L., Kramer, M.S., Block, G.A., & Silberstein, S.D. (1997). Improvement in migraine-specific quality of life in a clinical trial of rizatriptan. *Cephalalgia, 17,* 867–872.

Schein, J.R. (1995). Cigarette smoking and clinically significant drug interactions. *Annals of Pharmacotherapy, 29,* 1139–1148.

Scheinin, H., Anttila, M., Dahl, M., Karnani, H., Nyman, L., Taavitsainen, P., Pelkonen, O., & Bertilsson, L. (1998). CYP2D6 polymorphism is not crucial for the disposition of selegiline. *Clinical Pharmacology and Therapeutics, 64,* 402–411.

Schneider, J.K., Mion, L.C., & Frengley, J.D. (1992). Adverse drug reactions in an elderly outpatient population. *American Journal of Hospital Pharmacy, 49,* 90–96.

Schneider, P.J., Gift, M.G., Lee, Y.P., Rothermich, E.A., & Sill, B.E. (1995). Cost of medication-related problems at a university hospital. *American Journal of Health-System Pharmacology, 52,* 2415–2418.

Schoenen, J. (1997). Acute migraine therapy: The newer drugs. *Current Opinion in Neurology, 10,* 237–243.

Schumock, G.T., & Thornton, J.P. (1992). Focusing on the preventability of adverse drug reactions. *Hospital Pharmacy, 27,* 538.

Sciberras, D.G., Polvino, W.J., Gertz, B.J., Cheng, H., Stepanavage, M., Wittreich, J., Olah, T., Edwards, M., & Mant, T. (1997). Initial experience with MK-462 (rizatriptan): A novel 5-HT1D agonist. *British Journal of Clinical Pharmacology, 43,* 49–54.

Seaber, E., On, N., Dixon, R.M., Gibbens, M., Leavens, W.J., Liptrot, J., Chittick, G., Posner, J., Rolan, P.E., & Peck, R.W. (1997). The absolute bioavailability and metabolic disposition of the novel antimigraine compound zolmitriptan (311C90). *British Journal of Clinical Pharmacology, 43,* 579–587.

Sheiner, L.B., Benet, L.Z., & Pagliaro, L.A. (1981). A standard approach to compiling clinical pharmacokinetic data. *Journal of Pharmacokinetics and Biopharmaceutics, 9*, 59–127.

Shvaloff, A., Neuman, E., & Guez, D. (1996). Lines of therapeutics research in Alzheimer's disease. *Psychopharmacology Bulletin, 32*, 343–352.

Slattery, J.R., Nelson, S.D., & Thummel, K.E. (1996). The complex interaction between ethanol and acetaminophen. *Clinical Pharmacology & Therapeutics, 60*, 241–246.

Smiley, R.M., & Finster, M. (1996). Do receptors get pregnant too? Adrenergic receptor alterations in human pregnancy. *Journal of Maternal-Fetal Medicine, 5*(3), 106–114.

Some drugs that cause psychiatric symptoms. (1998). *The Medical Letter, 40*, 21–24.

Spaldin, V., Madden, S., Adams, D.A., Edwards, R.J., Davies, D.S., & Park, B.K. (1995). Determination of human hepatic cytochrome P4501A2 activity in vitro use of tacrine as an isoenzyme-specific probe. *Drug Metabolism and Disposition, 23*, 929–934.

Stanton, J.M. (1995). Weight gain associated with neuroleptic medication: A review. *Schizophrenia Bulletin, 21*, 463–472.

Stolley, P.D. (1990). How to interpret studies of adverse drug reactions. *Clinical Pharmacology & Therapeutics, 48*, 337–339.

Stopforth, J. (1997). Overdose with gabapentin and lamotrigine (letter). *South African Medical Journal, 87*, 1388.

Stowe, C.D., Ivey, M.M., Kuhn, R.J., & Piecoro, J.J. (1995). Administering intravenous drugs to infants and children. In L.A. Pagliaro & A.M. Pagliaro (Eds.), *Problems in pediatric drug therapy* (3rd ed., pp. 541–675). Hamilton, IL: Drug Intelligence.

Taddio, A., Nulman, I., & Reid, E. (1992). Effect of lidocaine-prilocaine cream (EMLA®) on pain of intramuscular Fluzone® injection. *The Canadian Journal of Hospital Pharmacy, 45*, 227–230.

Tasmar revised labeling. (1998). *Prescriber's Letter, 5*, 71.

Tatro, D.S. (1991). Food-drug interactions – Part I. *Facts and Comparisons Drug Newsletter, 10*(6), 41–42.

Tatro, D.S. (1997). Oral contraceptive drug interactions. *Prescriber's Letter, 4*, 10.

Tatro, D.S., Ow-Wing, S.D., & Huie, D.L. (1986). Drug toxicity. In A.M. Pagliaro & L.A. Pagliaro (Eds.), *Pharmacologic aspects of nursing* (pp. 180–187). St Louis, MO: Mosby.

Taylor, C.P., Gee, N.S., Su, T.Z., Kocsis, J.D., Welty, D.F., Brown, J.P., Dooley, D.J., Boden, P., & Singh, L. (1998). A summary of mechanistic hypotheses of gabapentin pharmacology. *Epilepsy Research, 29*, 233–249.

Taylor, D., & Lader, M. (1996). Cytochromes and psychotropic drug interactions. *British Journal of Psychiatry, 168*, 529–532.

Teall, J., Tuchman, M., Cutler, N., Gross, M., Willoughby, E., Smith, B., Jiang, K., Reines, S., & Block, G. (1998). Rizatriptan (MAXALT) for the acute treatment of migraine and migraine recurrence: A placebo-controlled, outpatient study. *Headache, 38*, 281–287.

Thomas, N.R. (1986). Review of the anatomy, physiology, and assessment of the central nervous system. In A.M. Pagliaro & L.A. Pagliaro (Eds.), *Pharmacologic aspects of nursing* (pp. 207–222). St Louis, MO: Mosby.

Tiagabine for epilepsy. (1998). *The Medical Letter, 40*, 45–46.

Tohgi, H., Abe, T., & Yamazaki, K. (1995). Effects of the catechol-O-methyltransferase inhibitor tolcapone in Parkinson's disease: Correlations between concentrations of dopaminergic substances in the plasma and cerebrospinal fluid and clinical improvement. *Neuroscience Letters, 192,* 165–168.

Tolcapone for Parkinson's disease. (1998). *The Medical Letter, 40,* 60–61.

Tolcapone (Tasmar). (1998). *Facts and Comparisons Drug Link, 2,* 17.

Touchon, J., Bertin, L., Pilgrim, A.J., Ashford, E., & Bos, A.A. (1996). A comparison of subcutaneous sumatriptan and dihydroergotamine nasal spray in the acute treatment of migraine. *Neurology, 47,* 361–365.

Tulloch, I.F. (1997). Pharmacologic profile of ropinirole: A nonergoline dopamine agonist. *Neurology, 49*(Suppl. 1), S58–S62.

Ueda, C.T., & Hoie, E.B. (1995). Pediatric pharmacokinetics. In A.M. Pagliaro & L.A. Pagliaro (Eds.), *Problems in pediatric drug therapy* (3rd ed.) (pp. 713–735). Hamilton, IL: Drug Intelligence.

Van Den Brink, M.A., Reekers, M., Bax, W.A., Ferrari, M.D., & Saxena, P.R. (1998). Coronary side-effect potential of current and prospective antimigraine drugs. *Circulation, 98,* 25–30.

Varhe, A., Olkkola, K.T., & Neuvonen, P.J. (1994). Pharmacokinetics and drug disposition: Oral triazolam is potentially hazardous to patients receiving systemic antimycotics ketoconazole or itraconazole. *Clinical Pharmacology and Therapeutics, 56,* 601–607.

Vauzelle-Kervroedan, F., Rey, E., Pons, G., d'Athis, P., Chiron, C., Dulac, O., Dumas, C., & Olive, G. (1996). *British Journal of Clinical Pharmacology, 42,* 779–781.

Visser, W.H., Terwindt, G.M., Reines, S.A., Jiang, K., Lines, C.R., & Ferrari, M.D. (1996). Rizatriptan vs sumatriptan in the acute treatment of migraine: A placebo-controlled, dose-ranging study. *Archives of Neurology, 53,* 1132–1137.

Volkow, N.D., Ding, Y., Fowler, J.S., Wang, G., Logan, J., Gatley, J.S., Dewey, S., Ashby, C., Liebermann, J., Hitzemann, R., & Wolf, A.P. (1995). *Archives of General Psychiatry, 52,* 456–463.

Walker, M.C., & Patsalos, P.N. (1995). Clinical pharmacokinetic of new antiepileptic drugs. *Pharmacology and Therapeutics, 67,* 351–384.

Watsky, E.J., & Salzman, C. (1991). Psychotropic drug interactions. *Hospital and Community Psychiatry, 42,* 247–256.

Weinstock, M. (1995). The pharmacotherapy of Alzheimer's disease based on the cholinergic hypothesis: An update. *Neurodegeneration, 4,* 349–356.

Williams, L., Davis, J.A., & Lowenthal, D.T. (1993). The influence of food on the absorption and metabolism of drugs. *Medical Clinics of North America, 77,* 815–829.

Wilson, J.M., Cohen, R.I., Kezer, E.A., Schange, S.J., & Smith, E.R. (1995). Single- and multiple-dose pharmacokinetics of dezocine in patients with acute or chronic pain. *Journal of Clinical Pharmacology, 35,* 398–403.

Winner, P., Ricalde, O., & LeForce, B. (1996). A double-blind study of subcutaneous dihydroergotamine versus subcutaneous sumatriptan in the treatment of acute migraine. *Archives of Neurology, 53,* 180–184.

Wong, Y.N., King, S.P., Laughton, W.B., McCormick, G.C., & Grebow, P.E. (1998). Single-dose pharmacokinetics of modafinil and methylphenidate given alone or in combination in healthy male volunteers. *Journal of Clinical Pharmacology, 38,* 276–282.

World Health Organization (1992). *The ICD-10 classification of mental and behavioural disorders: Clinical descriptions and diagnostic guidelines* (10th ed.). Geneva, Switzerland: World Health Organization.

Wright, C.E., Sisson, T.L., Ichhpurani, A.K., & Peters, G.R. (1997). Steady-state pharmacokinetic properties of pramipexole in healthy volunteers. *Journal of Clinical Pharmacology, 37,* 520–525.

Yee, L.Y., & Lopez, J.R. (1992). Transdermal fentanyl. *The Annals of Pharmacotherapy, 26,* 1393–1399.

Zagami, A. (1997). 311C90: Long-term efficacy and tolerability profile for the acute treatment of migraine. *Neurology, 48*(Suppl. 3), S25–S28.

Zolmitriptan for migraine. (1998). *The Medical Letter, 40,* 27–28.

Appendix A: Pharmacologic Classification and Listing of the Neuropsychotropic Drugs Included in This Text[1]

ANTICONVULSANTS

Barbiturates

butabarbital
mephobarbital
pentobarbital
phenobarbital
primidone

Benzodiazepines

alprazolam
bromazepam
chlordiazepoxide
clonazepam
clorazepate
diazepam
estazolam
flurazepam
lorazepam
nitrazepam
oxazepam
quazepam
temazepam
triazolam

[1] Pharmacologic classifications other than the one presented here can be used. However, the one selected for use in this text was developed by the authors and has been found, over the past two decades of publishing, researching, and teaching clinical neuropsychotropic pharmacology at the University of Alberta, to be both parsimonious and correct.

Some neuropsychotropics, because of the nature of their action, chemical structure, or therapeutic indication, may be classified into more than one category. For example, valproic acid (Depakene®) may be classified as: 1) an anticonvulsant prescribed for the prophylactic and symptomatic management of seizure disorders; 2) a drug used for the treatment of vascular headache (i.e., antimigraine drug); or 3) an antimanic prescribed for the adjunctive management of bipolar disorder. For clarity and convenience of use, this reference text discusses the neuropsychotropics in relation to their approved indications for neuropsychologic disorders (e.g., migraine headaches, seizure disorders). For discussion of other approved indications for use (e.g., bipolar disorder), readers are referred to the *PPDR: Psychologists' Psychotropic Drug Reference* (Pagliaro & Pagliaro, 1999). Although this classification scheme is somewhat arbitrary, we reasoned that it was the most appropriate for this text. For additional discussion regarding the pharmacologic classifications used in this text, the individual pharmacologic classes of the psychotropics, and the basic principles of clinical pharmacopsychology, see *The Pharmacologic Basis of Psychotherapeutics: An Introduction for Psychologists* (Pagliaro & Pagliaro, 1998).

Miscellaneous Anticonvulsants

acetazolamide (carbonic anhydrase inhibitor)
carbamazepine (iminostilbene derivative)
ethosuximide (succinimide derivative)
ethotoin (hydantoin derivative)
felbamate (dicarbamate)
fosphenytoin (phenytoin prodrug)
gabapentin (GABA structural analogue)
lamotrigine (phenyltriazine)
magnesium sulfate (inorganic salt)
mephenytoin (hydantoin derivative)
methsuximide (succinimide derivative)
paraldehyde (acetaldehyde polymer)
phenytoin (hydantoin derivative)
tiagabine (selective GABA uptake inhibitor)
topiramate (sulfamate substituted monosaccharide)
valproic acid (carboxylic acid derivative)
vigabatrin (GABA structural analogue)

ANTIDOTES

Benzodiazepine Antidote

flumazenil (imidazobenzodiazepine derivative and benzodiazepine receptor antagonist)

Opiate Analgesic Antidote

naloxone (opiate receptor antagonist)

ANTIPARKINSONIANS

amantadine (adamantane derivative)
benztropine (tertiary amine antimuscarinic)
biperiden (tertiary amine antimuscarinic)
bromocriptine (ergot alkaloid derivative)
ethopropazine (phenothiazine derivative and tertiary amine antimuscarinic)
levodopa (metabolic precursor to dopamine)
levodopa and benserazide (combination of a metabolic precursor to dopamine and a peripheral decarboxylase inhibitor)
levodopa and carbidopa (combination of a metabolic precursor to dopamine and a peripheral decarboxylase inhibitor)
pergolide (synthetic ergot derivative and dopamine receptor agonist)
pramipexole (benzothiazolamine derivative and non-ergot dopamine D2 receptor agonist)
procyclidine (tertiary amine antimuscarinic)
ropinirole (benzothiazolamine derivative and non-ergot dopamine D2 receptor agonist)
selegiline (selective type-B MAOI)
tolcapone (reversible COMT inhibitor)
trihexyphenidyl (tertiary amine antimuscarinic)

DRUGS USED FOR THE TREATMENT OF AMYOTROPHIC LATERAL SCLEROSIS

riluzole (aryl-substituted benzothiazolamine and glutamatergic transmission blocker)

DRUGS USED FOR THE TREATMENT OF HYPERKINETIC MOVEMENT DISORDERS

tetrabenazine (centrally acting monoamine depletor)

DRUGS USED FOR THE TREATMENT OF NARCOLEPSY

CNS Stimulants

Amphetamine and amphetamine derivatives

amphetamines, general monograph
amphetamines, mixed
dextroamphetamine
methylphenidate

Non-amphetamine derivatives

modafinil

DRUGS USED FOR THE TREATMENT OF VASCULAR HEADACHES (ANTIMIGRAINE DRUGS)

dihydroergotamine (ergot alkaloid)
naratriptan (vascular serotonin receptor agonist)
rizatriptan (vascular serotonin receptor agonist)
sumatriptan (vascular serotonin receptor agonist)
valproic acid (carboxylic acid derivative)
zolmitriptan (vascular serotonin receptor agonist)

NOOTROPICS (DRUGS USED FOR THE TREATMENT OF ALZHEIMER'S DISEASE)

donepezil (piperidine derivative and centrally active, reversible acetylcholinesterase inhibitor)
tacrine (monoamine acridine and centrally active, reversible cholinesterase inhibitor)

OPIATE ANALGESICS (DRUGS USED FOR THE TREATMENT OF PAIN DISORDERS)

anileridine
buprenorphine
butorphanol
codeine
dezocine
fentanyl
heroin
hydrocodone
hydromorphone
levomethadyl acetate
levorphanol
meperidine
methadone
morphine
nalbuphine
oxycodone
oxymorphone
pentazocine
propoxyphene
tramadol (opiate analgesic congener)

Appendix B: United States Drug Enforcement Agency Schedule Designations

USDEA SCHEDULE DESIGNATIONS[1]

Schedule I

No currently accepted medical use in the United States. Drugs in Schedule I are considered to have a high potential for abuse and cannot be legally prescribed. Examples of Schedule I drugs include heroin, LSD, and methaqualone.

Schedule II

Approved for medical use but are considered to have a high potential for abuse and a severe liability to produce physical and psychological dependence. Several states require that prescriptions for these abusable psychotropics be handwritten on special "triplicate" prescription pads. The prescriber writes the prescription, keeping a copy for his or her files, and gives two copies (an original and a carbon copy) to the patient, who then must have the prescription filled within a certain specified number of days or it becomes invalid. The pharmacist retains the original copy of the prescription for the pharmacy files and forwards the carbon copy to the state regulatory agency, where it is put into a special database for purposes of monitoring and regulation. Prescriptions for drugs included in Schedule II cannot be renewed (i.e., refilled). A new prescription must be handwritten each time that it is needed. Examples of Schedule II drugs include methylphenidate (Ritalin®), morphine (M.O.S.®), and secobarbital (Seconal®).

Schedule III

Potential for abuse and physical or psychological dependence exists but is thought to be less severe than for Schedule I or II. Generally, this schedule contains abusable psychotropics from the same pharmacologic categories as found in Schedule II but often in combination products (e.g., codeine and aspirin, codeine and acetaminophen). Other examples from Schedule III include benzphetamine (Didrex®), butabarbital (Butisol®), and phendimetrazine (Prelu-2®).

---

[1] These categories are specified in the *Code of Federal Regulations,* Title 21, Volume 9, Part 1308 (revised as of April 1, 1996). They were first delineated in and remain a part of the Comprehensive Drug Abuse Prevention and Control Act of 1970. Note that these categories are legal classifications and, as such, must be considered by all prescribers in the United States. However, they are *not* pharmacologic classifications. For detailed information and discussion of the pharmacologic classification of the "controlled substances" (i.e., abusable psychotropics), readers are referred to the first text in this series, *The Pharmacologic Basis of Psychotherapeutics: An Introduction for Psychologists* (Pagliaro & Pagliaro, 1998) and the reference text, *Substance Use Among Children and Adolescents: Its Nature, Extent, and Effects from Conception to Adulthood* (Pagliaro & Pagliaro, 1996).

Schedule IV

Potential for abuse and dependence is considered to be low and is less than for drugs in Schedule III. The various benzodiazepines (e.g., chlordiazepoxide [Librium®], diazepam [Valium®]) are all included in Schedule IV. Other examples of abusable psychotropics from Schedule IV include chloral hydrate (Noctec®), meprobamate (Equanil®, Miltown®), phentermine (Fastin®), phenobarbital (Luminal®), and propoxyphene (Darvon®).

Schedule V

Potential for abuse and dependence is considered to be limited and is less than for drugs in Schedule IV. In some states, limited quantities of Schedule V drugs may be dispensed by a pharmacist *without* a prescription. In these cases, the purchaser must be at least 18 years of age and present valid identification. The pharmacist must limit the quantity of the drug dispensed and keep a permanent record of these transactions, including the name and address of the purchaser, date dispensed, and quantity of drug dispensed. Schedule V drugs consist primarily of mixed-formulation (i.e., multi-ingredient) anticough and antidiarrheal products containing relatively low doses of opiates.

Appendix C: Food and Drug Administration Pregnancy Categories

FDA PREGNANCY CATEGORIES

Category A

Controlled studies show no significant risk. Human studies have failed to demonstrate a risk in the first or later trimesters of pregnancy. The possibility of fetal harm is remote.

Category B

No available evidence of significant risk in humans. Animal studies have not demonstrated a fetal risk, and human studies are lacking. Alternatively, animal studies have demonstrated adverse effects, but these effects have not been confirmed by first trimester human studies, and there is no evidence of adverse effects in later trimesters.

Category C

Risk cannot be adequately ruled out. Animal and human studies have shown an adverse effect (i.e., teratogenic or embryo-lethal), but there are no adequate human studies.

Category D

Positive evidence of risk exists. There is evidence of a risk of harm to the human fetus, but benefits from use might outweigh the risk.

Category X

Contraindicated in pregnancy. Animal or human studies have demonstrated a significant risk of teratogenesis and that the risk is clearly greater than the benefits.

Appendix D: Abbreviations and Symbols

5-HT	5-hydroxytryptamine; serotonin
ADH	antidiuretic hormone
AD-H/D	attention-deficit/hyperactivity disorder
ADR	adverse drug reaction
ALT	alanine aminotransferase
ALS	amyotrophic lateral sclerosis
APA	American Psychological Association
AV	atrioventricular
BAN	British Adopted Name(s)
BZD	benzodiazepine (receptor)
cm	centimeter(s); one-hundredth of one meter
CNS	central nervous system
COMT	catechol-O-methyltransferase
CSF	cerebrospinal fluid
CTZ	chemoreceptor trigger zone
CYP	cytochrome P-450
DSM-IV	*Diagnostic and Statistical Manual of Mental Disorders*, 4th ed.
EAA	excitatory amino acid
EEG	electroencephalogram
F	fraction of the administered dose that is available to the systemic circulation
FDA	Food and Drug Administration
FD & C	Food, Drug and Cosmetic
GABA	gamma-aminobutyric acid
GI	gastrointestinal
HPB	Health Protection Branch
HVA	homovanillic acid
ICD	International Classification of Diseases
kg	kilogram(s); one thousand grams
lb	pound(s)
LD_{50}	average dose that *is* lethal for 50% of the population

MAO	monoamine oxidase
MAOI	monoamine oxidase inhibitor
mEq	milliequivalent(s)
mg	milligram(s); one-thousandth of one gram
ml	milliliter(s); one-thousandth of one liter
mmol	millimole(s); one-thousandth of one mole
ng	nanogram(s); one-billionth of one gram
PCA	patient-controlled analgesia
PE	phenytoin equivalent(s)
PEMA	phenylethylmalonamide
pH	potential of hydrogen; degree of acidity or alkalinity of a solution
PNDR	*Psychologists' Neuropsychotropic Drug Reference*
PPDR	*Psychologists' Psychotropic Drug Reference*
PTP	post-tetanic potential
SA	sinoatrial
SIAHS	syndrome of inappropriate antidiuretic hormone secretion
SSRI	selective serotonin re-uptake inhibitor
$T_{1/2}$	half-life of elimination
TCA	tricyclic antidepressant
TDM	therapeutic drug monitoring
USAN	United States Adopted Name(s)
USDEA	United States Drug Enforcement Agency
★	drug or dosage form only available, at the time of publication, in the United States
⚜	drug or dosage form only available, at the time of publication, in Canada
®	registered trademark symbol
°C	degree(s) Centigrade
°F	degree(s) Fahrenheit
~	approximately
≃	approximately equals
=	equals
≤	less than or equal to
≥	greater than or equal to
<	less than
>	greater than
α	alpha
β	beta
δ	delta
θ	theta
μg	microgram; one-millionth of one gram
μmole	micromole; one-millionth of one mole

Index

A

ABOUT THE BOOK

This comprehensive neuropsychotropic drug reference is designed with prescribing psychologists and psychology students in mind. An accurate and authoritative reference, the *PNDR: Psychologists' Neuropsychotropic Drug Reference* details drug monographs for over 80 different neuropsychotropic drugs available for clinical prescription in North America.

Each neuropsychotropic drug monograph is written clearly and concisely to reflect essential and important data that are commonly required by prescribing psychologists and psychology students. Thus, whenever possible and appropriate, each monograph includes: a phonetic pronunciation guide; up to five common trade or brand names; pharmacologic or therapeutic classification and subclassification; approved indications for DSM-IV diagnoses; USDEA schedule designation for abuse potential; recommended dosages for adults, including pregnant and breast-feeding women, elderly adults, and adults who have renal or hepatic dysfuntion; recommended dosages for infants, children, and adolescents; and many other critical data.

The form, style, and content of each monograph has been reviewed by members of an Editorial Advisory Committee of distinguished psychologists. With this quality assurance, this text is certain to become an asset to prescribing psychologists and psychology students as they strive to provide the maximal benefit of neuropsychotropic pharmacotherapy to their patients and clients with minimal adverse drug effects.

ABOUT THE AUTHORS

Louis A. Pagliaro, MS, PharmD, PhD, FPPR, is a professor in the Department of Educational Psychology and past president of the College of Alberta Psychologists in Edmonton. Ann Marie Pagliaro, BSN, MSN, FPPR, and PhD candidate, is a professor in the Faculty of Nursing and director of the Substance Abusology Research Unit at the University of Alberta. Both authors received their professional degrees from the University of California at San Francisco. Forthcoming books with Taylor & Francis include *Clinical Pharmacopsychotherapeutics for Psychologists* and *Substance Use Among Women: Its Nature, Consequences, and Treatment*. The Pagliaros have authored 10 other books, notably *The Pharmacologic Basis of Psychotherapeutics: An Introduction for Psychologists*, *PPDR: Psychologists' Psychotropic Drug Reference*, and *Substance Use Among Childen and Adolescents: Its Nature, Extent, and Effects from Conception to Adulthood*.